An Update on Mechanisms and Treatments for Thyroid Cancer in Current Oncology

An Update on Mechanisms and Treatments for Thyroid Cancer in Current Oncology

Guest Editor

Zhilong Ai

MDPI

Basel • Beijing • Wuhan • Barcelona • Belgrade • Novi Sad • Cluj • Manchester

Guest Editor
Zhilong Ai
Department of Surgery
(Thyroid & Breast)
Fudan University
Shanghai
China

Editorial Office
MDPI AG
Grosspeteranlage 5
4052 Basel, Switzerland

This is a reprint of the Special Issue, published open access by the journal *Biomedicines* (ISSN 2227-9059), freely accessible at: https://www.mdpi.com/journal/biomedicines/special_issues/926C826QRM.

For citation purposes, cite each article independently as indicated on the article page online and as indicated below:

Lastname, A.A.; Lastname, B.B. Article Title. *Journal Name* **Year**, *Volume Number*, Page Range.

ISBN 978-3-7258-4715-0 (Hbk)
ISBN 978-3-7258-4716-7 (PDF)
https://doi.org/10.3390/books978-3-7258-4716-7

Contents

About the Editor

Zhilong Ai

Zhilong Ai is a Chief Physician at the Department of Thyroid and Breast Surgery, Zhongshan Hospital, Fudan University in Shanghai, China. His clinical and research interests focus on thyroid and parathyroid surgery, particularly the management of complex cases, including locally advanced thyroid cancer and reoperative surgery. He is actively involved in multidisciplinary approaches to treating aggressive thyroid cancers like anaplastic and medullary thyroid carcinoma. As a principal investigator, Dr. Ai leads several projects exploring novel biomarkers and therapeutic strategies for thyroid cancer, including the National Natural Science Foundation of China, Shanghai Natural Science Foundation, Shanghai Municipal Commission of Economy and Informatization et al. His contributions to the field have earned him leadership roles, including Vice Chairman of the Thyroid Cancer Committee at the Chinese Anti-Cancer Association. Through his clinical expertise and research endeavors, Dr. Ai aims to advance precision medicine and improve outcomes for patients with thyroid disorders.

Preface

In recent years, the global incidence of thyroid cancer has shown a significant upward trend. The diversity in pathological types, molecular mechanisms, and clinical management strategies has driven increasingly in-depth research in this field. To consolidate the latest scientific advancements and foster multidisciplinary collaboration, this volume compiles the key research literature on thyroid cancer, spanning fundamental discoveries to clinical applications. It aims to serve as a comprehensive and cutting-edge reference for researchers, clinicians, and graduate students.

This Reprint is structured around the following core considerations:

Scope and Themes: The focus encompasses molecular subtyping, diagnostic innovations (e.g., liquid biopsy and AI-assisted imaging), personalized therapies (including targeted drugs and immunotherapy), and prognostic management, with a particular emphasis on breakthroughs in treating poorly differentiated and anaplastic thyroid carcinoma.

Purpose and Motivation: Current thyroid cancer research is highly fragmented, necessitating a consolidated work to map knowledge gaps and emerging paradigms. This volume seeks to bridge that need while inspiring future investigations.

Intended Readership: Designed for oncologists, endocrinologists, pathologists, and senior clinicians, it also serves as an educational resource for advanced trainees.

Curated by an international panel of thyroid cancer specialists and meticulously reviewed by the Guest Editors, this compilation reflects rigorous scholarship. We extend our deepest gratitude to all contributors and the publishing team for their expertise. While every effort was made to ensure relevance, some cutting-edge developments may inevitably lie beyond this edition's scope—we anticipate incorporating these in future updates.

Zhilong Ai
Guest Editor

biomedicines

MDPI

Case Report

Treatment Outcomes and Toxicities of Multiple Tyrosin Kinase Inhibitors for Metastatic Medullary Thyroid Cancer: A Case Series

Marilda Mormando [1], Rosa Lauretta [1], Giulia Puliani [1], Marta Bianchini [1], Maria Elena Spoltore [2] and Marialuisa Appetecchia [1,*]

[1] Oncological Endocrinology Unit, IRCCS Regina Elena National Cancer Institute, Via Elio Chianesi 53, 00144 Rome, Italy; marilda.mormando@ifo.it (M.M.); rosa.lauretta@ifo.it (R.L.); giulia.puliani@ifo.it (G.P.); marta.bianchini@ifo.it (M.B.)

[2] Section of Medical Pathophysiology, Food Science and Endocrinology, Department of Experimental Medicine, Sapienza University of Roma, 00185 Rome, Italy; mariaelena.spoltore@uniroma1.it

* Correspondence: marialuisa.appetecchia@ifo.it; Tel.: +39-06-5266-6026

Abstract: Background: The current possible treatments of advanced medullary carcinoma (MTC) include different drugs belonging to the class of tyrosine kinase inhibitors (TKIs): vandetanib, cabozantinb, and selpercatinib. Although the effects of these TKIs have been well described in clinical trials, the real-practice evidence of the effectiveness and safety of these treatment is scant. This real-world case series aims to describe a niche of patients with advanced MTC treated with more than one TKI by focusing on treatment responses and any reported adverse events (AEs) and to provide additional insight on the individualized approach to the management of metastatic MTC. **Methods**: Five patients with a diagnosis of metastastic MTC, treated with at least two different molecules of TKIs, were retrospectively selected. **Results**: Three patients obtained a partial response (one with cabozantinb, one with selpercatinib, and one with vandetanib), and two patients obtained disease stability (both of them treated with all three TKIs, the first two lines discontinued for AEs). The AE profile agreed with the known clinical trials AEs except for non-neoplastic ascites related to selpercatinib and lung cavitations of non-neoplastic tissue related to cabozantinb. The latter was an AE never described so far in patients receiving TKIs. **Conclusions**: The best management of MTC relies on an individualized approach, keeping in mind and dealing with the potential toxicity in order to minimize the treatment withdrawal.

Keywords: medullary thyroid cancer; cabozantinib; vandetanib; selpercatinib; adverse events; lung cavitations

1. Introduction

Medullary thyroid carcinoma (MTC) is a rare neuroendocrine tumor and represents 3–4% of all thyroid cancer types. It is derived from the parafollicular cells of thyroid (C cells) producing calcitonin (CT); therefore, it is biologically distinct from more common differentiated thyroid cancer. MTC can appear as a sporadic (75%) or as an inherited tumor (25%) due to a germ-line mutation of the proto-oncogene rearranged during transfection (*RET*) coding for a receptor tyrosin kinase [1]. Its most common presentation is a solitary thyroid nodule without any symptoms. The first-line therapy and the only curative option for MTC is thyroidectomy associated with cervical lymph node dissection [2]. Different options are available in patients with recurrent MTC and distant metastases, but there is no agreement on which is the best therapeutic approach and on the right timing of starting treatment, because many patients with metastatic disease have indolent disease courses for a long time. Therefore, treatment management in these patients depends on the clinical conditions, presence of the symptoms, disease location, volume or burden, location of the metastatic lesion, and possibility of disease progression. Recurrent or metastatic MTC can be treated with surgical resection, external beam radiation therapy (EBRT), and directed local therapies when disease is localized. In the case of systemic disease, with a high disease burden, the first-line options are either vandetanib or cabozantinb, both belonging to the class of TKIs. A new target drug, selpercatinib, has been recently introduced, and the good results of the clinical trial will have an impact on the treatment scheme [3–5]. Figure 1 shows the molecular structures of vandetanib, cabozantinib, and selpercatinib and the receptors to which they bind, thereby inhibiting their respective intracellular pathways. The safety profile of the available TKIs should be considered in the treatment strategy, especially for patients treated with different lines of treatment. In this case series we analyzed the outcomes and side effects of different treatments for advanced MTC in patients treated with multiple lines, with the aim of providing useful information for increasingly personalized and patient-tailored medicine.

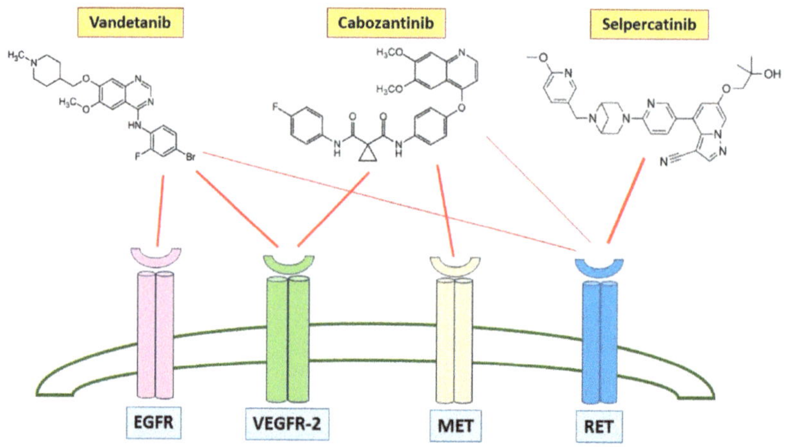

Figure 1. Vandetanib and cabozantinib inhibit different tyrosine kinase receptors. Vandetanib blocks EGFR (Epidermal Growth Factor Receptor), VEGFR-2 (Vascular Endothelial Growth Factor Receptor 2), and RET (Rearranged During Transfection). Cabozantinib acts on VEGFR-2, RET, and MET (Mitogen-Activated Protein Kinase). Selpercatinib is a selective RET inhibitor with higher affinity for RET compared with vandetanib and cabozantinib (the thickness of the red arrows is proportional to the affinity for the receptor).

2. Patients and Results

We selected, from our cohort of patients with MTC, five patients who had been treated with at least two different molecules of TKIs, excluding patients who had received only one line of therapy. The order of treatment with the different lines of drugs was not equal for all patients, according to the different start times of systemic therapy for each patient and related also to the different availability of these therapies over time. For each patient the clinical case description was reported, underlining all the AEs related to each therapy, as well as the efficacy in term of disease response. The study was conducted following the ethical principles of the revised version of the Declaration of Helsinki. All patients provided informed consent to the treatment and publication of clinical data.

Below, we describe the cases of the five patients and report in Table 1 the therapies performed along with their respective AEs, duration, and reasons for therapy discontinuation.

Table 1. Summary of the therapy sequences administered to each patient, including their associated adverse events, duration, and reasons for discontinuation.

	I Line Therapy (Duration and Efficacy)	Adverse Events	Reason for Stop	II Line Therapy (Duration and Efficacy)	Adverse Events	Reason for Stop	III Line Therapy (Duration and Efficacy)	Adverse Events	Current Therapy	Last Follow up/Death
Patient 1	Vandetanib (46 months; SD)	Hypertension (G2) Transient hypoadrenalism (G2)	Drug unavailable	Cabozantinib (9 months; SD)	Hypocalcemia (G3) Diarrhea (G2) Weight loss (G1) Inappetence (G2)	Hypocalcemia (G3)	Selpercatinib (2 months; NA)	Face and limbs edema (G1) Renal failure (G2)	Vandetanib	SD
Patient 2	Vandetanib (18 months; SD)	Hemoglobin increased (G1)	Drug unavailable	Cabozantinib (14 months; PR)	Weight loss (G2) Hemoglobin increased (G2)	Weight loss (G2) Pneumonia	–	–	–	Death
Patient 3	Cabozantinib (3 months; NA)	Proteinuria (G2)	Proteinuria (G2)	Selpercatinib (21 months-ongoing; PR)	Renal failure (G2) QTc prolongation (G2)	–	–	–	Selpercatinib	PR
Patient 4	Cabozantinib (18 months; PD)	Hypertension (G2) Dry skin (G1) Proteinuria (G1) Weight loss (G2)	PD	Selpercatinib (18 months; PD)	Ascites (G2) Hypertension (G2) Dry skin (G1)	PD	Vandetanib (14 months-ongoing; PR)	None	Vandetanib	PR
Patient 5	Vandetanib (1 month; NA)	None	Drug unavailable	Cabozantinib (10 months; SD)	Weight loss (G3)	Weight loss (G3)	Selpercatinib (21 months; SD)	Lower limbs edema (G2)	Selpercatinib	SD

Abbreviations: NA, not applicable due to the short duration of therapy; SD, stable disease; PR, partial response; G1, grade 1 CTCAE; G2, grade 2 CTCTA; G3, grade 3 CTCAE.

2.1. Case 1: Optimal Safety Profile of Vandetanib in Patient Developing Severe Adverse Events with Cabozantinib and Selpercatinib

In 2001, a 36-year-old man underwent total thyroidectomy with a diagnosis of MTC. Afterward, seven surgical revisions were performed for the involvement of the latero-cervical lymph nodes. The 6-[18F]-fluoro-L-dopa (F-DOPA) PET imaging showed the recurrence of disease in different bone segments, for which the patient underwent therapy with denosumab 120 mg monthly from June 2017 to May 2019. In July 2018, due to disease progression to the liver, chemotherapy with vandetanib at a dosage of 300 mg daily was started. The treatment was well tolerated, with the exception of a rise in blood pressure leading to the modification of antihypertensive therapy. The patient also developed transient primary hypoadrenalism, treated with cortisone acetate from November 2020 to May 2022. Vandetanib therapy determined a stable disease and led to a reduction in the serum CT. The patient was treated with vandetanib until May 2022 when, due to unavailability of the drug, he was switched to cabozantinib therapy 140 mg per day. A few days after starting the new therapy, the patient experienced severe hypocalcemia, diarrhea, and an acute rise in blood pressure, requiring hospitalization. Hypocalcemia occurred in the context of pre-existing hypoparathyroidism, already being treated with calcium and calcitriol. After increasing calcium carbonate therapy and despite normalized serum calcium levels, the inappetence and the weight loss persisted; then cabozantinib was first reduced and subsequently discontinued. The *RET* mutation in the surgical sample revealed the C618S mutation. In February 2023, CT values were increasing, and also taking into account the *RET* mutation, we switched to selpercatinib therapy at the dose of 160 mg twice daily. After only a few days, the patient experienced the onset of pronounced edemas mainly in the lower limbs and face; therefore, after 10 days, the dose was reduced to 120 mg twice a day. The blood tests showed a mild increase in the creatinine value (1.22 mg/dL) with a GFR of 64 mL/min/1.73 m^2 and a calcium value of 9.4 mg/dL but no protein in 24 h urine. Due to worsening of the declivous edemas, a new blood assessment was performed showing a creatinine value of 1.61 mg/dL with an estimated glomerular filtration rate (eGFR) of 47 mL/min/1.73 m^2. The hepatic and thyroid function, blood glucose, complete blood count, and urine test were within normal limits, and albumin was slightly reduced to 3.2 g/dL (normal value 3.4–4.6) with increased calcium levels (11.3 mg/dL). A color doppler ultrasound of the lower limbs showed bilateral superficial venous insufficiency, without phlebo-thrombosis, while the echocardiogram was within limits. Therefore, selpercatinib therapy was discontinued in March 2023. Since vandetanib was available again, it was decided to switch the patient back to this therapy as it was the one best tolerated by the patient. Later follow-ups showed fair tolerance to vandetanib. Creatinine values improved with the reduced vandetanib dose of 200 mg, assessing at 1.04 mg/dL with eGFR of 78 mL/min/1.73 m^2 at the latest follow-up visit.

2.2. Case 2: Partial Response to Cabozantinib with an Unusual Side Effect: Cavitation in Normal Lung

A 45-year-old patient in March 2019 underwent thyroidectomy and lymphadenectomy for a multifocal MTC with neoplastic diffusion at cervical nodes and paratracheal fibrous and muscle tissue (pT4aN1b). Pre-surgical CT was 4953 pg/mL, and carcino-embryonic antigen (CEA) was 69 ng/mL (normal value < 5 ng/mL). After surgery, CT and CEA levels persisted as elevated with a severe paraneoplastic syndrome characterized by diarrhea, for which therapy with somatostatin analogues was started without benefit. The computed tomography (TC) scan showed a metastatic high-burden disease localized in the neck and mediastinum with a greatest lymphadenopathy of 4.5 cm located in the jugular region. The germinal mutational assessment of the *RET* oncogene showed a wild-type condition. Because of the patient's refusal of another surgery, a first-line therapy with vandetanib was started in September 2019 with a stable disease until February 2021. Vandetanib therapy at the full dose of 300 mg daily was well tolerated without significant side effects, but paraneoplastic severe diarrhea persisted. The scheduled staging with a TC scan showed the dimensional increase in the mediastinal lymphadenopathies; then the patient was initiated to second-line therapy with cabozantinb 140 mg daily. CT levels decreased in five months from 18,943 pg/mL to 2864 pg/mL, and CEA levels decreased from 221 ng/mL to 86 ng/mL. The cabozantinb dose was reduced to 100 mg/daily due to increased hematocrit and hemoglobin levels. The patient experienced a progressive worsening of inappetence with a subsequent further weight loss (from 58 kg to 50 kg). The TC scan performed 6 months after starting cabozantinb showed a mediastinal lymph node shrinkage with a partial response (PR) (Figure 2) but a concomitant appearance of multiple bilateral lung cavitations, resulting as negative at bronchowashing for bacteria, mycobacteria, and viruses (Figure 3). However, the patient was treated with antibiotic therapy, and the TC scan imaging 4 months later showed a reduction in lung cavitations and a further shrinkage of all the mediastinal adenopathies with a necrotic reaction. Cabozantinib therapy was continued until April 2022 because the patient was unable to perform scheduled visits at our institution for progressive worsening of performance status complicated by SARS-CoV2 infection. At the same time, the molecular analysis of thyroid tissue excluded oncogene *RET* somatic mutation; hence, a switch therapy with selpercatinib had to be excluded. The last whole-body TC scan performed in September 2022 showed a stable mediastinic disease and a dimensional increase in lung cavitations characterized by thickened and irregular walls. The patient's clinical condition progressively worsened due to persistent anorexia and recurrent lung infections; then palliative care was started up to the exitus 6 months later.

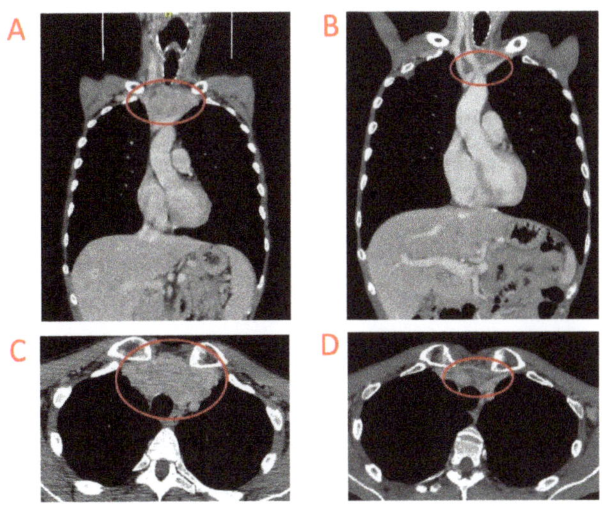

Figure 2. Coronal and axial scans (**A**,**C**) show the mediastinal metastatic lymphadenopathies in patient 2; in (**B**) (coronal scan) and (**D**) (axial scan), a significant shrinkage of the mass is clearly visible 6 months after cabozantinib therapy. The red circles indicate the tumor mass and its reduction.

2.3. Case 3: High Efficacy and Safety of Selpercatinib in an Older Adult Female Patient

In June 2022, a 76-year-old female patient came to our clinic for increases in CT and CEA values (CT > 2000 pg/mL and CEA 939 ng/mL). She underwent total thyroidectomy and central lymphadenectomy in 2014 with a post-surgical diagnosis of MTC (pT2pN0), but she did not have any subsequent clinical, laboratory, and instrumental follow-up for 8 years. The F-DOPA PET showed a huge buildup of radiopharmaceuticals in both lung fields, the liver with almost complete replacement of normal parenchyma, the abdominal lymph nodes, and also the left breast. The breast biopsy showed the simultaneous presence of an infiltrating ductal breast carcinoma; therefore, a differential diagnosis on the nature of the metastatic lesions was necessary. The hepatic biopsy confirmed a localization of MTC. Breast surgery was excluded, and a therapy with aromatase inhibitors was started;

in the meantime, due to the commercial unavailability of Vandetanib, in December 2022, treatment with cabozantinib was started at a reduced dose of 60 mg daily, considering both the patient's age and the liver failure. After 20 days, proteinuria increased to more than 3 g/24 h; then treatment was discontinued. Nevertheless, proteinuria persisted for three months and in March 2023 decreased to 400 mg/24 h; the biomolecular analysis of the surgical thyroid sample showed a mutation of the *RET* oncogene (M918T) making the patient eligible for selpercatinib, a RET-selective tyrosine kinase inhibitor (TKI). Considering the patient's age and the liver failure, selpercatinib was started in March 2023 at a reduced dose of 120 mg twice daily. In the meantime, the patient's clinical conditions were worsening, with the presence of liver enlargement and abdominal swelling; the abdominal TC confirmed abundant peritoneal effusion for which an evacuative paracentesis was necessary, but the cytology examination excluded the presence of neoplastic cells in peritoneal fluid. Due to the increased blood creatinine levels (grade 2 of "Common Terminology Criteria for Adverse Events", CTCAE) and QT prolongation, selpercatinib therapy was discontinued in June 2023 and restarted one month later at a reduced dose of 80 mg twice daily. Calcitonin and CEA levels progressively reduced over 11 months of selpercatinib therapy (CT from >7000 to 100 pg/mL and CEA from about 2700 to 100 ng/mL), the ascitic effusion was slightly reduced, and the CT scan in October 2023 showed a PR at the lung and abdominal lymph nodes.

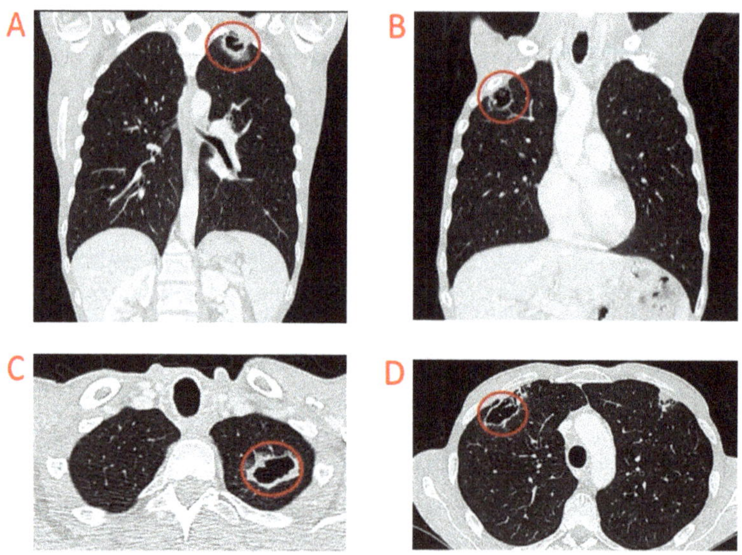

Figure 3. Bilateral apical lung cavitations indicated by the red circles in the normal lung parenchyma, free of metastatic lesions, were evident after 6 months of therapy with cabozantinib, as shown in the coronal (**A**,**B**) and axial (**C**,**D**) scans of patient 2.

2.4. *Case 4: Non-Neoplastic Ascites During Selpercatinib Therapy*

In July 2019, a 71-year-old patient with suspicious MTC with cervical lymph nodes and mediastinal and pulmonary metastasis underwent total thyroidectomy with surgical removal of neck and mediastinal lesions and an atypical left lung resection. The histological examination confirmed a diagnosis of MTC (pT2 (m)pN1b), while the pulmonary nodule was found to be an amartocondroma. The surgery was complicated by a non-neoplastic pleural effusion for which the patient was treated with drainage and pleural surface. The genetic analysis of the germinal *RET* mutation was negative. CT levels never normalized, and 18 months after surgery, they reached about 50 pg/mL, while CEA was normal. The TC scan, performed in September 2020, showed mediastinal lymphadenopathies and suspected liver lesions. The specific F-DOPA PET, in December 2020, detected an increased radionuclide uptake of the mediastinal lymphadenopathies. The mutational analysis of the thyroid specimen found the M918T *RET* proto-oncogene somatic mutation. Therefore, the patient was enrolled in a phase 3, randomized trial (J2G-MC-JZJB) involving *RET*-mutant patients affected by metastatic MTC TKI-naive, comparing selpercatinib, as the first-line therapy, with cabozantinb or vandetanib. Our patient was randomized to cabozantinib therapy at a daily dose of 140 mg. The adverse events that occurred during cabozontinib therapy were measured with CTCAE and were as follows: hypertension (grade 2), dry skin (grade 1), proteinuria (grade 1), weight loss (grade 2), nausea (grade 1–2), vomiting (grade 1), hypocalcemia, and hypothyroidism. Before starting cabozantinib, CT levels were 13.7 pg/mL, and CEA was 75 ng/mL, but about one year later, in March 2022, because of disease progression of the liver and mediastinal target lesions, cabozantinib was discontinued, although CT was reduced to 1.9 pg/mL and CEA to 49 ng/mL. The patient started selpercatinib treatment at a dose of 160 mg twice daily, achieving a good recovery of body weight and complete resolution of nausea and vomiting. Unfortunately, after 9 months of therapy, in December 2022, the patient developed ascites for which a cytological investigation was performed and excluded the presence of neoplastic cells in peritoneal cavity. Hypertension and dry skin persisted during selpercatinib treatment. After 18 months the TC scan showed a further progression of the liver lesions, which was the reason why, in October 2023, the patient started a third-line TKI therapy with vandetanib at a daily dose of 300 mg. After 3 months of therapy, this treatment was well tolerated by the patient, without significant adverse events. After six months, the abdominal ultrasound and TC examination documented the complete disappearance of the ascitic effusion and PR on liver metastasis (Figure 4).

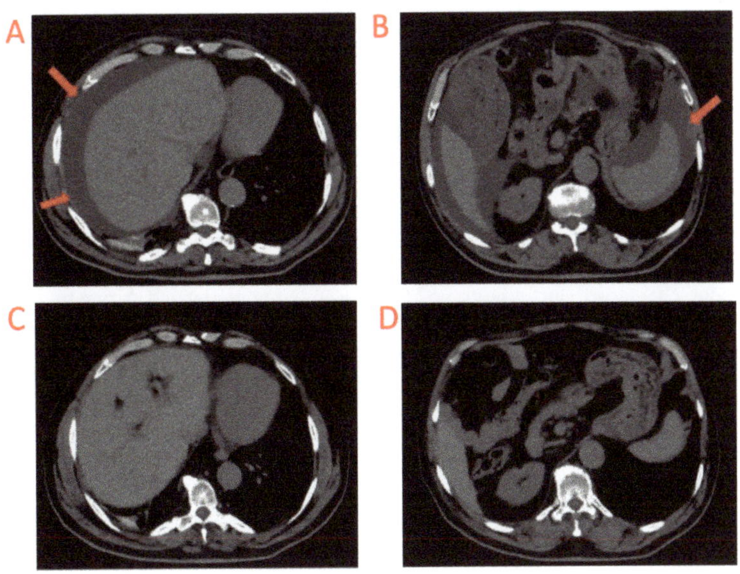

Figure 4. Axial scans of ascitic effusion indicated by red arrows during selpercatinib therapy (peri-hepatic in (**A**) and peri-splenic in (**B**)) and its complete disappearance 6 months after selpercatinib discontinuation (**C**,**D**) in patient 4.

2.5. Case 5: The Treatment of MTC with Bone Metastasis

In a 51-year-old female patient, MTC appeared with multiple metastatic lesions at the spine, skull, and pelvic bone. The bone biopsy confirmed the thyroid origin of the neoplastic cells; then the patient, in February 2022, underwent total thyroidectomy and jugular and left laterocervical lymphadenectomy. The histological examination confirmed a

5 cm MTC and 6 out of 15 metastatic lymph nodes, with extracapsular extension (pT3N1b). Two months after surgery, the patient started systemic therapy with vandetanib at a dose of 300 mg daily with a satisfying tolerance, but only one month later, due to vandetanib's commercial unavailability, the patient switched to cabozantinib starting at a reduced dose of 100 mg daily due to transaminases elevation caused by the strong painkiller therapy that the patient was taking for bone pain. During the 9 months of cabozantinib therapy, the dose was further reduced to 80 mg per day, and some periods of suspension were required due to the debilitating lack of appetite and weight loss. The patient lost 15 kg in 9 months. The mutational analysis of the thyroid specimen found the M918T *RET* proto-oncogene somatic mutation, although germinal *RET* mutation was negative; then selpercatinib therapy in March 2023 was initiated at a dose, by weight, of 120 mg twice daily. The patient experienced only lower limb edemas, and the dose was further reduced to 80 mg twice daily, with an excellent tolerance profile. At the same time, in May 2023, after solving dental problems, the patient started therapy with denosumab for bone metastases at a scheduled dose of 120 mg monthly. The patient gradually recovered the lost 15 kg, and to date, she is in good general condition with a dose of selpercatinib of 120 mg twice daily. The TC scans over time showed a stable disease, but CT and CEA levels reduced only with selpercatinib therapy. Before therapies, CT blood levels were 101 pg/mL (<10), while CEA was 850 ng/mL (<5). During cabozantinib therapy, CT dropped to 47 pg/mL, but CEA was unchanged; during selpercatinib therapy instead, CT normalized to 10 pg/mL, and CEA dropped to 357 ng/mL.

3. Discussion

MTC is one of the thyroid tumors that most frequently may present with distant metastases or that undergo progression after the initial surgical treatment. The management of metastatic MTC is challenging, especially until a few years ago, when cytotoxic chemotherapy was the only therapeutic option and had very poor outcomes [5]. Promising results in the treatment of advanced and progressive MTC were obtained 10 years ago with the development of the first multikinase inhibitors, targeting different tyrosin kinase receptors. Vandetanib and cabozantinib are the first-line therapeutic options approved for patients with advanced and progressive MTC [3,5,6], but two new targeted drugs, selpercatinib and pralsetinib, have been recently introduced, following promising results in clinical trials. The first TKI approved by the Food and Drug Administration (FDA) on April 2011 for the treatment of advanced and progressive and/or symptomatic MTC was vandetanib, which blocks signaling of epidermal growth factor receptor (EGFR), of vascular endothelial growth factor receptor-2 (VEGFR2), and of rearranged during transfection (RET). Meanwhile, cabozantinib blocks the hepatocyte growth factor receptor (MET), RET, and VEGFR2. The main activity of both drugs is versus VEGF receptors (particularly VEGFR2), while the affinity for RET is lower [1,7,8]. Both vandetanib and cabozantinib are shown to increase progression-free survival (PFS) in patients with symptomatic and progressive MTC [9,10]. Regarding the overall survival (OS), the best results appear to be related to the use of cabozantinib in patients with *RET* M918T-positive MTC (44.3 months vs. 18.9 months in those treated with placebo) [11]. More recently, highly selective RET kinase inhibitors, including selpercatinib and pralsetinib, have been approved in oncology, but the second drug has not yet been approved in Italy. Selpercatinib has been approved for adult patients with metastatic RET fusion–positive NSCLC and adult and pediatric patients $\geq$ 12 years of age with advanced or metastatic *RET*-mutant MTC or metastatic *RET* fusion–positive thyroid cancer who require systemic therapy and who are radioactive iodine refractory. In the registration studies (phase I–II trial, LIBRETTO-001 trial), at the dose of 160 mg twice daily, selpercatinib showed efficacy in MTC with a 1-year PFS of 82% in patients with *RET* mutant MTC who had previously been treated with vandetanib, cabozantinib, or both and of 92% in patients with *RET*-mutant MTC without previous treatment [12]. Selpercatinib, approved by the FDA in 2020 and in 2021 by the European Medicines Agency (EMA), has also been approved by the Italian Pharmaceutical Agency

(AIFA) in August 2022, after the results of the phase III randomized trial (Libretto-531) comparing selpercatinib as a first-line therapy with cabozantinib or vandetanib (control group) in patients with progressive MTC. The study showed a PFS at 12 months of 86.8% (95% CI, 79.8–91.6) in the selpercatinib group and 65.7% (95% CI, 51.9–76.4) in the control group; the overall response rate (ORR) was 69.4% (95% CI, 62.4–75.8) in the selpercatinib group and 38.8% (95% CI, 29.1–49.2) in the control group [4]. Although vandetanib and cabozantinib have been associated with increased AEs due to their wide antiangiogenetic activity with a frequent dose reduction or possible discontinuation, to date, there is still no clear evidence as to which systemic regimen should be used as the first-line treatment. The potential toxicity of all the drugs above, if severe, may lead in some cases to an early discontinuation of treatment; then, a proper management of side effects is essential to ensure the patient's compliance over the long term and thus to see the beneficial effects of the treatment, which should be continued as long as possible. We still do not know why some patients tolerate medications better than others, even if genetic makeup appears to play a role, but it is clear that higher doses are associated with more frequent and intense side effects [13]. In ZETA trial [10], vandetanib caused an AE in 55% of the patients (24% having at least grade 3 toxicities). The most common AEs were diarrhea (56%); skin abnormalities like rash, acne, and folliculitis (~50%); nausea (30%); hypertension (30%); abdominal pain, fatigue, headaches, and decreased appetite (20–25%); and proteinuria (10%). Fourteen percent of the patients had prolongation of the QT interval, a potentially life-threatening condition because it can predispose to torsade des pointes. Due to the side effects, 35% of the patients needed dose reductions, and 12% discontinued treatment. Five patients (2%) had treatment-related lethal toxicity, but their causes of death were not clearly related to prolongation of the QT interval. Rare but serious AEs included interstitial lung disease, Stevens–Johnson syndrome, cerebrovascular accidents, congestive heart failure, and reversible posterior leukoencephalopathy. The AEs of cabozantinib were reported in the EXAM trial [11]. The most common were diarrhea (63%), hypothyroidism, hypocalcemia, stomatitis, hand–foot syndrome, weight loss, nausea, lack of appetite, fatigue (40–50%), and hypertension (30%). Of the patients, 79% percent needed dose reductions, and 16% discontinued treatment. Of the patients, 69% had grade 3 or 4 AEs, and 6% experienced a fatal AE. Rare but serious AEs included gastrointestinal perforation, fistula formation, bleeding, thromboembolic phenomena, osteonecrosis of the jaw, poor wound healing, and reversible posterior leukoencephalopathy. The LIBRETTO-001 trial [14] described the efficacy and safety of selpercatinib in 702 patients, 143 of them *RET*-mutant, 55 previously treated with cabozantinib or vandetanib, and 88 patients naive. The most common severe AEs were hypertension (grades 1–4: 35% any grade, 18% grade 3–4), increased alanine aminotransferase (ALT) (45% any grade, 9% grades 3–4), increased aspartate aminotransferase (AST) (51% any grade, 8% grade 3–4), increased creatinine levels (37% any grade, 1% grade 3–4), and edemas (33% any grade, 0.3% grade 3–4). The LIBRETTO 531 comparing selpercatinib with vandetanib or cabozantinb as a first-line therapy confirmed the same AEs, including among the most common (>20%) also diarrhea (26%), dry mouth (32%), and fatigue (19%). In the LIBRETTO 531 trial, the AEs led to a dose reduction in 38.9% of the patients in the selpercatinib group, as compared with 77.3% in the control group, and to treatment discontinuation in 4.7% and 26.8%, respectively.

Due to the relatively recent introduction of these drugs, no consistent real-world data are available. A real-world multicenter retrospective experience conducted on 12 metastatic patients with locally advanced MTC treated with vandetanib demonstrated a PR in five patients (42%) and stable disease for $\geq$24 weeks in an additional five patients (83%) with a median PFS of 25.9 months [15]. Only one larger real-world study involving 48 progressive MTC patient treated with vandetanib and/or cabozantinib [16] confirmed their efficacy in this patient setting. A total of 47 patients (98%) were treated with vandetanib and 23 (48%) with cabozantinib (first- or second-line treatment), and a PR was observed in 26% of patients treated with vandetanib and 22% with cabozantinib. The median PFSs for vandetanib and cabozantinib were 17 months and 4 months, respectively. Both in patients treated with vandetanib and in those treated with cabozantinib, the PFS was significantly longer in patients experiencing AEs and in patients aged ≤60 years. In the vandetanib group the PFS was longer in the absence of bone metastases, but in this patient setting, vandetanib was more effective than cabozantinib (PR in 28% vs. none). The poorer prognosis of cabozantinib-treated patients was likely due to its use as a second-line treatment after vandetanib failure and in rapidly progressive diseases.

In our experience, described in this case series, we are aware that this is a very small cohort, but given the rarity of the disease, we wanted to describe our monocentric experience with recently introduced drugs for which there are still limited real-life data on efficacy and all potential side effects. Three out of five patients were treated, in a different order, with all of the three drugs currently available in Europe for metastatic MTC (vandetanib, cabozantinb, and selpercatinib) and two of them with only two drugs (vandetanib/cabozantinib and cabozantinib/selpercatinib). Three patients obtained a PR, one of these with cabozantinb (patient 2), one with selpercatinib (patient 3), and one with vandetanib (patient 4); all these responses were evident after 6 months of therapy. Disease progression occurred in patient 2 with the first-line therapy with vandetanib (PFS of 17 months) and in patient 4 with cabozantinib and selpercatinib (with PFS of 12 months and 18 months, respectively). Disease stability was evident in two patients, both of them with bone metastases (patients 1 and 5). A *RET* somatic mutation was observed in four of five patients (M918T mutation in three cases and C618S in one case). A disease PR was achieved in the wild-type *RET* patient with cabozantinb and in the two patients with M918T mutations with selpercatinib and vandetanib. Although responses to therapy were seen in a relatively short time (6 months), in some cases it was not possible to evaluate the real efficacy of selpercatinib and cabozantinib, due to early discontinuation for the AEs that were mostly in line with those reported in clinical trials and all reversible. In three of the patients, the first-line therapy with vandetanib was interrupted due to the drug's unavailability, without significant side effects or disease progression. It is worth mentioning that patient 5 was only on vandetanib for one month, so its efficacy could not be evaluated. For the second-line therapy, three out of five patients were treated with cabozantinib, and in all cases, treatment was discontinued due to side effects. Two patients received selpercatinib as a second-line therapy; in one case, treatment continued with a partial response, while in the other, it was stopped due to disease progression (Table 1).

From our experience we must point out two AEs not described in clinical trials probably due to the low prevalence: the lung cavitations on non-neoplastic tissue developed during cabozantinib therapy and the non-neoplastic ascites associated with selpercatinib therapy.

Regarding the lung cavitations, the antiangiogenetic agents have been associated with the development of cavitations of lung neoplastic lesions that can be explained with the necrosis treatment-related, cyst formation or desquamation/liquefaction of tumor cells within the lesion [17]. Several authors reported tumoral cavitations in advanced lung cancer during antiangiogenetic therapy [18,19]. To date, pulmonary cavitations are an unexpected AE in patients with metastatic thyroid cancer, but a recent retrospective cohort study conducted on 83 patients affected by thyroid cancer and lung metastases treated with multi-targeted antiangiogenic TKIs described 10 cases of lung cavitations (12%), two of them complicated with pneumothorax although without effects on survival [20]. The impact of tumor cavitation on survival in lung cancer patients treated with antiangiogenetic drugs remains controversial: studies conducted on different lung cancer histotypes have been associated with a better or worse PFS [21,22]. To the best of our knowledge, we described for the first time the case of lung cavitations arising on healthy tissue in a patient treated with a TKI drug, specifically with cabozantinib. The pathogenic mechanism underlying this event remains difficult to explain: we could consider the possible cumulative anti-angiogenic mechanism of the two drugs since the patient had been treated with vandetanib before cabozantinib, or we could consider the possibility of unknown genetic predisposing factors. Certainly, our findings will need to be confirmed by further studies. It is essential to take into account this AE since it compromised the patient's outcome and predisposed him to recurrent pneumonia and infections, which did not allow the continuation of oncological treatment. Unfortunately, the pulmonary cavitations were not responsive to antibiotic treatments, so this AE contributed, together with anorexia and severe weight loss, to the cabozantinb discontinuation, despite a satisfactory response on the other target lesions.

Currently, most of the information regarding the AEs associated with selpercatinib is derived from clinical trials, but long-term or rare AEs could be encountered from the clinical practice. The occurrence of effusions during selpercatinib treatment, although not reported in LIBRETTO-001 trials [14], has been recently described in a study using the FDA Adverse Event Reporting System Database [23]. In this study, three new significant AEs were described in a total of 464 reports and 1007 selpercatinib-related AEs: dysphagia, pericardial effusion, and hemiparesis. A retrospective multicenter study reported spontaneous chylous effusions associated with selpercatinib with an incidence of 7%, more than other TKIs [24]. Furthermore, a retrospective study evaluating MCT patients enrolled in the LIBRETTO-201 clinical trial (ClinicalTrial.gov Identifier NCT03906331) described the presence of effusions in 8/10 MTC patients treated with selpercatinib. Five of them had no effusions before starting selpercatinib, and three had some effusions already present before selpercatinib but developed new effusions in other sites (pleural, pericardial, abdominal, or pelvic) and/or worsened those that were already present. Fluid aspiration, performed in symptomatic and/or moderate/severe cases, demonstrated the chylous nature of the effusions and the absence of malignant cells. The dose reduction has proven effective on related symptoms [25]. Several etiologies of chylothorax or chylous ascites have been described, but in that cohort [25], congenital, traumatic, and obstructive causes have been excluded. Although the mechanism underlying chylous effusions remains unclear, given the potential role of the RET protein in the migration of lymphatic endothelial cells [26], a possible hypothesis is that RET inhibition could alter the integrity of lymphatic endothelial cells, leading to increased lymphatic endothelial permeability and ultimately resulting in chylous effusions. Also, in our experience the ascitic effusion was considered a selpercatinib-related AE in patient 4 but not certainly in patient 3, since the presence of ascites was found simultaneously with the start of selpercatinib therapy, and we can suppose a possible role of the previous cabozantinib therapy. In patient 4, the cytological analysis excluded the presence of malignant cells, although it did not analyze the nature of the effusion, and this AE was shown to be reversible with discontinuation of the drug.

In our clinical experience, vandetanib demonstrated an optimal efficacy profile in terms of disease stabilization and long-term tolerability, with a treatment duration of up to 48 months in one patient and mostly at the maximum dose of 300 mg daily without a dose reduction requirement. Undoubtedly, the longer-lasting experience on vandetanib may have led to better management of AEs, compared with cabozantinib and selpercatinib, which, however, demonstrated good efficacy in terms of response to treatment, and consequently, they may be more effective in patients with rapidly progressing MTC. Due to the little consensus available on how to select a specific treatment as the first line [5], actually, each of the three drugs can be chosen. Mutation analyses are yet not useful to indicate which patients are most likely to benefit from targeted treatment, although current evidence favors vandetanib and selpercatinib in cases of *RET* oncogene mutation. The selection of the first-line systemic therapy for MTC must be individualized, considering patients' characteristics, such as their performance status, age, physical examination, comorbidities, other treatment, social aspects, disease progression, tumor features, and medication availability. Advanced MTC with bone metastases remains one of the most urgent challenges since the objective response in these patients is very poor, and studies to date have not demonstrated the superiority of any treatment over another. In our patients with bone metastases, stable disease was observed during vandetanib, cabozantinib, and selpercatinib, but a significant reduction in CT and CEA levels was obtained only with selpercatinib. Our limited case series comparing different treatment regimens does not allow us to determine the most effective therapy for patients with metastatic MTC. What stands out from our experience is the importance of preventing severe side effects that could lead to therapy discontinuation. Specifically, with cabozantinib, it is crucial to closely monitor proteinuria, electrolyte imbalances (especially hypocalcemia), and weight loss. Therefore, nutritional support and adequate supplementation of calcium and magnesium are essential, particularly in patients with post-surgical hypoparathyroidism.

4. Conclusions

TKIs are valuable treatments in patients with non-resectable symptomatic, rapidly progressive MTC because they can extend PFS and provide long-term disease stabilization. However, complete responses are uncommon, and TKIs have many significant adverse effects, which can lead to poor quality of life. The best option for the management of MTC must be an individualized approach, keeping in mind the patient's characteristics, the potential toxicity, and the effects of the treatment on their quality of life in order to minimize the dose reduction or treatment withdrawal. Specifically, cabozantinib should be used with caution in patients with post-surgical hypoparathyroidism and malabsorption issues. In the case of selpercatinib, special attention should be given to patients with hepatic metastases or cardiovascular diseases due to the risk of ascites and pericardial effusion. Lung cavitations in the absence of pulmonary metastases should be considered as a possible adverse event with cabozantinib therapy.

Author Contributions: M.M., conception and design of the work; M.M., R.L., G.P. and M.B., data collection and interpretation; M.M., writing of the first draft; R.L. and M.E.S., writing of the article's sections; G.P. and M.A., review of the article. All authors have read and agreed to the published version of the manuscript.

Funding: This work was financially supported through funding from the institutional "Ricerca Corrente" granted by the Italian Ministry of Health.

Institutional Review Board Statement: The study was conducted in accordance with the Declaration of Helsinki and approved by the local ethics committee of Regina Elena National Cancer Institute on 3 December 2024 (reference number 271/24).

Informed Consent Statement: All the participants signed an informed consent form.

Data Availability Statement: All data generated or analyzed in this case series are included in this article. Further inquiries can be directed to the corresponding author.

Conflicts of Interest: M.A. declares consultancy and research grants from Bayer, Eisai, and Eli-Lilly. G.P. declares consultancy for Bayer. The other authors declare no conflicts of interest.

References

1. Fugazzola, L. Medullary thyroid cancer—An update. *Best Pract. Res. Clin. Endocrinol. Metab.* **2023**, *37*, 101655. [CrossRef] [PubMed]
2. Jin, L.X.; Moley, J.F. Surgery for lymph node metastases of medullary thyroid carcinoma: A review. *Cancer* **2016**, *122*, 358–366. [CrossRef] [PubMed]
3. Filetti, S.; Durante, C.; Hartl, D.; Leboulleux, S.; Locati, L.D.; Newbold, K.; Papotti, M.G.; Berruti, A.; the ESMO Guidelines Committee. Thyroid cancer: ESMO Clinical Practice Guidelines for diagnosis, treatment and follow-updagger. *Ann. Oncol.* **2019**, *30*, 1856–1883. [CrossRef]
4. Hadoux, J.; Elisei, R.; Brose, M.S.; Hoff, A.O.; Robinson, B.G.; Gao, M.; Jarzab, B.; Isaev, P.; Kopeckova, K.; Wadsley, J.; et al. Phase 3 Trial of Selpercatinib in Advanced RET-Mutant Medullary Thyroid Cancer. *N. Engl. J. Med.* **2023**, *389*, 1851–1861. [CrossRef] [PubMed]
5. Wells, S.A., Jr.; Asa, S.L.; Dralle, H.; Elisei, R.; Evans, D.B.; Gagel, R.F.; Lee, N.; Machens, A.; Moley, J.F.; Pacini, F.; et al. Revised American Thyroid Association guidelines for the management of medullary thyroid carcinoma. *Thyroid* **2015**, *25*, 567–610. [CrossRef] [PubMed]
6. Eisenhauer, E.A.; Therasse, P.; Bogaerts, J.; Schwartz, L.H.; Sargent, D.; Ford, R.; Dancey, J.; Arbuck, S.; Gwyther, S.; Mooney, M.; et al. New response evaluation criteria in solid tumours: Revised RECIST guideline (version 1.1). *Eur. J. Cancer* **2009**, *45*, 228–247. [CrossRef] [PubMed]
7. Yakes, F.M.; Chen, J.; Tan, J.; Yamaguchi, K.; Shi, Y.; Yu, P.; Qian, F.; Chu, F.; Bentzien, F.; Cancilla, B.; et al. Cabozantinib (XL184), a novel MET and VEGFR2 inhibitor, simultaneously suppresses metastasis, angiogenesis, and tumor growth. *Mol. Cancer Ther.* **2011**, *10*, 2298–2308. [CrossRef]

8. Wedge, S.R.; Ogilvie, D.J.; Dukes, M.; Kendrew, J.; Chester, R.; Jackson, J.A.; Boffey, S.J.; Valentine, P.J.; Curwen, J.O.; Musgrove, H.L.; et al. ZD6474 inhibits vascular endothelial growth factor signaling, angiogenesis, and tumor growth following oral administration. *Cancer Res.* **2002**, *62*, 4645–4655.
9. Elisei, R.; Schlumberger, M.J.; Muller, S.P.; Schoffski, P.; Brose, M.S.; Shah, M.H.; Licitra, L.; Jarzab, B.; Medvedev, V.; Kreissl, M.C.; et al. Cabozantinib in progressive medullary thyroid cancer. *J. Clin. Oncol.* **2013**, *31*, 3639–3646. [CrossRef] [PubMed]
10. Wells, S.A., Jr.; Robinson, B.G.; Gagel, R.F.; Dralle, H.; Fagin, J.A.; Santoro, M.; Baudin, E.; Elisei, R.; Jarzab, B.; Vasselli, J.R.; et al. Vandetanib in patients with locally advanced or metastatic medullary thyroid cancer: A randomized, double-blind phase III trial. *J. Clin. Oncol.* **2012**, *30*, 134–141. [CrossRef]
11. Schlumberger, M.; Elisei, R.; Muller, S.; Schoffski, P.; Brose, M.; Shah, M.; Licitra, L.; Krajewska, J.; Kreissl, M.C.; Niederle, B.; et al. Overall survival analysis of EXAM, a phase III trial of cabozantinib in patients with radiographically progressive medullary thyroid carcinoma. *Ann. Oncol.* **2017**, *28*, 2813–2819. [CrossRef]
12. Wirth, L.J.; Sherman, E.; Robinson, B.; Solomon, B.; Kang, H.; Lorch, J.; Worden, F.; Brose, M.; Patel, J.; Leboulleux, S.; et al. Efficacy of Selpercatinib in RET-Altered Thyroid Cancers. *N. Engl. J. Med.* **2020**, *383*, 825–835. [CrossRef] [PubMed]
13. Kiyota, N.; Schlumberger, M.; Muro, K.; Ando, Y.; Takahashi, S.; Kawai, Y.; Wirth, L.; Robinson, B.; Sherman, S.; Suzuki, T.; et al. Subgroup analysis of Japanese patients in a phase 3 study of lenvatinib in radioiodine-refractory differentiated thyroid cancer. *Cancer Sci.* **2015**, *106*, 1714–1721. [CrossRef]
14. Bradford, D.; Larkins, E.; Mushti, S.L.; Rodriguez, L.; Skinner, A.M.; Helms, W.S.; Price, L.S.L.; Zirkelbach, J.F.; Li, Y.; Liu, J.; et al. FDA Approval Summary: Selpercatinib for the Treatment of Lung and Thyroid Cancers with RET Gene Mutations or Fusions. *Clin. Cancer Res.* **2021**, *27*, 2130–2135. [CrossRef]
15. Kim, M.; Yoon, J.H.; Ahn, J.; Jeon, M.J.; Kim, H.K.; Lim, D.J.; Kang, H.C.; Kim, I.J.; Shong, Y.K.; Kim, T.Y.; et al. Vandetanib for the Management of Advanced Medullary Thyroid Cancer: A Real-World Multicenter Experience. *Endocrinol. Metab.* **2020**, *35*, 587–594. [CrossRef] [PubMed]
16. Koehler, V.F.; Adam, P.; Frank-Raue, K.; Raue, F.; Berg, E.; Hoster, E.; Allelein, S.; Schott, M.; Kroiss, M.; Spitzweg, C. Real-World Efficacy and Safety of Cabozantinib and Vandetanib in Advanced Medullary Thyroid Cancer. *Thyroid* **2021**, *31*, 459–469. [CrossRef] [PubMed]
17. Dodd, G.D.; Boyle, J.J. Excavating pulmonary metastases. *Am. J. Roentgenol. Radium Ther. Nucl. Med.* **1961**, *85*, 277–293.
18. Marom, E.M.; Martinez, C.H.; Truong, M.T.; Lei, X.; Sabloff, B.S.; Munden, R.F.; Gladish, G.W.; Herbst, R.S.; Morice, R.C.; Stewart, D.J.; et al. Tumor cavitation during therapy with antiangiogenesis agents in patients with lung cancer. *J. Thorac. Oncol.* **2008**, *3*, 351–357. [CrossRef] [PubMed]
19. Crabb, S.J.; Patsios, D.; Sauerbrei, E.; Ellis, P.M.; Arnold, A.; Goss, G.; Leighl, N.B.; Shepherd, F.A.; Powers, J.; Seymour, L.; et al. Tumor cavitation: Impact on objective response evaluation in trials of angiogenesis inhibitors in non-small-cell lung cancer. *J. Clin. Oncol.* **2009**, *27*, 404–410. [CrossRef] [PubMed]
20. Datar, S.; Cabanillas, M.; Dadu, R.; Ost, D.; Grosu, H.B. Pulmonary cavitation in patients with thyroid cancer receiving antiangiogenic agents. *BMC Cancer* **2020**, *20*, 1181. [CrossRef] [PubMed]
21. Chen, D.; Xu, J.; Zhao, Y.; Chu, T.; Zhong, H.; Han, B.; Zhong, R. Prognostic value of tumor cavitation in extensive-stage small-cell lung cancer patients treated with anlotinib. *J. Cancer Res. Clin. Oncol.* **2020**, *146*, 401–406. [CrossRef]
22. Zhou, F.; Ma, W.; Li, W.; Ni, H.; Gao, G.; Chen, X.; Zhang, J.; Shi, J. Thick-wall cavity predicts worse progression-free survival in lung adenocarcinoma treated with first-line EGFR-TKIs. *BMC Cancer* **2018**, *18*, 1033. [CrossRef] [PubMed]
23. Qian, J.; Zhang, S.; Jiang, C. Adverse event profiles of selpercatinib: A real-world pharmacovigilance analysis based on FAERS database. *BMC Cancer* **2024**, *24*, 1486. [CrossRef]
24. Kalchiem-Dekel, O.; Falcon, C.J.; Bestvina, C.M.; Liu, D.; Kaplanis, L.A.; Wilhelm, C.; Eichholz, J.; Harada, G.; Wirth, L.J.; Digumarthy, S.R.; et al. Brief Report: Chylothorax and Chylous Ascites During RET Tyrosine Kinase Inhibitor Therapy. *J. Thorac. Oncol.* **2022**, *17*, 1130–1136. [CrossRef]
25. Prete, A.; Gambale, C.; Cappagli, V.; Bottici, V.; Rossi, P.; Caciagli, M.; Papini, P.; Taddei, D.; Ortori, S.; Gabbrielli, L.; et al. Chylous effusions in advanced medullary thyroid cancer patients treated with selpercatinib. *Eur. J. Endocrinol.* **2022**, *187*, 905–915. [CrossRef] [PubMed]
26. Williams, S.P.; Odell, A.F.; Karnezis, T.; Farnsworth, R.H.; Gould, C.M.; Li, J.; Paquet-Fifield, S.; Harris, N.C.; Walter, A.; Gregory, J.L.; et al. Genome-wide functional analysis reveals central signaling regulators of lymphatic endothelial cell migration and remodeling. *Sci. Signal.* **2017**, *10*, eaal2987. [CrossRef]

biomedicines

Review

The SUMO Family: Mechanisms and Implications in Thyroid Cancer Pathogenesis and Therapy

Bahejuan Jiaerken [1,2], Wei Liu [1], Jiaojiao Zheng [1], Weifeng Qu [1], Qiao Wu [1,*] and Zhilong Ai [1,*]

1 Department of Surgery (Thyroid & Breast), Zhongshan Hospital, Fudan University, Shanghai 200032, China
2 School of Basic Medical Sciences, Fudan University, Shanghai 200032, China
* Correspondence: wqiao_@fudan.edu.cn (Q.W.); ai.zhilong@zs-hospital.sh.cn (Z.A.); Tel.: +86-15001937355 (Q.W.); +86-13916210622 (Z.A.)

Abstract: (1) Background: Small ubiquitin-like modifiers (SUMOs) are pivotal in post-translational modifications, influencing various cellular processes, such as protein localization, stability, and genome integrity. (2) Methods: This review explores the SUMO family, including its isoforms and catalytic cycle, highlighting their significance in regulating key biological functions in thyroid cancer. We discuss the multifaceted roles of SUMOylation in DNA repair mechanisms, protein stability, and the modulation of receptor activities, particularly in the context of thyroid cancer. (3) Results: The aberrant SUMOylation machinery contributes to tumorigenesis through altered gene expression and immune evasion mechanisms. Furthermore, we examine the therapeutic potential of targeting SUMOylation pathways in thyroid cancer treatment, emphasizing the need for further research to develop effective SUMOylation inhibitors. (4) Conclusions: By understanding the intricate roles of SUMOylation in cancer biology, we can pave the way for innovative therapeutic strategies to improve outcomes for patients with advanced tumors.

Keywords: SUMOylation; thyroid cancer; therapeutic targets; SUMO inhibitor; TAK-981; drug sensitivity

1. Introduction

With over 821,000 cases worldwide in 2022 [1], thyroid cancer ranks as the seventh most common cancer in terms of overall incidence and fifth in women. The incidence rate is three times higher in women than in men. China alone accounted for over half of the global incidence burden, with 466,000 new cases in 2022. Thyroid cancer is classified into three main histological types: (1) differentiated thyroid cancer (DTC), which includes papillary, follicular, and oncocytic carcinomas; (2) medullary thyroid cancer (MTC), sometimes linked with multiple endocrine neoplasia type 2 syndromes; and (3) anaplastic thyroid cancer (ATC), often evolving from differentiated thyroid cancer and associated with high mortality [2]. A study across 25 countries found that the increase in thyroid cancer was primarily confined to papillary carcinomas, which are often detected through intensive thyroid gland screening [3]. For many years, the primary approach to treating thyroid cancer has been the surgical removal of the thyroid gland.

In some cases, particularly for DTC, this surgery is followed by post-operative treatment with radioactive iodine (RAI) and suppressive doses of thyroid replacement hormones. Surgery often results in a cure for most patients with well-differentiated thyroid cancer. Additionally, RAI therapy after surgery has been shown to enhance overall survival in patients who are at a high risk of recurrence. In the management of metastatic thyroid cancer, there is a growing use of antiangiogenic multikinase inhibitors and targeted therapies aimed at specific genetic mutations responsible for the cancer [4].

Protein post-translational modification (PTM) by small ubiquitin-like modifiers (SUMOs) involves the wide-spread regulation of many cellular functions inside the cell of eukaryotic organisms. The SUMO protein is a member of the ubiquitin-like modifier (UbL) protein superfamily: These proteins are composed of analogous small protein domains that are conjugated to target proteins by creating an isopeptidic linkage between the lysine groups of the substrate and the C-terminal end of the UbL protein. This linkage is characterized by the presence of a distinctive diglycine motif at the C-terminus of the UbL protein [5–9]. Since their initial identification in 1996 [10], SUMO proteins have been found to exist in five isoforms in mammalian cells: SUMO1, SUMO2, SUMO3, SUMO4, and SUMO5. While SUMO1–3 are broadly expressed across human tissues, SUMO4 and SUMO5 exhibit more restricted expression patterns, particularly in the testis and lymphocytes [11]. The dynamic nature of SUMO modification (SUMOylation), a reversible modification process, plays a critical role in modulating protein localization, stability, and function, thereby influencing key biological pathways such as DNA repair, transcriptional regulation, and cellular stress responses [12,13]. Recent studies have highlighted the multifaceted roles of SUMOylation in cancer biology, particularly in thyroid cancer, where aberrant SUMOylation patterns contribute to tumorigenesis and progression [14,15]. This review explores the intricate mechanisms of SUMOylation and its implications in thyroid cancer, emphasizing potential therapeutic strategies that target the SUMOylation pathway to improve patient outcomes.

2. SUMO Proteins and SUMO Catalytic Cycle

2.1. SUMO Family in Human

Essential for cellular homeostasis, SUMO proteins regulate various biological processes via a dynamic SUMOylation–deSUMOylation cycle. SUMO proteins, first discovered in 1996, play a pivotal role in PTM in eukaryotic cells, with five isoforms—SUMO1–5—that structurally resemble ubiquitin [16].

SUMO proteins, which come in five isoforms (SUMO1, SUMO2, SUMO3, SUMO4, and SUMO5), are crucial in post-translational modification across human tissues. While SUMO1–3 are ubiquitously expressed, SUMO4 and SUMO5 follow tissue-specific patterns, with SUMO5 being particularly abundant in testis and blood lymphocytes [11]. SUMO2 and SUMO3, due to their high amino acid sequence similarity, are collectively referred to as SUMO-2/3 [17,18]. SUMO1 typically modifies proteins related to physiological status, while SUMO-2/3 is involved in stress-responsive protein modifications [19]. It is hypothesized that SUMO-2/3 may compensate for SUMO1 in its typical protein targets [20]. Current research on SUMO4 and SUMO5 suggests potential associations with diabetes and leukemia, respectively, though further investigation is ongoing [21].

2.2. SUMO Catalytic Cycle

SUMO proteins, initially present as inactive precursors with a molecular weight of around 11 kDa, undergo activation via proteolytic cleavage catalyzed by enzymes such as ULP1 in yeast or Sentrin/SUMO-specific protease 1 (SENP1) in humans. This cleavage exposes a crucial diglycine motif for subsequent interactions [22,23]. SUMO activation is mediated by the heterodimeric E1-activating enzyme (SAE1/SAE2), which forms a thioester bond between the SUMO and its internal cysteine residue (Cys593) through ATP hydrolysis [24–26]. Subsequently, the activated SUMO is transferred to the cysteine residue at position 93 of UBC9, the sole E2-conjugating enzyme, via a transesterification reaction, generating an E2-SUMO thioester [27–32]. UBC9 catalyzes the conjugation of SUMO to lysine residues of target proteins, completing the SUMOylation process. This process is facilitated by E3 ligases, which stabilize the E2-SUMO thioester conformation, enabling its conjugation to the substrate lysine residue within a SUMO-interacting motif (SIM) [33–35]. This multi-step enzymatic cascade ensures the accurate and efficient modification of target proteins by the SUMO [36–38].

DeSUMOylation, a reversible and dynamic process, is terminated by SUMO proteases known as SENPs or Sentrin/SUMO-specific proteases, Figure 1. Six SENPs have been identified in humans, with unique cellular locations and substrate specificities [39]. SENP1 and SENP2, localized primarily at the nuclear pore, can process all three SUMO isoforms

(SUMO1, 2, and 3) and remove both mono- and polymeric SUMOylated proteins. By contrast, SENP3 to SENP7 exclusively process SUMO-2/3, with SENP6 and SENP7 exhibiting sole hydrolase activity [40]. These proteases play a pivotal role in embryonic development, reflecting their distinct functions [41–43]. Recent discoveries include SUMO proteases deSUMOylating isopeptidase 1 (DESI1), DESI2, and USPL1, which have little sequence identity with the ULP/SENP family [44,45]. Each SENP exhibits various cellular locations and substrate specificities [39,46,47].

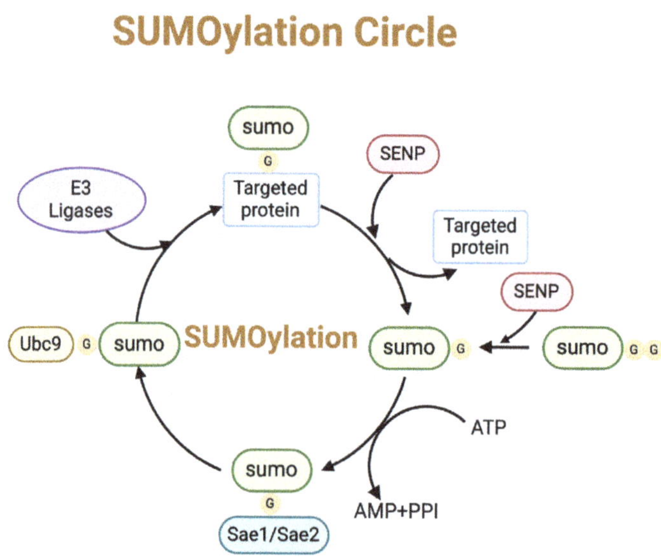

Figure 1. The visualization of SUMOylation circle. SUMO precursors are processed by Sentrin-specific protease 1 (SENP1), SENP2, and SENP5 to yield SUMO-GG, which is activated by SUMO E1 (SAE1/SAE2), transferred to SUMO E2 (UBC9), and assisted by a SUMO E3 ligase to conjugate to substrates. SUMO can be removed from SUMO-conjugated substrates through SENPs.

3. The Multifaceted Functions of SUMOylation in Protein Localization, Stability, and Genome Integrity

Over the past few years, SUMOylation has become a crucial regulator of diverse cellular processes, including protein localization, stability, and genome integrity, with important roles in transcriptional regulation.

3.1. SUMOylation in DNA End Resection and Genome Stability

Zhang et al. showed that MRE11 SUMOylation and ubiquitylation are dynamically controlled by PIAS1 and SENP3 to facilitate DNA end resection and genome stability [12]. Additionally, the SUMOylation of MORC2, a chromatin-remodeling enzyme, is crucial for chromatin remodeling and DNA repair in response to DNA damage [13]. These findings underscore the importance of post-translational modifications, particularly SUMOylation, in regulating DNA repair mechanisms and genome stability.

3.2. Role of SUMOylation in Maintaining Protein Stability

The dysregulation of the SUMOylation process can lead to the loss of HNF4α and hepatic function, underscoring its vital role in maintaining the hepatocellular phenotype. It has been established that the SUMOylation of HNF4α regulates its protein stability and potentially its transcriptional activity [48]. Furthermore, the pathogenic mutations in the TRAIP gene are associated with primordial dwarfism in patients [49]. SUMOylation has been demonstrated as critical for ensuring the proper subcellular localization and protein stability of TRAIP, which exhibits various functions in the nucleus [50]. Notably, Hamard, P.J., et al. discovered that the ATF7 transcription factor undergoes SUMOylation both in vitro and in vivo. SUMOylation affects the intranuclear localization and transcriptional activity of the ATF7 transcription factor by interfering with its interaction with TAF12, thus impeding its access to specific promoters [51]. These findings underscore the significance of SUMOylation in various biological processes.

3.3. Impact of SUMOylation on Receptors

In the intricate landscape of cellular regulation, SUMOylation emerges as a crucial mechanism modulating the activities of various proteins. Among these, peroxisome-proliferator-activated receptor γ (PPARγ) and pregnane X receptor (PXR) are pivotal players in lipid metabolism and xenobiotic responses, respectively.

PPARγ, a ligand-activated nuclear receptor regulating sugar and lipid metabolism, can be SUMOylated to modulate its activity [52]. The SUMOylation of PPARγ can inhibit its activity, thus affecting lipid metabolism. In lung cancer cells, SUMO modification of PPARγ induces lipid-metabolism-related gene expression, promoting lipid synthesis and NADPH consumption. This process enhances β-oxidation and mitochondrial reactive oxygen species (ROS) production, leading to tumor suppression [53].

In the liver, SUMOylation and ubiquitination of the nuclear receptor pregnane X receptor (PXR/NR1I2) regulate its biological functions, particularly in response to xenobiotic or inflammatory stimuli. The nuclear receptor PXR/NR1I2 is a key regulator in xenobiotic responses, involved in the metabolism and clearance of toxic substances, as well as inflammatory reactions. Specifically, ubiquitination promotes inflammatory responses, while SUMOylation inhibits them [54].

3.4. Regulatory Role of SUMOylation in Ras Proteins

Recent research has shed light on the regulatory impact of Ras proteins via SUMOylation, a process in which all three isoforms of Ras proteins (HRas, KRas, and NRas) are modified by SUMO3 [55]. Identifying lysine 42 as the key site responsible for this modification is of particular significance. Studies involving the KRas V12/r42 mutant discovered that the mutation impedes the activation of the Raf/MEK/ERK signaling pathway, resulting in a decrease in cell migration and invasion rates in diverse in vitro cell models [56]. Additionally, blocking SUMO E2 in pancreatic cells undergoing transformation was found to reduce cell migration dependent on the dosage, corresponding to diminished levels of KRas SUMOylation and the expression of mesenchymal cell markers. Further evidence from experiments using mice as model organisms has shown that introducing SUMO-resistant mutants can impede tumor growth in vivo. Collectively, these findings support the idea that SUMOylation plays a vital role in regulating the functions of Ras in processes such as cell proliferation, differentiation, and malignant transformation. Thus, targeting the SUMO modification system of Ras oncoproteins may offer a promising and innovative therapeutic strategy for addressing various human malignancies.

4. SUMOylation and Thyroid Cancer

4.1. CCDC6 and SUMOylation

Cyclic AMP (cAMP)-response-element-binding protein 1 (CREB) is a 43 kDa stimulus-induced transcription factor (TF) [57]. The overexpression of CREB is associated with aberrant signal transduction caused by the deregulated expression of downstream genes that control the hallmarks of cancer, such as proliferation, apoptosis, angiogenesis, metastasis, immune surveillance, and metabolism, and the generation of tumor stem cells, which lead to the initiation and progression of tumors. These different CREB activities result in increased tumor growth, resistance to antiproliferative signals, decreased apoptosis, enhanced angiogenesis, increased metabolism, and reduced immunogenicity.

The RET/papillary thyroid carcinoma 1 (PTC1) oncogene, frequently found in human papillary thyroid carcinomas, involves the fusion of RET's kinase domain with the initial

101 amino acids of CCDC6, leading to allelic expression loss and influencing thyroid cancer development [58]. This fusion reduces the CCDC6-mediated inhibition of CREB1, resulting in increased CREB1 activity and the upregulation of its target genes, such as AREG and cyclin A, thereby promoting thyroid tumorigenesis [59]. CCDC6, a tumor repressor known for its pro-apoptotic effects [60,61], undergoes SUMOylation, influencing its tumor-suppressive functions. SUMOylation leads to the cytoplasmic sequestration of CCDC6 and a decrease in its interaction with CREB1 (Figure 2), thereby promoting CREB1-dependent transcriptional activity and cellular proliferation [14]. This mechanism highlights the dual role of SUMOylation in regulating tumor suppressor activity and promoting thyroid cancer progression (Figure 2).

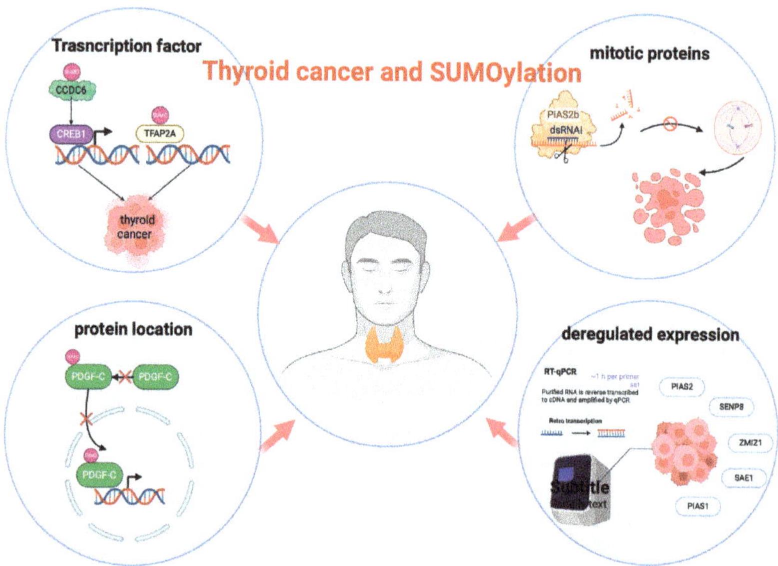

Figure 2. SUMOylation and Thyroid cancer.

4.2. *PDGF-C and SUMOylation*

Platelet-derived growth factor-C (PDGF-C), a key growth factor in cancer progression, plays a crucial role in promoting growth, angiogenesis, and tumorigenesis in various types of cancers [62–64]. Recent studies have shown that in thyroid cancer cells, the levels of SUMOylated PDGF-C in the nucleus are significantly lower than normal thyroid cells [65] (Figure 2). This decrease in SUMOylation may play a role in the development of thyroid cancer by impacting growth, angiogenesis, and tumor formation. However, further research is needed to fully understand the mechanisms involved, whether through inhibited SUMOylation or increased deSUMOylation.

4.3. *TFAP2A and SUMOylation*

Recent findings indicate that the progression from papillary to anaplastic thyroid cancer in cell models may be driven by the SUMOylation of transcription factor TFAP2A, which alters gene expression patterns linked to anaplastic thyroid cancer [15]. Follow-up studies using SUMO inhibitors, PYR-41 and anacardic acid, in murine models of anaplastic thyroid cancer demonstrated reductions in tumor size and enhanced tumor-free survival (Figure 2), suggesting that targeting this post-translational modification could potentially ameliorate outcomes in anaplastic thyroid cancer. However, these promising outcomes from cell and animal models need further validation and cautious interpretation before clinical application.

4.4. Deregulation of SUMOylation Machinery in Thyroid Cancer

A comprehensive analysis of the expression of SUMOylation machinery components in papillary thyroid cancer (PTC) reveals the significant deregulation of SENP8, ZMIZ1, SAE1, PIAS1, and PIAS2 in most cases [66] (Figure 2). Although these alterations do not correlate with clinicopathological parameters, they likely contribute to the PTC phenotype, underscoring the complex role of SUMOylation in thyroid cancer pathogenesis.

4.5. The Role of PIAS2b in Anaplastic Thyroid Carcinomas

The PIAS family (PIAS1-4) comprises nuclear, zinc-binding proteins distinguished by a Siz/PIAS (SP)-RING domain that functions as an E3 SUMO ligase [67]. Among these, PIAS2 is highly expressed in differentiated papillary thyroid carcinomas but significantly reduced in anaplastic thyroid carcinomas (ATC), a highly lethal, undifferentiated cancer. Recent research [68] identified PIAS2b as essential for mitosis in ATC cells. Silencing PIAS2b with dsRNAi selectively induces cell death in these aggressive cancer cells by disrupting spindle assembly, impairing chromosome–microtubule attachment, and enhancing proteasome activity (Figure 2). This silencing leads to reduced levels and the SUMOylation of key mitotic proteins (e.g., Tubulin gamma, PLK1, CDK1, PSMC5, TUBB3, and PPP2CA), culminating in mitotic catastrophe. Notably, PIAS2b-dsRNAi specifically targets anaplastic cancer cells, both thyroid and non-thyroid, while sparing normal or hyperplastic cells, underscoring its potential as a therapeutic strategy for these aggressive cancers.

5. The Potential Application of SUMOylation in the Treatment of Thyroid Cancer

Thyroid cancer is a prevalent form of endocrine malignancy worldwide, showing an increased incidence rate in recent years. While conventional treatment options like surgery and radiation therapy are commonly used, some patients do not respond well to these methods or face recurrence and metastasis after initial treatment. Differentiated thyroid cancer (DTC) constitutes the majority of thyroid malignancies, representing roughly 80–90% of diagnosed cases [69]. This category predominantly includes papillary and follicular carcinomas. Total thyroidectomy (TT) and thyroid lobectomy (TL) are the main surgical approaches to DTC, with low to intermediate risk of recurrence. Complications arising from these procedures, notably injury to the recurrent laryngeal nerve and hypocalcemia due to parathyroid gland dysfunction, can significantly affect the patient's overall well-being. In the pediatric population, as observed in adults, there has been a documented increase in the incidence of thyroid cancer over the past few decades [70]. The risk of surgical complications in children is elevated compared with the adult patient cohort. Given the exceedingly low disease-specific mortality rate in pediatric DTC patients, it is of the utmost importance to minimize the morbidity associated with treatment [71]. To enhance the effectiveness of thyroid cancer treatment, it is imperative to delve into innovative therapeutic approaches and molecular targets. The SUMOylation pathway, a crucial cellular modification process, has emerged as a promising target for thyroid cancer therapy. By focusing on this pathway, researchers aim to develop new strategies that may revolutionize the outcomes of thyroid cancer treatment and offer hope to patients battling this disease.

The dual roles of SUMOylation on substrates disrupt normal cellular processes, thereby playing a significant role in cancer promotion and suppression. On the one hand, SUMOylation primarily promotes oncogenic effects, driven by the deregulation of SUMO machinery components and the abnormal SUMOylation of key oncoproteins and tumor suppressors. Conversely, while SUMOylation does have tumor-suppressive effects, these are relatively minor, indicating a need for further research in this area. Thus, a comprehensive investigation into the targets and effects of SUMOylation will bolster confidence in the efficacy of SUMOylation-based cancer therapies. A growing body of research strongly supports the oncogenic roles of SUMOylation in tumor invasion, metastasis, angiogenesis, DNA damage and repair, and metabolic reprogramming. These oncogenic mechanisms offer potential targets and avenues for SUMOylation-based cancer therapies.

5.1. Potential Therapeutic Targets in the SUMOylation Pathway

5.1.1. Targeting Tumor Invasion and Metastasis

The hallmark of tumor cell dissemination is the invasive metastatic cascade, the most lethal aspect of tumors. Notably, the SUMOylation cascade regulates tumor metastasis by promoting tumor angiogenesis and the epithelial–mesenchymal transition (EMT). Tumor angiogenesis refers to the forming of new blood vessels that supply tumors with essential oxygen and nutrients for growth and metastasis. Various angiogenic signaling pathways regulate this process. Although the role of SUMOylation in tumor angiogenesis remains unclear, evidence suggests its involvement. HEY1 (hairy/enhancer of split related with YRPW motif), a transcription factor from the basic helix–loop–helix family, is recognized as a key player in developmental angiogenesis. Researchers have found that SUMOylation facilitates the formation of the HEY1 transcriptional complex and enhances its DNA-binding capacity in endothelial cells. Consequently, SUMOylation preserves HEY1's role as a repressive transcription factor that regulates numerous angiogenic genes, including receptor tyrosine kinases (RTKs) and components of the Notch pathway [72]. Another study involving HCC stem cells found that the deSUMOylation of hypoxia-inducible factor (HIF-1α) and Oct4 reduced their nuclear accumulation, thereby inhibiting tumor angiogenesis and maintaining stemness [73].

The EMT, characterized by enhanced invasiveness and metastatic potential, is regulated by SUMOylation across various types of cancers. For example, ginkgolic acid inhibits the proliferation, migration, and EMT of gastric cancer cells by blocking the SUMOylation of IGF-1R (insulin-like growth factor 1 receptor), which is significantly upregulated in these cells [74]. Conversely, SUMOylation can inhibit the EMT and tumor metastasis. Specifically, the SUMOylation of annexin A6 slows cell migration and tumor growth by suppressing the RHOU/AKT1-mediated EMT in hepatocellular carcinoma [75].

5.1.2. Targeting the DNA Damage Response

The DNA damage response (DDR) is crucial for maintaining genomic stability. The inherent genomic instability of rapidly proliferating tumors presents therapeutic opportunities to target DDR pathways, enabling the selective destruction of cancer cells through additional replication stress, exogenous DNA damage, or DDR inhibition. Two primary pathways, non-homologous end joining (NHEJ) and homologous recombination (HR), are used by cells to repair the most severe form of DNA damage known as double-strand breaks (DSBs). Studies have shown that post-translational modifications of proteins play a critical role in regulating double-strand break repair. In the NHEJ repair pathway, the ubiquitin E3 ligase RNF168 acts as a key protein that responds promptly to DNA double-strand break damage. SENP1 has been identified as a specific deSUMOylase of RNF168 and is highly expressed in colorectal adenocarcinoma. SENP1 reduces the SUMOylation of RNF168 in response to DNA damage, limiting its recruitment to damaged DNA sites and enhancing repair efficiency, leading to cancer cell resistance against DNA-damaging agents [76]. Conversely, TIP60 is rapidly deSUMOylated by SENP3, facilitating its interaction with DNA-PKcs after irradiation, which promotes NHEJ repair. It is suggested that leaking SENP3 levels increase tumor cell sensitivity to various DNA damage treatments [77].

5.1.3. Targeting RNA Transcription

Several transcription factors and co-transcriptional regulators have been reported as SUMOylated proteins. The relationship between SUMOylation and RNA transcription is primarily reflected in the regulatory effects of SUMOylation modifications on transcription factors and the functional impact on RNA polymerase. Understanding the impact of SUMOylation on RNA metabolism may yield new therapeutic strategies for cancer treatment. Since most SUMOylation substrate proteins are localized in the nucleus, SUMOylation mainly inhibits global transcription activity [78]. Specifically, DAXX, a key regulator of gene expression, interacts with core histones and various proteins to function as a transcriptional co-repressor or co-activator [79], influencing genes involved in cell death, survival, and tumorigenesis. Its expression is elevated in several cancers, including prostate [80], ovarian [81], and gastric cancer [82]. Notably, the SUMO1 modification of DAXX enhances its recruitment to PML-NBs and promotes apoptosis in cancer cells [83]. Transcription profiling indicates that SUMOylation represses global transcription by inhibiting transcriptional elongation. SUMOs and MYC exert opposing effects on global gene expression by modulating the dynamic processes of the SUMOylation and deSUMOylation of CDK9, the catalytic subunit of the P-TEFb kinase, which is crucial for effective transcriptional elongation. Specifically, the SUMOylation of CDK9 leads to transcriptional repression, while MYC enhances global transcription by counteracting CDK9 SUMOylation [84]. As an oncogene, MYC belongs to a superfamily of genes that encode frequently activated oncoproteins in human cancers [85]. Since MYC promotes gene expression by inhibiting CDK9 SUMOylation, targeting CDK9 SUMOylation may represent a viable therapeutic strategy, especially since there are currently no approved direct inhibitors of MYC.

5.1.4. Targeting Immune Evasion

Many cancers evade the immune system through distinct immune evasion strategies [86]. Targeting the SUMOylation cascade inhibits tumor immune evasion by altering the tumor microenvironment and reconstituting immune surveillance. ROS, central factors in regulating the tumor microenvironment, also contribute to tumor immune evasion [87,88]. Cytotoxic T-cells (CTLs) are key players in cellular defense within the adaptive immune response. CTLs recognize foreign antigens processed and presented by the MHC class I (MHC-I) antigen processing and presentation machinery (APM) of target cells. The loss or down-regulation of the MHC-I APM is a common cause of primary and acquired resistance to cancer immunotherapies. The pharmacological inhibition of SUMOylation (SUMOi) not only drives the activation and IFN-γ secretion of CTLs but also amplifies the IFN-γ-induced restoration of tumor-intrinsic MHC-I suppression, thereby reconstituting immune surveillance [89]. In addition to immune cells, SUMOylation in tumor cells can also facilitate tumor immune evasion. Specifically, the SUMOylation of programmed cell death protein-1 ligand (PD-L1) by TRIM28, an E3 ubiquitin ligase and SUMO ligase, stabilizes PD-L1 by hampering its ubiquitination and enhancing its SUMOylation, leading to T-cell inactivation and immune evasion in gastric cancer [90]. Emerging data demonstrate that protein modification by SUMO represents a novel target for activating antitumor immunity. Combining tumor immunotherapy with SUMOylation inhibitors may provide a promising strategy for overcoming resistance to immunotherapy.

5.1.5. Targeting Metabolic Reprogramming

Metabolic reprogramming is a hallmark of tumor cells, characterized by alterations in metabolic pathways during their proliferation and progression [91]. The SUMOylation cascade plays a crucial role in metabolic reprogramming, including the Warburg effect and fatty acid metabolism [92]. Therefore, targeting the SUMOylation cascade presents a promising strategy to suppress metabolic reprogramming, improve the tumor microenvironment, inhibit tumor growth, and enhance the sensitivity to antitumor drugs. The Warburg effect, also known as aerobic glycolysis, represents a typical abnormality in glucose metabolism within tumors and is regulated by SUMOylation. Specifically, the SUMO1-induced SUMOylation of PKM2, through binding to the SUMO-interacting motif site IKII265-268, promotes PKM2 dimerization and nuclear translocation, thereby facilitating glycolysis in hepatocellular carcinoma (HCC) [93]. However, the SUMOylation cascade can also inhibit glycolysis in tumors. Hexokinase 2 (HK2), the first rate-limiting enzyme of glycolysis, is SUMOylated at K315 and K492 in prostate cancer cells, which inhibits its binding to mitochondria and consequently reduces glycolysis in tumor cells [94]. In addition to aerobic glycolysis, SUMOylation may disrupt fatty acid metabolism in tumors. Specifically, SENP2, a deSUMOylating protease, enhances fatty acid degradation and consumption by increasing the expression of PPARγ, CPT1A, ACSL1, and CD36 through deSUMOylating

SETDB1, thereby generating more energy to support esophageal squamous cell carcinoma (ESCC) proliferation [95].

5.2. Therapeutic Potential and Development of SUMOylation Inhibitors

The E1 enzyme plays a crucial role in the SUMOylation process. It is emerging as a promising therapeutic target due to its involvement in essential biological functions that support cancer cell survival and progression, such as proliferative signaling, cell cycle regulation, and DNA damage response [96]. Preclinical studies have demonstrated that inhibiting E1 enzymes can restrict tumor growth and enhance antitumor immune responses, suggesting that targeting E1 enzymes represents a viable and rational approach for cancer therapy [97]. Inhibition of SUMOylation has been shown to promote the production of type I interferons (IFNs) and IFNγ [98], which is significant because activation of type I IFN expression can stimulate dendritic cells, leading to immune-mediated tumor rejection through CD8+ T-cell responses [99]. In addition to its immune-modulating effects, direct targeting of SAE has been found to inhibit tumor cell proliferation. Genome-wide RNAi screens have identified the genes encoding the SAE subunits (SAE1 and SAE2) as having the strongest synthetic lethal interactions with c-Myc [100]. Researchers indicated that inhibiting SAE activates the expression of the tumor suppressor miR-34, which targets the mRNA of c-Myc and other oncogenic pathways [101]. Furthermore, SAE is also a critical target for reducing cancer cell stemness [102].

The most successful approach in developing inhibitors of UbL E1 enzymes involves targeting their ATP-binding sites. MLN-4924 (or pevonedistat) is the first molecule resulting from this strategy, highly potent and specific in inhibiting E1 for UbL Nedd8, showing efficacy in treating acute myeloid leukemia [103,104]. The success of MLN-4924 has paved the way for the development of structurally related inhibitors specific to UbL E1 and SUMO E1. For example, the SUMO E1 inhibitor ML-792 displays selective cytotoxicity in c-Myc-overexpressing cells in preclinical studies [105]. ML-93, a derivative of ML-792, demonstrates strong selectivity in inhibiting SUMOylation through a similar mechanism of action in pancreatic cancer, which leads to G2/M phase arrest and promotes apoptosis [106]. Several natural products have also been identified that inhibit SUMO E1 activity, including ginkgolic acid [74,107,108], davidiin [109], tannic acid [110], and kerriamycin B [111]. However, the effectiveness and specificity of these natural compounds are limited, as indicated by their half maximal inhibitory concentration (IC50) values in the micromolar range and their broad range of targets. A newly discovered SAE inhibitor, COH000, targets a cysteine residue in the AAD without affecting the catalytic cysteine [112].

TAK-981, a first-in-class small molecule SUMOylation inhibitor, inhibits SAE similarly to ML-792 by forming an irreversible adduct with SUMO protein in an enzyme-catalyzed, ATP-dependent process. TAK-981 has been found to activate IFN1 signaling to promote antitumor immune responses and is currently undergoing phase I clinical trials [113]. Specifically, an in vivo study revealed that TAK-981 enhanced the proportions of activated CD8 T-cells and natural killer (NK) cells [114]. Furthermore, pretreatment with TAK-981 enhanced macrophage phagocytosis or NK cell cytotoxicity against CD20+ target cells in combination with the anti-CD20 antibody rituximab [115]. TAK-981 also provokes apoptosis and cell cycle arrest in acute myeloid leukemia [116].

The broad application of TAK-981 faces significant challenges, particularly regarding the potential toxicity risks linked to the widespread presence of SUMO modifications. Both systemic and local injections of TAK-981 can cause undesirable inflammation in normal tissues, resulting in adverse events such as diarrhea and ulceration [117]. Furthermore, its poor solubility and low bioavailability further restrict its clinical utility. Another challenge is the inability of systemic or local injections to provide sustained release. Notably, recent research proposes an injectable PDLLA-PEG-PDLLA (PLEL) nanocomposite hydrogel that incorporates self-assembled TAK-981 and BSA nanoparticles for localized treatment of residual tumors following iRFA. The sustained release of TAK-981 from this hydrogel inhibits the expansion of residual tumors and significantly stimulates dendritic cell and cytotoxic lymphocyte-mediated antitumor immune responses while ensuring biosafety. The development of an injectable drug delivery hydrogel holds promise for enhancing the efficacy and expanding the clinical applications of the SUMOylation inhibitor [118] (Table 1).

Table 1. SUMOylation Inhibitors.

Inhibitor [1]	Target	Cancer Type	Refs.
ZHAWOC8697	SENP1 and SENP2	-	[119]
Ursolic acid	SENP1	Hepatocellular carcinoma	[120]
SENP12-(4-Chlorophenyl)-2-oxoethyl 4-benzamidobenzoate derivatives	SENP1	Prostate cancer	[120]
1-[4-(N-benzylamino) phenyl]-3-phenylurea derivatives	SENP1	Cervical carcinoma	[120]
Gallic acid	SENP1	Colorectal cancer	[121,122]
BW467C60	SENP1	-	[123]
Triptolide	SENP1	Prostate cancer	[124]
Momordin Ic	SENP1	Acute myeloid leukemia, colon cancer, prostate cancer	[125]
Ginkgolic acid	E1	Gastric cancer, Breast cancer, Uveal melanoma	[126]
Anacardic acid	E1	Thyroid cancer, nonpromyelocytic acute myeloid leukemia, breast cancer, colon cancer, B-cell lymphoma	[126]
Kerriamycin B	E1	-	[111]
Davidiin	E1	Gastric cancer	[109]
Tannic acid	E1	-	[110]
compound 15	E1	-	[127]
COH000	E1	-	[112]
ML-792	E1	Hepatocellular carcinoma, pancreatic cancer	[105]
ML-93	E1	Pancreatic cancer	[106]
TAK-981	E1	Leukemia, acute myeloid, hepatocellular carcinoma, chronic lymphocytic leukemia, glioblastoma, pancreatic cancer, multiple myeloma	[128]

[1] A plethora of natural and synthetic SUMOylation inhibitors have been identified.

Several studies have reported that SENPs' aberrant expression is associated with the development and progression of cancer [129–131]. SENPs are cysteine proteases with isopeptidase activity, play a crucial role in maintaining the balance between the pools of SUMOylated and unSUMOylated proteins and in SUMO recycling. MiR-145-mediated down-regulation of SENP1 induced quiescence of prostate cancer cells and reversed SENP1-promoted tumorigenesis in mice. This highlights the potential of miR-145 as a therapeutic molecule against cancer [132]. Thus, targeting SENPs could offer a promising strategy in cancer treatment by modulating the SUMOylation process.

Knockdown of SENP6 has been found to induce the radiosensitization of liver cancer cells, highlighting its potential to enhance the sensitivity of cancer cells to anticancer therapy [133]. In addition to impeding tumor growth, the silencing of SENP can play a crucial role in enhancing the effectiveness of anticancer treatments. The current research focuses on the discovery of SENP inhibitors with a specific emphasis on developing isoform-selective inhibitors, which poses a significant challenge. Various strategies have been employed in the design and development of SENP inhibitors, including non-peptidyl low-molecular-weight inhibitors [134], virtual-screening-assisted low-molecular-weight inhibitors [135], and natural compounds extracted from plants [124]. Despite these efforts, developing effective SENP inhibitors continues to be a complex and challenging task of cancer research.

Furthermore, a study identifies BMP8A, RGS8, and SERPIND1 as key biomarkers associated with SUMOylation in PTC, suggesting potential targets for therapeutic intervention and prognosis in PTC research [136]. Developing a nomogram based on the SUMOylation score could provide valuable insights for individualized treatment strategies in thyroid cancer. In lung adenocarcinoma, high SUMOylation scores correlate with poor prognosis [137], emphasizing the significance of understanding SUMOylation patterns in predicting patient outcomes. Their connection to immune response and drug sensitivity further underscores the importance of these biomarkers in PTC research. According to a recent study, protein SUMOylation levels in thyroid tumor tissues were higher than those in paired nontumor tissues, and the higher the SUMOylation in tumor tissues, the shorter the overall survival time of the patients, especially among males [138].

6. Conclusions and Future Perspective

The study of SUMOylation in thyroid cancer has illuminated its pivotal role in tumorigenesis and progression, opening up promising avenues for therapeutic intervention. Our comprehensive review underscores the dual nature of SUMOylation, highlighting its capacity to both promote and suppress oncogenic processes. This complexity suggests that nuanced strategies targeting SUMOylation could yield significant therapeutic benefits.

Key findings of this review emphasize the aberrant SUMOylation patterns in thyroid cancer, particularly in differentiated and anaplastic subtypes, and the potential to exploit these modifications for targeted therapies. The involvement of SUMOylation in crucial cellular processes—such as DNA repair, transcription regulation, and protein stability—underscores its broad impact on cancer biology and its potential as a therapeutic target. The deregulation of SUMO machinery components and the SUMOylation of specific proteins like CCDC6, PDGF-C, and TFAP2A offer novel insights into thyroid cancer pathogenesis and progression.

Future research should focus on elucidating the detailed molecular networks and pathways modulated by SUMOylation in thyroid cancer, considering the heterogeneity among different subtypes. Additionally, developing specific inhibitors of the SUMOylation pathway, including SUMO E1 enzyme inhibitors and SENP protease modulators, could provide innovative therapeutic options. It is crucial to integrate these strategies with existing treatment modalities to enhance efficacy and overcome resistance.

Furthermore, preclinical and clinical trials are necessary to validate the safety and effectiveness of targeting SUMOylation in thyroid cancer patients. Such trials will pave the way for personalized treatment approaches, taking into account individual SUMOylation profiles and tumor characteristics. By advancing our understanding of SUMOylation's role in thyroid cancer, we can develop more precise and effective therapies, ultimately improving patient outcomes and quality of life. The potential of SUMOylation-based therapies to revolutionize the treatment landscape underscores the need for continued exploration and innovation in this promising field.

Author Contributions: Conceptualization, Q.W. and Z.A.; methodology, Q.W.; software, B.J., W.L. and J.Z.; validation, B.J. and Q.W.; formal analysis, Q.W.; investigation, B.J.; resources, Z.A.; data curation, Q.W.; writing—original draft preparation, B.J.; writing—review and editing, Q.W. and Z.A.; visualization, B.J. and W.Q.; supervision, Z.A.; project administration, Z.A.; funding acquisition, Z.A. All authors have read and agreed to the published version of the manuscript.

Funding: This research was funded by Shanghai Innovation Medical Device Application Demonstration Project 2023, grant number 23SHS05200, Medical and Health Guided Project of Xiamen (No. 3502Z20224ZD1093), and 2022 Key Clinical Specialty Discipline Construction Program of Fujian.

Conflicts of Interest: The authors declare no conflicts of interest.

Abbreviations

APM, antigen processing and presentation machinery; ATC, anaplastic thyroid carcinomas; cAMP, cyclic AMP; CREB, cAMP-response-element-binding protein; CTLs, cytotoxic T-cells; DDR, DNA damage response; DESI1, deSUMOylating isopeptidase 1; DSBs, double-strand breaks; DTC, differentiated thyroid cancer; EMT, epithelial–mesenchymal transition; ESCC, esophageal squamous cell carcinoma; HCC, hepatocellular carcinoma; HEY1, hairy/enhancer of split related with YRPW motif; HIF, hypoxia-inducible factor; HK2, hexokinase 2; HR, homologous recombination; IC50, half maximal inhibitory concentration; IFNs, interferons; IGF-1R, insulin-like growth factor 1 receptor; MTC, medullary thyroid cancer; NHEJ, non-homologous end joining; NK, natural killer; PDGF-C, platelet-derived growth factor-C; PD-L1, programmed cell death protein-1 ligand; PPARγ, peroxisome-proliferator-activated receptor γ; PTC, papillary thyroid cancer; PTC1, RET/papillary thyroid carcinoma 1; PTM, protein post-translational modification; PXR, pregnane X receptor; RAI, radioactive iodine; ROS, reactive oxygen species; RTKs, receptor tyrosine kinases; SAE1/SAE2, SUMO-activating enzyme subunit 1/2; SENPs, Sentrin/SUMO-specific proteases; SIM, SUMO-interacting motif; SUMO, small ubiquitin-like modifier; SUMOi, pharmacological inhibition of SUMOylation; SUMOylation, SUMO modification; TF, transcription factor; TL, thyroid lobectomy; TT, total thyroidectomy; UbL, ubiquitin-like modifiers.

References

1. Bray, F.; Laversanne, M.; Sung, H.; Ferlay, J.; Siegel, R.L.; Soerjomataram, I.; Jemal, A. Global cancer statistics 2022: GLOBOCAN estimates of incidence and mortality worldwide for 36 cancers in 185 countries. *CA Cancer J. Clin.* **2024**, *74*, 229–263. [CrossRef] [PubMed]
2. Chen, D.W.; Lang, B.H.H.; McLeod, D.S.A.; Newbold, K.; Haymart, M.R. Thyroid cancer. *Lancet* **2023**, *401*, 1531–1544. [CrossRef] [PubMed]
3. Miranda-Filho, A.; Lortet-Tieulent, J.; Bray, F.; Cao, B.; Franceschi, S.; Vaccarella, S.; Dal Maso, L. Thyroid cancer incidence trends by histology in 25 countries: A population-based study. *Lancet Diabetes Endocrinol.* **2021**, *9*, 225–234. [CrossRef] [PubMed]
4. Boucai, L.; Zafereo, M.; Cabanillas, M.E. Thyroid Cancer: A Review. *JAMA* **2024**, *331*, 425–435. [CrossRef] [PubMed]
5. Cappadocia, L.; Lima, C.D. Ubiquitin-like Protein Conjugation: Structures, Chemistry, and Mechanism. *Chem. Rev.* **2018**, *118*, 889–918. [CrossRef]
6. Flotho, A.; Melchior, F. Sumoylation: A regulatory protein modification in health and disease. *Annu. Rev. Biochem.* **2013**, *82*, 357–385. [CrossRef]
7. Geiss-Friedlander, R.; Melchior, F. Concepts in sumoylation: A decade on. *Nat. Rev. Mol. Cell Biol.* **2007**, *8*, 947–956. [CrossRef]
8. Hay, R.T. SUMO: A history of modification. *Mol. Cell* **2005**, *18*, 1–12. [CrossRef]
9. Rabut, G.; Peter, M. Function and regulation of protein neddylation. 'Protein modifications: Beyond the usual suspects' review series. *EMBO Rep.* **2008**, *9*, 969–976. [CrossRef]
10. Mahajan, R.; Delphin, C.; Guan, T.; Gerace, L.; Melchior, F. A small ubiquitin-related polypeptide involved in targeting RanGAP1 to nuclear pore complex protein RanBP2. *Cell* **1997**, *88*, 97–107. [CrossRef]
11. Mattoscio, D.; Medda, A.; Chiocca, S. Recent Highlights: Onco Viral Exploitation of the SUMO System. *Curr. Issues Mol. Biol.* **2020**, *35*, 1–16. [CrossRef] [PubMed]
12. Zhang, T.; Yang, H.; Zhou, Z.; Bai, Y.; Wang, J.; Wang, W. Crosstalk between SUMOylation and ubiquitylation controls DNA end resection by maintaining MRE11 homeostasis on chromatin. *Nat. Commun.* **2022**, *13*, 5133. [CrossRef] [PubMed]
13. Zhang, F.L.; Yang, S.Y.; Liao, L.; Zhang, T.M.; Zhang, Y.L.; Hu, S.Y.; Deng, L.; Huang, M.Y.; Andriani, L.; Ma, X.Y.; et al. Dynamic SUMOylation of MORC2 orchestrates chromatin remodelling and DNA repair in response to DNA damage and drives chemoresistance in breast cancer. *Theranostics* **2023**, *13*, 973–990. [CrossRef] [PubMed]

14. Luise, C.; Merolla, F.; Leone, V.; Paladino, S.; Sarnataro, D.; Fusco, A.; Celetti, A. Identification of sumoylation sites in CCDC6, the first identified RET partner gene in papillary thyroid carcinoma, uncovers a mode of regulating CCDC6 function on CREB1 transcriptional activity. *PLoS ONE* **2012**, *7*, e49298. [CrossRef]
15. De Andrade, J.P.; Lorenzen, A.W.; Wu, V.T.; Bogachek, M.V.; Park, J.M.; Gu, V.W.; Sevenich, C.M.; Cassady, V.C.; Beck, A.C.; Kulak, M.V.; et al. Targeting the SUMO pathway as a novel treatment for anaplastic thyroid cancer. *Oncotarget* **2017**, *8*, 114801–114815. [CrossRef]
16. Okura, T.; Gong, L.; Kamitani, T.; Wada, T.; Okura, I.; Wei, C.F.; Chang, H.M.; Yeh, E.T. Protection against Fas/APO-1- and tumor necrosis factor-mediated cell death by a novel protein, sentrin. *J. Immunol.* **1996**, *157*, 4277–4281. [CrossRef]
17. Kamitani, T.; Kito, K.; Nguyen, H.P.; Fukuda-Kamitani, T.; Yeh, E.T. Characterization of a second member of the sentrin family of ubiquitin-like proteins. *J. Biol. Chem.* **1998**, *273*, 11349–11353. [CrossRef]
18. Saitoh, H.; Hinchey, J. Functional heterogeneity of small ubiquitin-related protein modifiers SUMO-1 versus SUMO-2/3. *J. Biol. Chem.* **2000**, *275*, 6252–6258. [CrossRef]
19. Han, Z.J.; Feng, Y.H.; Gu, B.H.; Li, Y.M.; Chen, H. The post-translational modification, SUMOylation, and cancer (Review). *Int. J. Oncol.* **2018**, *52*, 1081–1094. [CrossRef]
20. Evdokimov, E.; Sharma, P.; Lockett, S.J.; Lualdi, M.; Kuehn, M.R. Loss of SUMO1 in mice affects RanGAP1 localization and formation of PML nuclear bodies, but is not lethal as it can be compensated by SUMO2 or SUMO3. *J. Cell Sci.* **2008**, *121 Pt 24*, 4106–4113. [CrossRef]
21. Liang, Y.C.; Lee, C.C.; Yao, Y.L.; Lai, C.C.; Schmitz, M.L.; Yang, W.M. SUMO5, a Novel Poly-SUMO Isoform, Regulates PML Nuclear Bodies. *Sci. Rep.* **2016**, *6*, 26509. [CrossRef] [PubMed]
22. Li, S.J.; Hochstrasser, M. A new protease required for cell-cycle progression in yeast. *Nature* **1999**, *398*, 246–251. [CrossRef] [PubMed]
23. Reverter, D.; Lima, C.D. A basis for SUMO protease specificity provided by analysis of human Senp2 and a Senp2-SUMO complex. *Structure* **2004**, *12*, 1519–1531. [CrossRef] [PubMed]
24. Walden, H.; Podgorski, M.S.; Schulman, B.A. Insights into the ubiquitin transfer cascade from the structure of the activating enzyme for NEDD8. *Nature* **2003**, *422*, 330–334. [CrossRef]
25. Lois, L.M.; Lima, C.D. Structures of the SUMO E1 provide mechanistic insights into SUMO activation and E2 recruitment to E1. *EMBO J.* **2005**, *24*, 439–451. [CrossRef]
26. Schulman, B.A.; Harper, J.W. Ubiquitin-like protein activation by E1 enzymes: The apex for downstream signalling pathways. *Nat. Rev. Mol. Cell Biol.* **2009**, *10*, 319–331. [CrossRef]
27. Johnson, E.S.; Blobel, G. Ubc9p is the conjugating enzyme for the ubiquitin-like protein Smt3p. *J. Biol. Chem.* **1997**, *272*, 26799–26802. [CrossRef]
28. Olsen, S.K.; Lima, C.D. Structure of a ubiquitin E1-E2 complex: Insights to E1-E2 thioester transfer. *Mol. Cell* **2013**, *49*, 884–896. [CrossRef]
29. Wang, J.; Hu, W.; Cai, S.; Lee, B.; Song, J.; Chen, Y. The intrinsic affinity between E2 and the Cys domain of E1 in ubiquitin-like modifications. *Mol. Cell* **2007**, *27*, 228–237. [CrossRef]
30. Wang, J.; Taherbhoy, A.M.; Hunt, H.W.; Seyedin, S.N.; Miller, D.W.; Miller, D.J.; Huang, D.T.; Schulman, B.A. Crystal structure of UBA2(ufd)-Ubc9: Insights into E1-E2 interactions in Sumo pathways. *PLoS ONE* **2010**, *5*, e15805. [CrossRef]
31. Liu, B.; Lois, L.M.; Reverter, D. Structural insights into SUMO E1-E2 interactions in Arabidopsis uncovers a distinctive platform for securing SUMO conjugation specificity across evolution. *Biochem. J.* **2019**, *476*, 2127–2139. [CrossRef] [PubMed]
32. Lv, Z.; Rickman, K.A.; Yuan, L.; Williams, K.; Selvam, S.P.; Woosley, A.N.; Howe, P.H.; Ogretmen, B.; Smogorzewska, A.; Olsen, S.K. *S. pombe* Uba1-Ubc15 Structure Reveals a Novel Regulatory Mechanism of Ubiquitin E2 Activity. *Mol. Cell* **2017**, *65*, 699–714.e6. [CrossRef] [PubMed]
33. Yunus, A.A.; Lima, C.D. Lysine activation and functional analysis of E2-mediated conjugation in the SUMO pathway. *Nat. Struct. Mol. Biol.* **2006**, *13*, 491–499. [CrossRef] [PubMed]
34. Pabst, S.; Doring, L.M.; Petreska, N.; Dohmen, R.J. Methods to study SUMO dynamics in yeast. *Methods Enzymol.* **2019**, *618*, 187–210. [CrossRef] [PubMed]
35. Pichler, A.; Fatouros, C.; Lee, H.; Eisenhardt, N. SUMO conjugation—A mechanistic view. *Biomol. Concepts* **2017**, *8*, 13–36. [CrossRef]
36. Zheng, N.; Shabek, N. Ubiquitin Ligases: Structure, Function, and Regulation. *Annu. Rev. Biochem.* **2017**, *86*, 129–157. [CrossRef]
37. Tozluoğlu, M.; Karaca, E.; Nussinov, R.; Haliloğlu, T. A mechanistic view of the role of E3 in sumoylation. *PLoS Comput. Biol.* **2010**, *6*, e1000913. [CrossRef]
38. Varejão, N.; Lascorz, J.; Li, Y.; Reverter, D. Molecular mechanisms in SUMO conjugation. *Biochem. Soc. Trans.* **2020**, *48*, 123–135. [CrossRef]
39. Hickey, C.M.; Wilson, N.R.; Hochstrasser, M. Function and regulation of SUMO proteases. *Nat. Rev. Mol. Cell Biol.* **2012**, *13*, 755–766. [CrossRef]
40. Claessens, L.A.; Vertegaal, A.C.O. SUMO proteases: From cellular functions to disease. *Trends Cell Biol.* **2024**. [CrossRef]
41. Cheng, J.; Kang, X.; Zhang, S.; Yeh, E.T. SUMO-specific protease 1 is essential for stabilization of HIF1alpha during hypoxia. *Cell* **2007**, *131*, 584–595. [CrossRef] [PubMed]

42. Kang, X.; Qi, Y.; Zuo, Y.; Wang, Q.; Zou, Y.; Schwartz, R.J.; Cheng, J.; Yeh, E.T. SUMO-specific protease 2 is essential for suppression of polycomb group protein-mediated gene silencing during embryonic development. *Mol. Cell* **2010**, *38*, 191–201. [CrossRef] [PubMed]
43. Li, J.; Lu, D.; Dou, H.; Liu, H.; Weaver, K.; Wang, W.; Li, J.; Yeh, E.T.H.; Williams, B.O.; Zheng, L.; et al. Desumoylase SENP6 maintains osteochondroprogenitor homeostasis by suppressing the p53 pathway. *Nat. Commun.* **2018**, *9*, 143. [CrossRef] [PubMed]
44. Schulz, S.; Chachami, G.; Kozaczkiewicz, L.; Winter, U.; Stankovic-Valentin, N.; Haas, P.; Hofmann, K.; Urlaub, H.; Ovaa, H.; Wittbrodt, J.; et al. Ubiquitin-specific protease-like 1 (USPL1) is a SUMO isopeptidase with essential, non-catalytic functions. *EMBO Rep.* **2012**, *13*, 930–938. [CrossRef] [PubMed]
45. Shin, E.J.; Shin, H.M.; Nam, E.; Kim, W.S.; Kim, J.H.; Oh, B.H.; Yun, Y. DeSUMOylating isopeptidase: A second class of SUMO protease. *EMBO Rep.* **2012**, *13*, 339–346. [CrossRef]
46. Nayak, A.; Muller, S. SUMO-specific proteases/isopeptidases: SENPs and beyond. *Genome Biol.* **2014**, *15*, 422. [CrossRef]
47. Kunz, K.; Piller, T.; Müller, S. SUMO-specific proteases and isopeptidases of the SENP family at a glance. *J. Cell Sci.* **2018**, *131*, jcs211904. [CrossRef]
48. Zhou, W.; Hannoun, Z.; Jaffray, E.; Medine, C.N.; Black, J.R.; Greenhough, S.; Zhu, L.; Ross, J.A.; Forbes, S.; Wilmut, I.; et al. SUMOylation of HNF4alpha regulates protein stability and hepatocyte function. *J. Cell Sci.* **2012**, *125 Pt 15*, 3630–3635. [CrossRef]
49. Harley, M.E.; Murina, O.; Leitch, A.; Higgs, M.R.; Bicknell, L.S.; Yigit, G.; Blackford, A.N.; Zlatanou, A.; Mackenzie, K.J.; Reddy, K.; et al. TRAIP promotes DNA damage response during genome replication and is mutated in primordial dwarfism. *Nat. Genet.* **2016**, *48*, 36–43. [CrossRef]
50. Park, I.S.; Han, Y.; Chung, H.J.; Jung, Y.W.; Kim, Y.; Kim, H. SUMOylation regulates nuclear localization and stability of TRAIP/RNF206. *Biochem. Biophys. Res. Commun.* **2016**, *470*, 881–887. [CrossRef]
51. Hamard, P.J.; Boyer-Guittaut, M.; Camuzeaux, B.; Dujardin, D.; Hauss, C.; Oelgeschläger, T.; Vigneron, M.; Kedinger, C.; Chatton, B. Sumoylation delays the ATF7 transcription factor subcellular localization and inhibits its transcriptional activity. *Nucleic Acids Res.* **2007**, *35*, 1134–1144. [CrossRef] [PubMed]
52. Dutchak, P.A.; Katafuchi, T.; Bookout, A.L.; Choi, J.H.; Yu, R.T.; Mangelsdorf, D.J.; Kliewer, S.A. Fibroblast growth factor-21 regulates PPARγ activity and the antidiabetic actions of thiazolidinediones. *Cell* **2012**, *148*, 556–567. [CrossRef] [PubMed]
53. Phan, A.N.H.; Vo, V.T.A.; Hua, T.N.M.; Kim, M.K.; Jo, S.Y.; Choi, J.W.; Kim, H.W.; Son, J.; Suh, Y.A.; Jeong, Y. PPARγ sumoylation-mediated lipid accumulation in lung cancer. *Oncotarget* **2017**, *8*, 82491–82505. [CrossRef] [PubMed]
54. Moreau, A.; Vilarem, M.J.; Maurel, P.; Pascussi, J.M. Xenoreceptors CAR and PXR activation and consequences on lipid metabolism, glucose homeostasis, and inflammatory response. *Mol. Pharm.* **2008**, *5*, 35–41. [CrossRef]
55. Choi, B.H.; Chen, C.; Philips, M.; Dai, W. RAS GTPases are modified by SUMOylation. *Oncotarget* **2018**, *9*, 4440–4450. [CrossRef]
56. Choi, B.H.; Philips, M.R.; Chen, Y.; Lu, L.; Dai, W. K-Ras Lys-42 is crucial for its signaling, cell migration, and invasion. *J. Biol. Chem.* **2018**, *293*, 17574–17581. [CrossRef]
57. Steven, A.; Friedrich, M.; Jank, P.; Heimer, N.; Budczies, J.; Denkert, C.; Seliger, B. What turns CREB on? And off? And why does it matter? *Cell Mol. Life Sci.* **2020**, *77*, 4049–4067. [CrossRef]
58. Puxeddu, E.; Zhao, G.; Stringer, J.R.; Medvedovic, M.; Moretti, S.; Fagin, J.A. Characterization of novel non-clonal intrachromosomal rearrangements between the H4 and PTEN genes (H4/PTEN) in human thyroid cell lines and papillary thyroid cancer specimens. *Mutat. Res.* **2005**, *570*, 17–32. [CrossRef]
59. Leone, V.; Mansueto, G.; Pierantoni, G.M.; Tornincasa, M.; Merolla, F.; Cerrato, A.; Santoro, M.; Grieco, M.; Scaloni, A.; Celetti, A.; et al. CCDC6 represses CREB1 activity by recruiting histone deacetylase 1 and protein phosphatase 1. *Oncogene* **2010**, *29*, 4341–4351. [CrossRef]
60. Celetti, A.; Cerrato, A.; Merolla, F.; Vitagliano, D.; Vecchio, G.; Grieco, M. H4(D10S170), a gene frequently rearranged with RET in papillary thyroid carcinomas: Functional characterization. *Oncogene* **2004**, *23*, 109–121. [CrossRef]
61. Merolla, F.; Pentimalli, F.; Pacelli, R.; Vecchio, G.; Fusco, A.; Grieco, M.; Celetti, A. Involvement of H4(D10S170) protein in ATM-dependent response to DNA damage. *Oncogene* **2007**, *26*, 6167–6175. [CrossRef] [PubMed]
62. Turrell, F.K.; Orha, R.; Guppy, N.J.; Gillespie, A.; Guelbert, M.; Starling, C.; Haider, S.; Isacke, C.M. Age-associated microenvironmental changes highlight the role of PDGF-C in ER(+) breast cancer metastatic relapse. *Nat. Cancer* **2023**, *4*, 468–484. [CrossRef] [PubMed]
63. Hurst, N.J., Jr.; Najy, A.J.; Ustach, C.V.; Movilla, L.; Kim, H.R. Platelet-derived growth factor-C (PDGF-C) activation by serine proteases: Implications for breast cancer progression. *Biochem. J.* **2012**, *441*, 909–918. [CrossRef] [PubMed]
64. Reigstad, L.J.; Varhaug, J.E.; Lillehaug, J.R. Structural and functional specificities of PDGF-C and PDGF-D, the novel members of the platelet-derived growth factors family. *Febs J.* **2005**, *272*, 5723–5741. [CrossRef] [PubMed]
65. Reigstad, L.J.; Martinez, A.; Varhaug, J.E.; Lillehaug, J.R. Nuclear localisation of endogenous SUMO-1-modified PDGF-C in human thyroid tissue and cell lines. *Exp. Cell Res.* **2006**, *312*, 782–795. [CrossRef]
66. Tuccilli, C.; Baldini, E.; Sorrenti, S.; Di Gioia, C.; Bosco, D.; Ascoli, V.; Mian, C.; Barollo, S.; Rendina, R.; Coccaro, C.; et al. Papillary thyroid cancer is characterized by altered expression of genes involved in the sumoylation process. *J. Biol. Regul. Homeost. Agents* **2015**, *29*, 655–662.
67. Rabellino, A.; Andreani, C.; Scaglioni, P.P. The Role of PIAS SUMO E3-Ligases in Cancer. *Cancer Res.* **2017**, *77*, 1542–1547. [CrossRef]

68. Rodrigues, J.S.; Chenlo, M.; Bravo, S.B.; Perez-Romero, S.; Suarez-Fariña, M.; Sobrino, T.; Sanz-Pamplona, R.; González-Prieto, R.; Blanco Freire, M.N.; Nogueiras, R.; et al. dsRNAi-mediated silencing of PIAS2beta specifically kills anaplastic carcinomas by mitotic catastrophe. *Nat. Commun.* **2024**, *15*, 3736. [CrossRef]
69. Husson, O.; Haak, H.R.; Buffart, L.M.; Nieuwlaat, W.A.; Oranje, W.A.; Mols, F.; Kuijpens, J.L.; Coebergh, J.W.; van de Poll-Franse, L.V. Health-related quality of life and disease specific symptoms in long-term thyroid cancer survivors: A study from the population-based PROFILES registry. *Acta Oncol.* **2013**, *52*, 249–258. [CrossRef]
70. Vaccarella, S.; Lortet-Tieulent, J.; Colombet, M.; Davies, L.; Stiller, C.A.; Schuz, J.; Togawa, K.; Bray, F.; Franceschi, S.; Dal Maso, L.; et al. Global patterns and trends in incidence and mortality of thyroid cancer in children and adolescents: A population-based study. *Lancet Diabetes Endocrinol.* **2021**, *9*, 144–152. [CrossRef]
71. Sosa, J.A.; Tuggle, C.T.; Wang, T.S.; Thomas, D.C.; Boudourakis, L.; Rivkees, S.; Roman, S.A. Clinical and economic outcomes of thyroid and parathyroid surgery in children. *J. Clin. Endocrinol. Metab.* **2008**, *93*, 3058–3065. [CrossRef] [PubMed]
72. Ren, R.; Ding, S.; Ma, K.; Jiang, Y.; Wang, Y.; Chen, J.; Wang, Y.; Kou, Y.; Fan, X.; Zhu, X.; et al. SUMOylation Fine-Tunes Endothelial HEY1 in the Regulation of Angiogenesis. *Circ. Res.* **2024**, *134*, 203–222. [CrossRef] [PubMed]
73. Jiang, Z.; Zhang, C.; Liu, X.; Ma, X.; Bian, X.; Xiao, X.; Gao, R.; Sun, Y.; Wu, W.; Zhao, P. Dexamethasone inhibits stemness maintenance and enhances chemosensitivity of hepatocellular carcinoma stem cells by inducing deSUMOylation of HIF-1α and Oct4. *Int. J. Oncol.* **2020**, *57*, 780–790. [CrossRef] [PubMed]
74. Liu, D.; Li, Z.; Yang, Z.; Ma, J.; Mai, S. Ginkgoic acid impedes gastric cancer cell proliferation, migration and EMT through inhibiting the SUMOylation of IGF-1R. *Chem. Biol. Interact.* **2021**, *337*, 109394. [CrossRef] [PubMed]
75. Yang, Y.; Huang, L.; Zhang, N.; Deng, Y.N.; Cao, X.; Liang, Y.; Hou, H.; Luo, Y.; Yang, Y.; Li, Q.; et al. SUMOylation of annexin A6 retards cell migration and tumor growth by suppressing RHOU/AKT1-involved EMT in hepatocellular carcinoma. *Cell Commun. Signal* **2024**, *22*, 206. [CrossRef] [PubMed]
76. Wei, M.; Huang, X.; Liao, L.; Tian, Y.; Zheng, X. SENP1 Decreases RNF168 Phase Separation to Promote DNA Damage Repair and Drug Resistance in Colon Cancer. *Cancer Res.* **2023**, *83*, 2908–2923. [CrossRef]
77. Han, Y.; Huang, X.; Cao, X.; Li, Y.; Gao, L.; Jia, J.; Li, G.; Guo, H.; Liu, X.; Zhao, H.; et al. SENP3-mediated TIP60 deSUMOylation is required for DNA-PKcs activity and DNA damage repair. *MedComm* **2022**, *3*, e123. [CrossRef]
78. Rouvière, J.O.; Geoffroy, M.C.; Palancade, B. Multiple crosstalks between mRNA biogenesis and SUMO. *Chromosoma* **2013**, *122*, 387–399. [CrossRef]
79. Mahmud, I.; Liao, D. DAXX in cancer: Phenomena, processes, mechanisms and regulation. *Nucleic Acids Res.* **2019**, *47*, 7734–7752. [CrossRef]
80. Tsourlakis, M.C.; Schoop, M.; Plass, C.; Huland, H.; Graefen, M.; Steuber, T.; Schlomm, T.; Simon, R.; Sauter, G.; Sirma, H.; et al. Overexpression of the chromatin remodeler death-domain-associated protein in prostate cancer is an independent predictor of early prostate-specific antigen recurrence. *Hum. Pathol.* **2013**, *44*, 1789–1796. [CrossRef]
81. Pan, W.W.; Zhou, J.J.; Liu, X.M.; Xu, Y.; Guo, L.J.; Yu, C.; Shi, Q.H.; Fan, H.Y. Death domain-associated protein DAXX promotes ovarian cancer development and chemoresistance. *J. Biol. Chem.* **2013**, *288*, 13620–13630. [CrossRef] [PubMed]
82. Xu, J.F.; Zhao, Z.G.; Ye, L.L.; Zhuge, W.; Han, Z.; Zhang, T.M.; Ye, S.S.; Chen, W.J.; Zhu, S.; Shi, L.; et al. Prognostic significance of Daxx NCR (Nuclear/Cytoplasmic Ratio) in gastric cancer. *Cancer Med.* **2017**, *6*, 2063–2075. [CrossRef] [PubMed]
83. Jang, M.S.; Ryu, S.W.; Kim, E. Modification of Daxx by small ubiquitin-related modifier-1. *Biochem. Biophys. Res. Commun.* **2002**, *295*, 495–500. [CrossRef] [PubMed]
84. Yu, F.; Shi, G.; Cheng, S.; Chen, J.; Wu, S.Y.; Wang, Z.; Xia, N.; Zhai, Y.; Wang, Z.; Peng, Y.; et al. SUMO suppresses and MYC amplifies transcription globally by regulating CDK9 sumoylation. *Cell Res.* **2018**, *28*, 670–685. [CrossRef] [PubMed]
85. Schaub, F.X.; Dhankani, V.; Berger, A.C.; Trivedi, M.; Richardson, A.B.; Shaw, R.; Zhao, W.; Zhang, X.; Ventura, A.; Liu, Y.; et al. Pan-cancer Alterations of the MYC Oncogene and Its Proximal Network across the Cancer Genome Atlas. *Cell Syst.* **2018**, *6*, 282–300.e2. [CrossRef]
86. Vinay, D.S.; Ryan, E.P.; Pawelec, G.; Talib, W.H.; Stagg, J.; Elkord, E.; Lichtor, T.; Decker, W.K.; Whelan, R.L.; Kumara, H.; et al. Immune evasion in cancer: Mechanistic basis and therapeutic strategies. *Semin. Cancer Biol.* **2015**, *35*, S185–S198. [CrossRef]
87. Wu, Z.; Huang, H.; Han, Q.; Hu, Z.; Teng, X.L.; Ding, R.; Ye, Y.; Yu, X.; Zhao, R.; Wang, Z.; et al. SENP7 senses oxidative stress to sustain metabolic fitness and antitumor functions of CD8+ T cells. *J. Clin. Investig.* **2022**, *132*, e155224. [CrossRef]
88. Yu, X.; Lao, Y.; Teng, X.L.; Li, S.; Zhou, Y.; Wang, F.; Guo, X.; Deng, S.; Chang, Y.; Wu, X.; et al. SENP3 maintains the stability and function of regulatory T cells via BACH2 deSUMOylation. *Nat. Commun.* **2018**, *9*, 3157. [CrossRef]
89. Demel, U.M.; Böger, M.; Yousefian, S.; Grunert, C.; Zhang, L.; Hotz, P.W.; Gottschlich, A.; Köse, H.; Isaakidis, K.; Vonficht, D.; et al. Activated SUMOylation restricts MHC class I antigen presentation to confer immune evasion in cancer. *J. Clin. Investig.* **2022**, *132*, e152383. [CrossRef]
90. Zhao, Y.; Chen, Y.; Jin, M.; Wang, J. The crosstalk between m(6)A RNA methylation and other epigenetic regulators: A novel perspective in epigenetic remodeling. *Theranostics* **2021**, *11*, 4549–4566. [CrossRef]
91. Sun, L.; Zhang, H.; Gao, P. Metabolic reprogramming and epigenetic modifications on the path to cancer. *Protein Cell* **2022**, *13*, 877–919. [CrossRef] [PubMed]
92. Zhu, S.; Gu, H.; Peng, C.; Xia, F.; Cao, H.; Cui, H. Regulation of Glucose, Fatty Acid and Amino Acid Metabolism by Ubiquitination and SUMOylation for Cancer Progression. *Front. Cell Dev. Biol.* **2022**, *10*, 849625. [CrossRef] [PubMed]

93. Zhou, Q.; Yin, Y.; Yu, M.; Gao, D.; Sun, J.; Yang, Z.; Weng, J.; Chen, W.; Atyah, M.; Shen, Y.; et al. GTPBP4 promotes hepatocellular carcinoma progression and metastasis via the PKM2 dependent glucose metabolism. *Redox Biol.* **2022**, *56*, 102458. [CrossRef] [PubMed]
94. Shangguan, X.; He, J.; Ma, Z.; Zhang, W.; Ji, Y.; Shen, K.; Yue, Z.; Li, W.; Xin, Z.; Zheng, Q.; et al. SUMOylation controls the binding of hexokinase 2 to mitochondria and protects against prostate cancer tumorigenesis. *Nat. Commun.* **2021**, *12*, 1812. [CrossRef]
95. Sun, L.; Ma, K.; Zhang, S.; Gu, J.; Wang, H.; Tan, L. SENP2 promotes ESCC proliferation through SETDB1 deSUMOylation and enhanced fatty acid metabolism. *Heliyon* **2024**, *10*, e34010. [CrossRef]
96. Gu, Y.; Fang, Y.; Wu, X.; Xu, T.; Hu, T.; Xu, Y.; Ma, P.; Wang, Q.; Shu, Y. The emerging roles of SUMOylation in the tumor microenvironment and therapeutic implications. *Exp. Hematol. Oncol.* **2023**, *12*, 58. [CrossRef]
97. Barghout, S.H.; Schimmer, A.D. E1 Enzymes as Therapeutic Targets in Cancer. *Pharmacol. Rev.* **2021**, *73*, 1–58. [CrossRef]
98. Decque, A.; Joffre, O.; Magalhaes, J.G.; Cossec, J.C.; Blecher-Gonen, R.; Lapaquette, P.; Silvin, A.; Manel, N.; Joubert, P.E.; Seeler, J.S.; et al. Sumoylation coordinates the repression of inflammatory and anti-viral gene-expression programs during innate sensing. *Nat. Immunol.* **2016**, *17*, 140–149. [CrossRef]
99. Fuertes, M.B.; Kacha, A.K.; Kline, J.; Woo, S.R.; Kranz, D.M.; Murphy, K.M.; Gajewski, T.F. Host type I IFN signals are required for antitumor CD8+ T cell responses through CD8{alpha}+ dendritic cells. *J. Exp. Med.* **2011**, *208*, 2005–2016. [CrossRef]
100. Luo, J.; Emanuele, M.J.; Li, D.; Creighton, C.J.; Schlabach, M.R.; Westbrook, T.F.; Wong, K.K.; Elledge, S.J. A genome-wide RNAi screen identifies multiple synthetic lethal interactions with the Ras oncogene. *Cell* **2009**, *137*, 835–848. [CrossRef]
101. Li, Y.J.; Du, L.; Aldana-Masangkay, G.; Wang, X.; Urak, R.; Forman, S.J.; Rosen, S.T.; Chen, Y. Regulation of miR-34b/c-targeted gene expression program by SUMOylation. *Nucleic Acids Res.* **2018**, *46*, 7108–7123. [CrossRef] [PubMed]
102. Du, L.; Li, Y.J.; Fakih, M.; Wiatrek, R.L.; Duldulao, M.; Chen, Z.; Chu, P.; Garcia-Aguilar, J.; Chen, Y. Role of SUMO activating enzyme in cancer stem cell maintenance and self-renewal. *Nat. Commun.* **2016**, *7*, 12326. [CrossRef] [PubMed]
103. Brownell, J.E.; Sintchak, M.D.; Gavin, J.M.; Liao, H.; Bruzzese, F.J.; Bump, N.J.; Soucy, T.A.; Milhollen, M.A.; Yang, X.; Burkhardt, A.L.; et al. Substrate-assisted inhibition of ubiquitin-like protein-activating enzymes: The NEDD8 E1 inhibitor MLN4924 forms a NEDD8-AMP mimetic in situ. *Mol. Cell* **2010**, *37*, 102–111. [CrossRef] [PubMed]
104. Soucy, T.A.; Smith, P.G.; Milhollen, M.A.; Berger, A.J.; Gavin, J.M.; Adhikari, S.; Brownell, J.E.; Burke, K.E.; Cardin, D.P.; Critchley, S.; et al. An inhibitor of NEDD8-activating enzyme as a new approach to treat cancer. *Nature* **2009**, *458*, 732–736. [CrossRef] [PubMed]
105. He, X.; Riceberg, J.; Soucy, T.; Koenig, E.; Minissale, J.; Gallery, M.; Bernard, H.; Yang, X.; Liao, H.; Rabino, C.; et al. Probing the roles of SUMOylation in cancer cell biology by using a selective SAE inhibitor. *Nat. Chem. Biol.* **2017**, *13*, 1164–1171. [CrossRef]
106. Biederstädt, A.; Hassan, Z.; Schneeweis, C.; Schick, M.; Schneider, L.; Muckenhuber, A.; Hong, Y.; Siegers, G.; Nilsson, L.; Wirth, M.; et al. SUMO pathway inhibition targets an aggressive pancreatic cancer subtype. *Gut* **2020**, *69*, 1472–1482. [CrossRef]
107. Brackett, C.M.; García-Casas, A.; Castillo-Lluva, S.; Blagg, B.S.J. Synthesis and Evaluation of Ginkgolic Acid Derivatives as SUMOylation Inhibitors. *ACS Med. Chem. Lett.* **2020**, *11*, 2221–2226. [CrossRef]
108. Liu, K.; Wang, X.; Li, D.; Xu, D.; Li, D.; Lv, Z.; Zhao, D.; Chu, W.F.; Wang, X.F. Ginkgolic Acid, a SUMO-1 Inhibitor, Inhibits the Progression of Oral Squamous Cell Carcinoma by Alleviating SUMOylation of SMAD4. *Mol. Ther. Oncolytics* **2020**, *16*, 86–99. [CrossRef]
109. Takemoto, M.; Kawamura, Y.; Hirohama, M.; Yamaguchi, Y.; Handa, H.; Saitoh, H.; Nakao, Y.; Kawada, M.; Khalid, K.; Koshino, H.; et al. Inhibition of protein SUMOylation by davidiin, an ellagitannin from Davidia involucrata. *J. Antibiot.* **2014**, *67*, 335–338. [CrossRef]
110. Suzawa, M.; Miranda, D.A.; Ramos, K.A.; Ang, K.K.; Faivre, E.J.; Wilson, C.G.; Caboni, L.; Arkin, M.R.; Kim, Y.S.; Fletterick, R.J.; et al. A gene-expression screen identifies a non-toxic sumoylation inhibitor that mimics SUMO-less human LRH-1 in liver. *Elife* **2015**, *4*, e09003. [CrossRef]
111. Fukuda, I.; Ito, A.; Uramoto, M.; Saitoh, H.; Kawasaki, H.; Osada, H.; Yoshida, M. Kerriamycin B inhibits protein SUMOylation. *J. Antibiot.* **2009**, *62*, 221–224. [CrossRef] [PubMed]
112. Lv, Z.; Yuan, L.; Atkison, J.H.; Williams, K.M.; Vega, R.; Sessions, E.H.; Divlianska, D.B.; Davies, C.; Chen, Y.; Olsen, S.K. Molecular mechanism of a covalent allosteric inhibitor of SUMO E1 activating enzyme. *Nat. Commun.* **2018**, *9*, 5145. [CrossRef] [PubMed]
113. Lightcap, E.S.; Yu, P.; Grossman, S.; Song, K.; Khattar, M.; Xega, K.; He, X.; Gavin, J.M.; Imaichi, H.; Garnsey, J.J.; et al. A small-molecule SUMOylation inhibitor activates antitumor immune responses and potentiates immune therapies in preclinical models. *Sci. Transl. Med.* **2021**, *13*, eaba7791. [CrossRef] [PubMed]
114. Kumar, S.; Schoonderwoerd, M.J.A.; Kroonen, J.S.; de Graaf, I.J.; Sluijter, M.; Ruano, D.; González-Prieto, R.; Verlaan-de Vries, M.; Rip, J.; Arens, R.; et al. Targeting pancreatic cancer by TAK-981: A SUMOylation inhibitor that activates the immune system and blocks cancer cell cycle progression in a preclinical model. *Gut* **2022**, *71*, 2266–2283. [CrossRef]
115. Nakamura, A.; Grossman, S.; Song, K.; Xega, K.; Zhang, Y.; Cvet, D.; Berger, A.; Shapiro, G.; Huszar, D. The SUMOylation inhibitor subasumstat potentiates rituximab activity by IFN1-dependent macrophage and NK cell stimulation. *Blood* **2022**, *139*, 2770–2781. [CrossRef]
116. Gabellier, L.; De Toledo, M.; Chakraborty, M.; Akl, D.; Hallal, R.; Aqrouq, M.; Buonocore, G.; Recasens-Zorzo, C.; Cartron, G.; Delort, A.; et al. SUMOylation inhibitor TAK-981 (subasumstat) synergizes with 5-azacytidine in preclinical models of acute myeloid leukemia. *Haematologica* **2024**, *109*, 98–114. [CrossRef]
117. Kroonen, J.S.; Vertegaal, A.C.O. Targeting SUMO Signaling to Wrestle Cancer. *Trends Cancer* **2021**, *7*, 496–510. [CrossRef]

118. Liu, J.; Li, X.; Chen, J.; Guo, J.; Guo, H.; Zhang, X.; Fan, J.; Zhang, K.; Mao, J.; Zhou, B. Targeting SUMOylation with an injectable nanocomposite hydrogel to optimize radiofrequency ablation therapy for hepatocellular carcinoma. *J. Nanobiotechnology* **2024**, *22*, 338. [CrossRef]
119. Brand, M.; Bommeli, E.B.; Rutimann, M.; Lindenmann, U.; Riedl, R. Discovery of a Dual SENP1 and SENP2 Inhibitor. *Int. J. Mol. Sci.* **2022**, *23*, 12085. [CrossRef]
120. Huang, Q.; Chen, H.; Ren, Y.; Wang, Z.; Zeng, P.; Li, X.; Wang, J.; Zheng, X. Anti-hepatocellular carcinoma activity and mechanism of chemopreventive compounds: Ursolic acid derivatives. *Pharm. Biol.* **2016**, *54*, 3189–3196. [CrossRef]
121. Taghvaei, S.; Sabouni, F.; Minuchehr, Z.; Taghvaei, A. Identification of novel anti-cancer agents, applying in silico method for SENP1 protease inhibition. *J. Biomol. Struct. Dyn.* **2022**, *40*, 6228–6242. [CrossRef] [PubMed]
122. Deng, B.; Yang, B.; Chen, J.; Wang, S.; Zhang, W.; Guo, Y.; Han, Y.; Li, H.; Dang, Y.; Yuan, Y.; et al. Gallic acid induces T-helper-1-like T(reg) cells and strengthens immune checkpoint blockade efficacy. *J. Immunother. Cancer* **2022**, *10*, e004037. [CrossRef] [PubMed]
123. Taghvaei, S.; Minuchehr, Z.; Sabouni, F. Computational drug repurposing of bethanidine for SENP1 inhibition in cardiovascular diseases treatment. *Life Sci.* **2022**, *292*, 120122. [CrossRef] [PubMed]
124. Huang, W.; He, T.; Chai, C.; Yang, Y.; Zheng, Y.; Zhou, P.; Qiao, X.; Zhang, B.; Liu, Z.; Wang, J.; et al. Triptolide inhibits the proliferation of prostate cancer cells and down-regulates SUMO-specific protease 1 expression. *PLoS ONE* **2012**, *7*, e37693. [CrossRef] [PubMed]
125. Wu, J.; Lei, H.; Zhang, J.; Chen, X.; Tang, C.; Wang, W.; Xu, H.; Xiao, W.; Gu, W.; Wu, Y. Momordin Ic, a new natural SENP1 inhibitor, inhibits prostate cancer cell proliferation. *Oncotarget* **2016**, *7*, 58995–59005. [CrossRef]
126. Fukuda, I.; Ito, A.; Hirai, G.; Nishimura, S.; Kawasaki, H.; Saitoh, H.; Kimura, K.; Sodeoka, M.; Yoshida, M. Ginkgolic acid inhibits protein SUMOylation by blocking formation of the E1-SUMO intermediate. *Chem. Biol.* **2009**, *16*, 133–140. [CrossRef]
127. Chen, Y.; Li, Y.J. Bicyclic and Tricyclic Inhibitors of Sumoylation Enzymes and Methods of Their Use. W.O. Patent PTC/US2011/060063, 18 May 2012.
128. Heynen, G.; Baumgartner, F.; Heider, M.; Patra, U.; Holz, M.; Braune, J.; Kaiser, M.; Schaffer, I.; Bamopoulos, S.A.; Ramberger, E.; et al. SUMOylation inhibition overcomes proteasome inhibitor resistance in multiple myeloma. *Blood Adv.* **2023**, *7*, 469–481. [CrossRef]
129. Guervilly, J.H.; Gaillard, P.H. SLX4: Multitasking to maintain genome stability. *Crit. Rev. Biochem. Mol. Biol.* **2018**, *53*, 475–514. [CrossRef]
130. Garvin, A.J.; Walker, A.K.; Densham, R.M.; Chauhan, A.S.; Stone, H.R.; Mackay, H.L.; Jamshad, M.; Starowicz, K.; Daza-Martin, M.; Ronson, G.E.; et al. The deSUMOylase SENP2 coordinates homologous recombination and nonhomologous end joining by independent mechanisms. *Genes. Dev.* **2019**, *33*, 333–347. [CrossRef]
131. Wang, Q.; Xia, N.; Li, T.; Xu, Y.; Zou, Y.; Zuo, Y.; Fan, Q.; Bawa-Khalfe, T.; Yeh, E.T.; Cheng, J. SUMO-specific protease 1 promotes prostate cancer progression and metastasis. *Oncogene* **2013**, *32*, 2493–2498. [CrossRef]
132. Wang, C.; Tao, W.; Ni, S.; Chen, Q.; Zhao, Z.; Ma, L.; Fu, Y.; Jiao, Z. Tumor-suppressive microRNA-145 induces growth arrest by targeting SENP1 in human prostate cancer cells. *Cancer Sci.* **2015**, *106*, 375–382. [CrossRef] [PubMed]
133. Qian, J.; Luo, Y.; Gu, X.; Wang, X. Inhibition of SENP6-induced radiosensitization of human hepatocellular carcinoma cells by blocking radiation-induced NF-κB activation. *Cancer Biother. Radiopharm.* **2013**, *28*, 196–200. [CrossRef] [PubMed]
134. Uno, M.; Koma, Y.; Ban, H.S.; Nakamura, H. Discovery of 1-[4-(N-benzylamino)phenyl]-3-phenylurea derivatives as non-peptidic selective SUMO-sentrin specific protease (SENP)1 inhibitors. *Bioorg. Med. Chem. Lett.* **2012**, *22*, 5169–5173. [CrossRef] [PubMed]
135. Zhao, Y.; Wang, Z.; Zhang, J.; Zhou, H. Identification of SENP1 inhibitors through in silico screening and rational drug design. *Eur. J. Med. Chem.* **2016**, *122*, 178–184. [CrossRef] [PubMed]
136. Li, X.; Ding, Z.; Tong, Y. Identification of SUMOylation-related biomarkers in papillary thyroid carcinoma. *Cancer Cell Int.* **2024**, *24*, 149. [CrossRef]
137. Chen, Z.; Yang, J.; Tang, L.; Sun, X.; Li, Y.; Sheng, Z.; Ding, H.; Xu, C.; Tong, X.; Zhao, J. SUMOylation patterns and signature characterize the tumor microenvironment and predict prognosis in lung adenocarcinoma. *Front. Cell Dev. Biol.* **2023**, *11*, 1094588. [CrossRef]
138. Wu, Q.; Liu, W.; Zheng, J.J.; Wang, C.; Ai, Z.L. Correlationship between total proteins SUMOylation and papillary thyroid carcinoma in males. *J. Surg. Concepts Pract.* **2024**, *in press*.

biomedicines

MDPI

Article

Management of Giant Thyroid Tumors in Patients with Multiple Comorbidities in a Tertiary Head and Neck Surgery Center

Daniela Vrinceanu [1], Mihai Dumitru [1,*], Andreea Marinescu [2], Crenguta Serboiu [3], Gabriela Musat [4], Mihai Radulescu [5], Matei Popa-Cherecheanu [6], Catalina Ciornei [7] and Felicia Manole [8]

1 ENT Department, Faculty of Medicine, Carol Davila University of Medicine and Pharmacy, 020021 Bucharest, Romania; vrinceanudana@yahoo.com

2 Imaging Department, Carol Davila University of Medicine and Pharmacy, 020021 Bucharest, Romania; andreea_marinescu2003@yahoo.com

3 Molecular Biology and Histology Department, Carol Davila University of Medicine and Pharmacy, 050474 Bucharest, Romania; crengutas@yahoo.com

4 ENT Department, Faculty of Dentistry, Carol Davila University of Medicine and Pharmacy, 020021 Bucharest, Romania; gabimusat@yahoo.com

5 Thoracic Surgery Department, Carol Davila University of Medicine and Pharmacy, 020021 Bucharest, Romania; iulianmihai@yahoo.com

6 Vascular Surgery Department, Carol Davila University of Medicine and Pharmacy, 020021 Bucharest, Romania; matei.cherecheanu@gmail.com

7 Physiology Department, Carol Davila University of Medicine and Pharmacy, 020021 Bucharest, Romania; catalina.ciornei@umfcd.ro

8 ENT Department, Faculty of Medicine, University of Oradea, 410073 Oradea, Romania; manole.felicia@gmail.com

* Correspondence: orldumitrumihai@yahoo.com

Abstract: Background/Objectives: The thyroid gland can represent the seat of development for giant tumors exceeding 10 cm in diameter. A retrospective analysis on 21 cases of giant thyroid tumors with comorbidities, operated in the ENT Department of the Bucharest University Emergency Hospital has been conducted. **Methods**: Giant benign tumors accounted for 28.57% of the cases studied and reached gigantic volumes in an average time interval of 3 years, with an average resection piece weight of 318 g. Malignant tumors accounted for 71.43%, with an average duration of evolution of 7 years, with an average resection piece weight of 581 g. **Results**: Dysphagia was present in all patients, dyspnea in 47.61% and dysphonia in 38.09% of cases. Total thyroidectomy is the gold standard in giant thyroid tumors, associated with radical neck dissection, extended to groups VI and VII in malignant tumors. In 10 of 11 cases of giant malignant thyroid tumors (90.90%), without anaplastic thyroid carcinoma, the survival at 5 years after multimodal oncologic treatment was favorable. Anticoagulant treatment increased the risk of postoperative reversible recurrent laryngeal nerve lesion. **Conclusions**: The management of giant thyroid tumors in patients with multiple comorbidities needs a multidisciplinary team including endocrinologist, radiologist, anesthesiologist, pathologist, ENT surgeon, thoracic surgeon, oncologist and radiotherapist.

Keywords: giant; thyroid tumors; comorbidities; multidisciplinary; challenges

1. Introduction

The thyroid gland, with its well-known butterfly shape, which typically weighs 30–50 g, can represent the seat of development for tumors that can reach impressive sizes. Usually, a cervical tumor can be categorized as giant or bulky if its diameter exceeds 10 cm [1].

Thyroid cancer is the most common endocrine malignancy, accounting for ~2.1% of all cancer diagnoses worldwide, with ~77% of these diagnoses occurring in women. Approximately 90% of all thyroid cancers are differentiated, meaning that they arise from thyroid follicular cells and are generally iodine-avid (able to "take up" iodine). Papillary thyroid carcinoma (PTC) is the most common histological type of differentiated thyroid cancer, followed by follicular thyroid carcinoma.

In the histological classification of thyroid gland tumors, epithelial tumors are the most numerous [2].

Among malignant epithelial tumors, the most common are papillary carcinoma (80–85%) and follicular carcinoma (15–18%). Among the rare forms of malignant epithelial tumors encountered are Hurthle cell carcinoma (3–5%), medullary carcinoma (3%) and undifferentiated, anaplastic carcinoma (1–2%) [3]. Thyroid tumor pathology is often interdisciplinary, being addressed equally by several specialties: endocrinology, the endocrinologist surgeon, the head and neck surgeon, the thoracic surgeon or even by the general surgeon. Diagnostic principles in thyroid gland tumors include endocrinological examination with thyroid hormone dosing in order to identify and preoperatively treat hyperthyroidism [4].

Thyroid and cervical ultrasound is a preoperative imaging exploration, often sufficient for simple poly nodular goiters, but which must be completed in the case of thyroid tumors, especially in large ones, with high-performance imaging. Fine needle aspiration (FNA) or ultrasound-guided core-biopsy is part of the routine preoperative assessment in a poly nodular goiter [5].

ENT clinical examination by fiberoptic laryngoscopy is necessary to highlight any recurrent paresis/paralysis. Thyroid scintigraphy provides information regarding cold nodules with high suspicion of malignant nodule, but it has limited use in the case of giant tumors. Imaging required for a giant thyroid tumor should be performed by a cervical CT with contrast or cervical MRI [6].

Regarding the management of malignant tumors of the thyroid gland, a multidisciplinary approach is required. The endocrinologist compensates for any preoperative hyperthyroidism, determines the optimal time of the surgical intervention, as well as the postoperative replacement treatment. He also monitors the patient clinically, sonographically and hormonally through TSH levels, in the postoperative period [7].

Surgical management of thyroid malignancies consists of total thyroidectomy with preservation of the recurrent laryngeal nerves and at least one parathyroid gland associated with radical neck dissection (RND) that must also include cervical ganglion groups V, VI and VII. There are studies that show that unilateral thyroid lobectomy in certain forms of thyroid nodules may be equivalent in terms of results and long-term prognosis, but this statement remains valid only for small nodules. In voluminous tumors with extracapsular extension, salvage surgery is performed with total thyroidectomy with neck dissection and ablation also of invaded adjacent structures like infrahyoid muscles. Surgery is correlated with TNM classification [8].

The pathologist has an essential input in the treatment team by formulating a preliminary diagnosis after FNA, but especially by formulating a diagnosis on frozen sections. Paraffin histopathological examination and immunohistochemical examination formulate a diagnosis of certainty and can certify the shift of a papillary carcinoma with a long evolution to an anaplastic carcinoma [9].

The radiologist provides the necessary acquisitions for a correct and complete preoperative assessment, providing essential details regarding relationships with the great cervical vessels, possible internal jugular vein thrombosis, mediastinal extension, or invasion of cavitary organs, such as the larynx, pharynx, esophagus. The cardiologist contributes by preoperative cardiac compensation. In the multimodal treatment of malignant thyroid tumors, postoperative radiotherapy intervenes. In differentiated (follicular or papillary) carcinomas, radioactive iodine therapy is useful, while in undifferentiated forms, external beam radiation therapy is applied, as in all head and neck cancers. The oncologist proves its usefulness by combining chemotherapy in forms of anaplastic carcinoma [10].

Data from Italy reveal that cardiovascular pathology seems higher as incidences in cases with enlarged thyroid nodules [11]. Metabolic syndrome is an increased public health problem as tends to be associated with a higher risk of developing aggressive thyroid carcinoma [12]. Older age is now increasing in the possible indications for preferring percutaneous radiofrequency ablation of thyroid carcinomas in cases ineligible for surgery [13].

All previously mentioned types of malignant tumors can develop as giant thyroid tumors that impose numerous challenges in surgical management.

In the present article, we aimed to present our experience in managing these challenges in the management of giant thyroid tumors in a tertiary head and neck surgery center within a multidisciplinary hospital.

2. Materials and Methods

We performed a retrospective analysis on 21 cases of giant thyroid tumors with comorbidities, operated in the ENT Department of the Bucharest University Emergency Hospital, between January 2012 and December 2021. Our department is a reference center for head and neck oncological surgery. Patients admitted to the study were referred to our department due to experience in oncological cervical surgery, as well as due to the presence of at least one comorbidity, with the need for monitoring and treatment in a multidisciplinary hospital. Inclusion criteria were patients with bulky thyroid tumors (more than 10 cm in craniocaudal dimension), located in at least one thyroid lobe and having at least one major comorbidity such as cardiovascular disease, vascular neurological disease, degenerative neurological disease and chronic lung disease. Patients with thyroid tumors smaller than 10 cm in cranio-caudal diameter, patients without comorbidities and patients with a histopathological result of lymphoma type were excluded. Patients were referred to our department, which is a tertiary head and neck surgery center in a multidisciplinary hospital, by other endocrinological surgery centers where they could not be approached surgically due to anesthetic and surgical risks, as well as of the impossibility of a multidisciplinary approach to cases. These are the aspects that increase the difficulty of such complex cases, because the patients scarcely controlled their associated pathology. Unfortunately, apparently controllable associated pathology presents an increased burden to the patient with giant thyroid tumors. The preoperative protocol consisted of endocrinological examination and full thyroid hormone profile dosage (TSH, free T3, free T4, calcitonin, parathormone, thyroglobulin); ENT clinical examination, with nasopharyngolaryngeal flexible endoscopy; thyroid ultrasound, cervical and thoracic CT with iv contrast agent; in cases that represented hyperthyroidism, cervical and thoracic CT examination was replaced by cervical and thoracic MRI examination; in one case, bilateral carotid and subclavian angiography was performed, with preoperative selective embolization; cardiological examination; preanesthetic exam. Patients who presented hyperthyroidism were appropriately treated and compensated preoperatively by the endocrinologist. All patients underwent total thyroidectomy with functional or radical neck dissection. All patients underwent extemporaneous intraoperative examination, with sections on ice, then histopathological examination with paraffin, with immunohistochemistry. All operated patients were admitted to the ATI postoperatively for a minimum of 48 h and received replacement therapy with synthetic thyroid hormones Euthyrox 100 micrograms/day and calcium preparations with vitamin D3 p.o., starting 48 h postoperatively. In the retrospective analysis, patients with a histopathological result of follicular adenoma, papillary carcinoma, follicular carcinoma, medullary carcinoma, or anaplastic carcinoma were included.

The long period of time of almost 10 years implied that some aspects from the records, such as all daily laboratory results, all daily measurements of temperature or blood pressure, were unavailable in some of the records. Therefore, we focused only on the data that were consistently available for all the cases included in the study.

3. Results

From the perspective of distribution by gender, there was a higher percentage of men than women, with practically 61.90% of the cases being represented by male patients.

The breakdown by age group reveals a classification of four cases in the 40–49 age group (19.05%), six cases corresponding to the 50–59 age group, six cases in the 60–69 age group (28.57%), respectively, and two cases in patients older than or at least 70 years old (9.52%). The 50–59 age group represented 42.85% of the cases, and the 40–49 and 50–59 age groups represented, cumulatively, 61.90% of the cases, Figure 1.

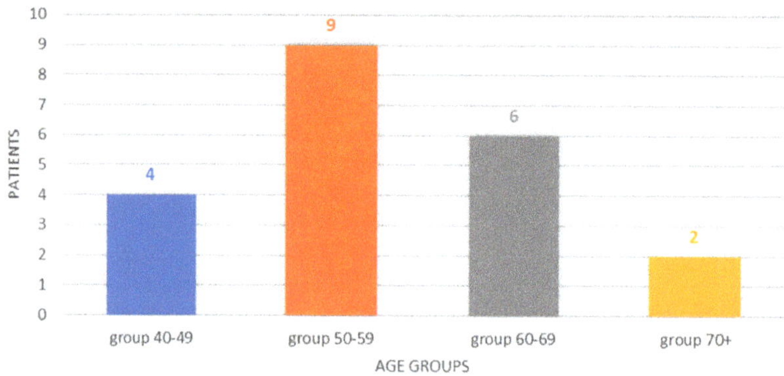

Figure 1. Chart showing the distribution of cases by age group.

Distribution according to the histopathological result confirmed by immunohistochemistry the following: giant follicular cyst on poly nodular goiter, with intracystic hemorrhage—one case; follicular adenoma on poly nodular goiter—five cases; papillary carcinoma—seven cases; follicular carcinoma—two cases; medullary carcinoma—two cases; anaplastic carcinoma—four cases. Rare forms of thyroid cancer represented eight cases in our group, while papillary carcinoma was present in seven cases. It is noteworthy that the patients with benign thyroid tumor pathology accounted for 28.57%. On the other hand, there were four patients with anaplastic carcinoma, representing 19.04% of the studied cases.

Distribution according to the clinical picture at presentation: appearance of goiter/bulky cervical tumor—21 cases; moderate/severe dysphagia—21 cases; dysphonia—eight cases; dyspnea—10 cases; unilateral recurrent paralysis, documented fibroscopically—eight cases; Gerhardt syndrome—two cases; pulmonary metastases at presentation—three cases; Figure 2.

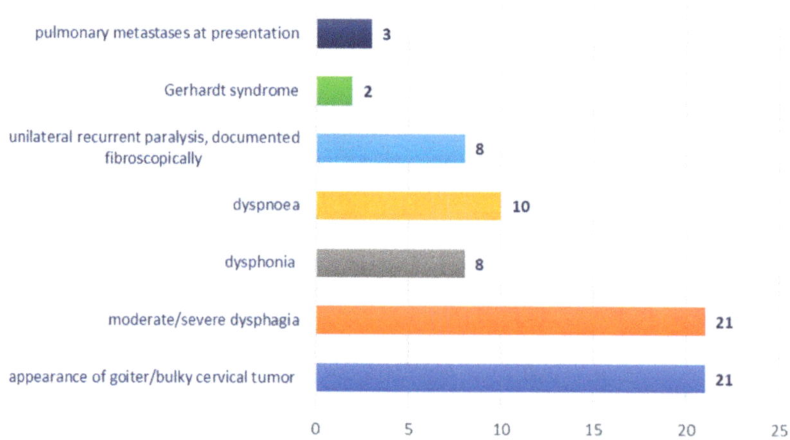

Figure 2. Chart depicting the distribution of cases according to clinical presentation.

Breakdown by type of comorbidities: hypertension—16 cases; ischemic coronary disease—11 cases, of which four cases were with coronary stents; stroke sequelae—four cases; pulmonary fibrosis—two cases; obesity—10 cases, type 2 diabetes—seven cases; hepatitis C virus—two cases; dementia—one case; depressive disorder—one case; Figure 3.

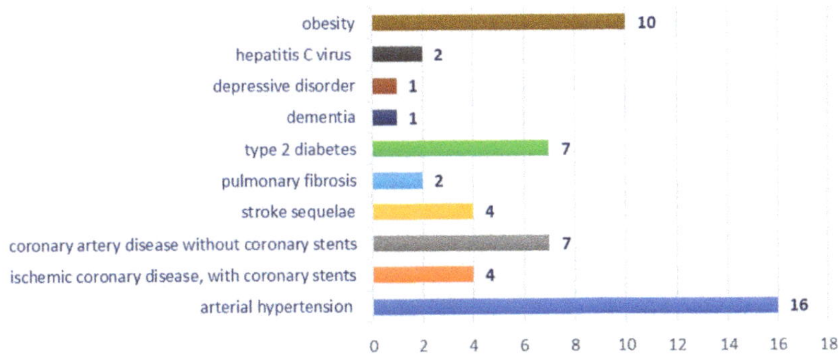

Figure 3. Chart showing the distribution of cases according to the associated comorbidity.

Distribution according to the type of surgical interventions performed: total left thyroid lobectomy—one case; total thyroidectomy—five cases; total thyroidectomy, with the infrahyoid muscle resection—three cases; total thyroidectomy + neck dissection (radical/functional)—12 cases, of which three cases were with radical neck dissection and nine cases were with functional neck dissection; sacrifice of recurrent laryngeal nerve without reconstruction—two cases with unilateral lesion; tracheostomy—two cases; gastrostomy—one case.

Distribution by type of multidisciplinary team of surgeons: head and neck surgeon—21 cases; thoracic surgeon—four cases; vascular surgeon—one case.

Distribution by type of orotracheal intubation: on videolaryngoscope—19 cases; awake intubation on the bronchoscope—two cases.

Distribution according to postoperative complications: recurrent unilateral postoperative paralysis—12 cases, of which eight cases were reversible, four cases were irreversible; postoperative Gerhardt syndrome—two cases, of which one case is reversible, one case is irreversible; parathyroid tetany—one case; malignant arterial hypertension—one case, Figure 4. In one case of medullary thyroid carcinoma, there was a right phrenic nerve paresis and a paralytic ileus, reversible after 72 h of cortisone treatment.

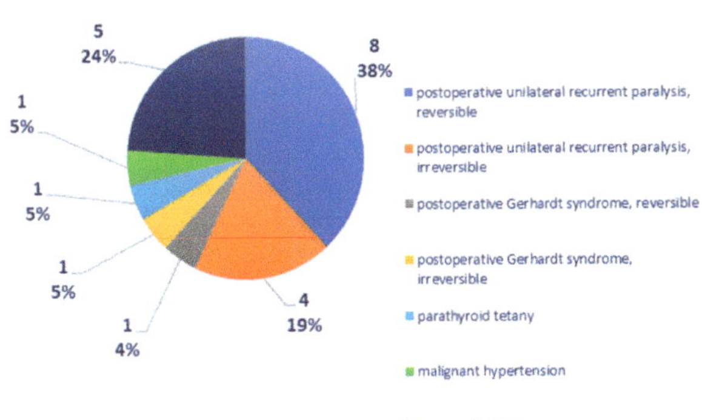

Figure 4. Chart depicting the distribution of cases according to postoperative complications.

Distribution of cases according to adjuvant treatment: endocrinological substitution treatment, under the supervision of the endocrinologist—21 cases; radioactive iodine—nine cases; external radiotherapy—two cases; chemotherapy—three cases; immunotherapy—two cases.

Breakdown by evolution: the LTS giant follicular cyst case was followed at 1 month and 3 months and then endocrinologically discharged, and the five poly nodular goiter follicular adenoma cases were followed at 1 month and 6 months and entered in the endocrinological dispensary. Among the 21 cases of the studied group, there were 16 survivors at 5 years, in oncological monitoring at 3 months. The four cases of anaplastic carcinoma resulted in death, as well as one case of papillary carcinoma with multiple metastatic disease. The outcome was through tracheal invasion—four cases, respectively, through multiple metastatic disease—one case. Among the four cases of anaplastic carcinoma, three cases followed chemotherapy, with resumption of evolution and exitus, respectively, and one case had a resumption of evolution 6 weeks postoperatively, with exitus, Figure 5.

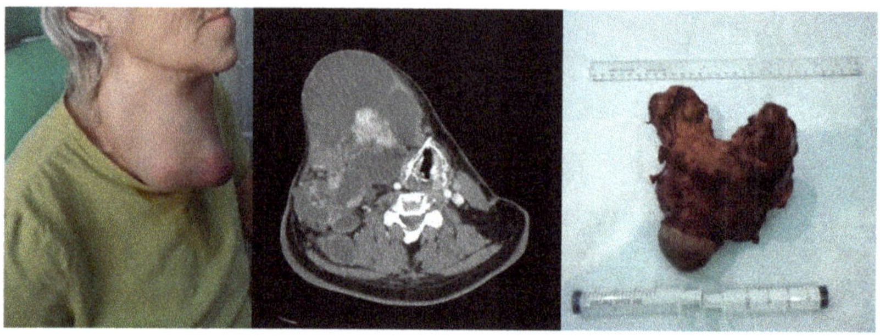

Figure 5. Anaplastic thyroid carcinoma. Left image—clinical aspect. Center image—axial CT scan with tumor displacement of the airway. Right image—resection piece 750 g.

4. Discussions

In the studied group, male patients were respondents, representing almost 2/3 (61.90%) of patients with bulky thyroid tumors and multiple comorbidities. The mean age of patients at presentation was 58 years, with an age range between 44 and 77 years. The most numerous were patients in the 50–59 age group, representing 42.85% of the cases, followed by the 60–69 age group, representing 28.57% of the cases. Basically, 61.90% of patients with giant thyroid tumors were between the ages of 40 and 59, representing younger ages than those of 60–69 and 70 and over, which accounted for 28.57% and, respectively, 9.52% of cases. The occurrence of giant thyroid tumors is correlated, rather, with a younger age. The duration of the evolution in time, until the first presentation to the doctor, had a median of 6 years, with a range between 3 months and 11 years. These aspects are in concordance with a similar study from Korea where 73% of the patients were between 40 and 69 years of age [14]. A history of autoimmune thyroid disease poses specific problems for patients in the 35–55 age group according to a study on 237 patients with Graves Disease with Synchronous Thyroid Nodules [15]. A study from Lithuania showed that a total of 5664 cases of thyroid cancer were registered in the entire Lithuanian population in the last 25 years; 817 cases in the age group from 0 to 19 years at the time of the Chernobyl accident, and 266 cases in the age group from 0 to 9 years, due to the exposure to the Chernobyl accident [16]. In China, age-standardized mortality rates decreased in specific age groups and genders, especially among women. Conversely, the age-standardized mortality rate significantly increased in groups aged over 70. The mortality/incidence ratio exhibited a declining trend, but this decrease was less noticeable in men and the group aged over 70 [17]. Thus, our findings show that the increased trend of a higher incidence of giant carcinoma of the thyroid gland is part of the general increased trend of general carcinoma of the thyroid gland incidence.

The clinical picture at presentation included a bulky cervical tumor, with skin invasion in three of the cases. It should be noted that the reason for presenting to the doctor was not the unaesthetic appearance of the tumor, but the appearance of another clinical sign such as dysphagia, dysphonia or dyspnea. Dysphagia was present in all cases and was objectively evaluated by pharyngoesophageal barite transit and functional endoscopic evaluation of swallowing (FEES). From a subjective point of view, swallowing disorders were subjectively assessed by the patients by completing an EAT-type questionnaire. This is an aspect also reported in other cases with a long-neglected evolution leading to extreme weight loss at the moment of admission to the hospital [18].

Dysphonia was present in eight cases (38.09%) and dyspnea in 10 cases (47.61%), so practically in half of the cases. In the six cases with benign tumor pathology, the clinical symptoms were limited to the presence of the thyroid tumor and dysphagia, except for the case of giant follicular cyst which also associated dysphonia and dyspnea and cervical pain, possibly also in a post-traumatic context (two episodes of syncope). The syncope can be generated through a direct compression mechanism on the major blood vessels of the neck as shown by other cases also reported [19].

Unilateral recurrent paralysis was present in eight cases, and Gerhardt's syndrome in two cases, including one female patient, 53 years old, with papillary carcinoma and one case of a female patient, 57 years old, with anaplastic carcinoma. There was no case of recurrent paralysis at presentation in patients with bulky benign thyroid tumors. The presence of this neurological disorder at admission is associated with a malignant histological diagnosis. Pulmonary metastases at presentation in three cases were associated with longer evolution and the large volume of the primary tumor. Sometimes, the involvement of the recurrent laryngeal nerve can be both in the intrathoracic course through goiter-like pressure and in the neck through sheer tumor mass displacement [20].

The comorbidities of the patients in the studied group fall into vascular and cerebrovascular diseases (hypertension, ischemic coronary disease with/without coronary stents, stroke sequelae, type 2 diabetes), neurological and psychiatric conditions (dementia, depressive disorder). A special remark deserves to be made on patients with antiplatelet and/or anticoagulant treatment who assume a risk of postoperative complications; therefore, the resumption of anticoagulant therapy with low molecular weight heparin was conducted 16 h postoperatively. Metabolic syndrome was reported as a negative predictor for the evolution of thyroid carcinoma [21].

A study on 21,509 patients with a median age of 72 years (range 66–106), revealed that 4168 (19.4%) died of other causes and 2644 (12.3%) died of thyroid cancer during the study period. For differentiated thyroid cancer patients, the likelihood of dying from other causes exceeds the likelihood of dying from thyroid cancer, whereas the opposite is true for anaplastic thyroid cancer. For medullary thyroid cancer, after 6.25 years, patients are more likely to die from other etiologies than thyroid cancer [22]. In a bigger cohort, after a median follow-up of 101 months, 23,040 (13.3%) deaths occurred, of which 29.1% and 21.7% were attributable to thyroid cancer and cardiovascular disease (CVD), respectively [23]. We cannot generalize our findings, but they are concurring with the findings in the general population of thyroid carcinoma patients. The added impact of the dimensions of the tumor, local impact on blood vessels and the airway increases the cardiovascular risk of the patients with giant thyroid carcinoma.

From the point of view of surgical interventions performed in giant thyroid tumors, total thyroidectomy is certainly the gold standard. One case of giant follicular cyst of the left thyroid lobe received total left thyroid lobectomy, in order not to expose the patient to additional risks, being a 77-year-old patient with dementia, who clinically presented dysphagia, dyspnea and dysphonia. In all surgical interventions, an extemporaneous examination was used with sections on ice, which facilitated our operative decision. Radical neck dissection included lymph node groups VI and VII in all cases with malignant extemporaneous examination. In four cases, a thoracic surgeon joined the operative team, to ensure the mediastinal dissection, and in one case the aid of a vascular surgeon in the team was solicited to ensure the dissection of the thoracic duct in the case of a patient with anaplastic carcinoma developed predominantly on the left side. The tumor-invaded recurrent laryngeal nerve was resected without reconstruction in two cases (unilateral lesion) [24].

There are still debates regarding the concept of extended neck dissection in cases with giant thyroid tumors. The cases in the study group tend to some of the characteristics of an extended neck dissection which refers to the excision of one or more additional lymph node clusters or nonlymphatic entities, or both, that are not covered by the radical neck dissection (examples of these lymph node clusters include parapharyngeal, superior mediastinal, paratracheal; examples of nonlymphatic entities include the recurrent laryngeal nerve and paraspinal muscles) [25]. Salvage surgery has a high risk of complications and it may be worthwhile when macroscopic curative resection is available. The decision should be made considering various factors including curability, risk of surgical procedure, functional outcome and life expectancy [26].

The surgical interventions were, except for cases with benign tumor pathology, of long duration, on average 428 min (over 7 h). The average bleeding in these procedures for giant malignant thyroid tumors was 335 mL and required intraoperative transfusion of labile blood products (erythrocyte mass, fresh frozen plasma). A case of voluminous anaplastic carcinoma received preoperative angiography with selective embolization of the superior thyroid artery and thyrocervical trunk, without operatively finding a significant change in bleeding, despite the embolization (in that case, with an intraoperative bleeding of approximately 500 mL). Large populational studies credit these types of tumors with only a 1.3% risk of bleeding [27].

It should be noted that postoperative complications recorded 12 cases of recurrent unilateral paralysis, of which eight were reversible and four irreversible, as well as two postoperative Gerhardt syndromes, of which one was reversible and one was irreversible. It is worth noting that two cases of reversible recurrent paralysis and one case of reversible Gerhardt syndrome were found in patients with benign tumors (three of six cases). In these cases of benign tumor pathology, the recurrent paralysis is explained by the large tumor volume that compresses the nerve that involves laborious dissection, and especially by the vascular status of the patient and the use of antiaggregant, oral anticoagulants that can cause microhemorrhages in the nerve sheath, which can be associated with a postoperative transient recurrent paralysis. One case developed postoperative Gerhardt syndrome in an obese patient with a history of acute myocardial infarction and coronary stents, who was being treated with oral anticoagulants. The occurrence of postoperative Gerhardt syndrome, after extubating, required the maintenance of intubation for another 48 h and treatment with systemic corticosteroids + group B vitamins, and later tracheotomy on the same thyroidectomy incision. Fortunately, the evolution was favorable, and the patient was able to be decannulated after 2 months. It is useful in preventing postoperative recurrent paralysis to avoid dissection and the use of monopolar electrocautery medial to the recurrent line without prior identification of the nerve [28].

Differentiated thyroid carcinoma has a promising prognosis if detected in early stages contrary to prognosis of the pathology subtypes included in the present group of giant thyroid tumors. The overall survival for patients with advanced or metastatic differentiated thyroid carcinoma resistant to radioactive iodine therapy is poor, with 5- and 10-years survival rates of 50% and 10%, respectively [29]. In a study on almost 300 cases of papillary thyroid carcinoma, recurrence occurred in 20 cases (7.3%) and lympho-vascular invasion and lateral cervical lymph node metastasis made significant independent contributions [30]. The major indicator in a low quality of life for the patients undergoing thyroid surgery is the necessity of tracheostomy. A study from Japan concluded that super-radical procedures may be indicated in select patients to avoid mortality due to locally uncontrolled disease at the expense of tracheostomy [31]. Our study focusing on giant thyroid tumors underlines that extensive surgeries are associated with a reserved prognosis, diminished survival rates and poor quality of life implied by salvage surgery procedures.

There was a single case of parathyroid tetany in a patient with anaplastic carcinoma. In these giant tumor cases, the preoperative identification of the parathyroid glands is very difficult [32].

Regarding the distant evolution, 16 (76.19%) of the 21 cases of giant thyroid tumors in patients with multiple comorbidities survived, following a program of oncological monitoring every 3 months. All cases of anaplastic carcinoma resulted in death (four of four) and one case of papillary carcinoma with multiple metastatic disease, confirming data from the literature regarding this type of neoplasia [33].

The molecular biology of thyroid carcinoma is very complex ranging from gene mutations, gene amplifications and copy-number gains, gene translocations, aberrant gene methylation, to altered signaling pathways and progressive molecular alterations [34]. Anaplastic thyroid carcinoma presents various subtypes: Type 1 *BRAF*-positive, with a genetic landscape similar to papillary thyroid carcinoma; Type 2 *NRAS*-positive which may originate from follicular thyroid carcinoma; Type 3 which carries *RAS* mutations or more atypical ones (e.g., *PTEN*, *NF1* and *RB1*) and is likely to originate from Hürthle cell carcinoma; and Type 4 mixed, which harbor loss-of-function genetic alterations and mutations in the genes of cell-cycle regulations (*CDKN2A* and *CDKN2B*) [35]. This leads to uncontrolled activity of various signaling pathways: the MAPK, PI3K–AKT, nuclear factor-κB (NF-κB), RASSF1–mammalian STE20-like protein kinase 1 (MST1)–forkhead box O3 (FOXO3), WNT–β-catenin, hypoxia-inducible factor 1α (HIF1α) and thyroid-stimulating hormone (TSH)–TSH receptor (TSHR) pathways [36].

For patients with locoregionally confined (stage IVA or IVB) anaplastic thyroid carcinoma, chemotherapy is applied as concurrent radiochemotherapy or adjuvant therapy. The drug candidates are taxanes, anthracyclines and platinum derivatives. Weekly regimens are recommended when administered concurrently with radiotherapy [37].

In summary, we consider the management of bulky thyroid tumors in patients with multiple comorbidities to be performed in a multidisciplinary team pre, intra and postoperatively. This multidisciplinary team necessarily includes the endocrinologist, the imager, the anesthetist, the anatomopathologist, the neck surgeon, sometimes the thoracic surgeon, the oncologist and the radiotherapist, which sometimes makes the timing difficult. The anesthetist's challenges relate to difficult intubation requiring video laryngoscopy or awake bronchoscope intubation, intraoperative transfusion, postoperative intensive care and cardiac monitoring. Surgical challenges relate to the preservation of the recurrent laryngeal nerves, preservation of at least one parathyroid gland, preservation of the integrity of the pharyngoesophageal axis and control of hemostasis. The surgical team involved in the ablation of bulky tumors of the thyroid gland must be physically and psychologically trained, because it is a long surgery, with experience gained over time. Just as functional outcomes differ between an occasional thyroid surgeon and a routine thyroid surgeon, the challenges of surgical management in bulky tumors are better addressed in multidisciplinary teams trained in this type of pathology.

Limitations

There are some limitations to the present study due to the fact that it is a transversal retrospective study design. The number of subjects in the study is limited because these types of tumors are rare. The complex team necessary to manage such difficult surgical cases is available only in few tertiary healthcare units. Future studies on a wider group of patients are still necessary for clearing the indication of salvage surgery in these advanced carcinoma cases.

5. Conclusions

The data presented in this study strengthen the hypothesis that the long evolution of a thyroid tumor is associated with malignancy. Total thyroidectomy is the gold standard in giant thyroid tumors, associated with neck dissection, extended to groups VI and VII in malignant tumors. Cardiological, neurological and endocrinological monitoring prevented major complications in the postoperative period. The presence of comorbidities did not negatively influence the postoperative evolution, but it was important to know them for investigation and specialized monitoring. The unfavorable prognosis was associated with the HP type of anaplastic carcinoma. Extending the research to larger study groups may help in generalizing the findings.

Author Contributions: Conceptualization, D.V. and M.D.; methodology, A.M. and C.S.; software, G.M. and M.R.; validation, D.V., M.D. and F.M.; formal analysis, M.P.-C. and C.C.; investigation, A.M. and C.S.; resources, G.M. and M.R.; data curation, M.P.-C. and C.C.; writing—original draft preparation, D.V.; writing—review and editing, M.D.; visualization, A.M. and C.C.; supervision, G.M.; project administration, C.S.; funding acquisition, F.M. All authors have read and agreed to the published version of the manuscript.

Funding: This research received no external funding.

Institutional Review Board Statement: The study was conducted in accordance with the Declaration of Helsinki, and approved by the Ethics Committee of Bucharest University Emergency Hospital (43690/2024).

Informed Consent Statement: Informed consent was obtained from all subjects involved in the study. Written informed consent has been obtained from the patients to publish this paper.

Data Availability Statement: All data are available from the corresponding author upon reasonable request due to the increased size of the dataset.

Acknowledgments: Publication of this article was supported by the 'Carol Davila' University of Medicine and Pharmacy (Bucharest, Romania) through the institutional program 'Publish not Perish'.

Conflicts of Interest: The authors declare no conflicts of interest.

References

1. Sak, S.D. Variants of Papillary Thyroid Carcinoma: Multiple Faces of a Familiar Tumor. *Turk. Patoloji Derg.* **2015**, *31* (Suppl. S1), 34–47. [CrossRef] [PubMed]
2. Kitahara, C.M.; Sosa, J.A. The changing incidence of thyroid cancer. *Nat. Rev. Endocrinol.* **2016**, *12*, 646–653. [CrossRef] [PubMed] [PubMed Central]
3. Salazar-Mejía, C.E.; Pérez-Arredondo, L.A. A giant mass in the neck of a young men: A case of anaplastic thyroid cancer. *Pan Afr. Med. J.* **2018**, *30*, 151. [CrossRef] [PubMed] [PubMed Central]
4. Xi, F.C.; Song, Y.Q.; Li, W.Q.; Yu, W.K. Extracorporeal membrane oxygenation would provide a new approach to anesthesia for giant thyroid tumor resection: A case report. *Asian J. Surg.* **2020**, *43*, 1123–1125. [CrossRef] [PubMed]
5. Vrînceanu, D.; Sajin, M.; Dumitru, M.; Mogoantă, C.A.; Cergan, R.; Georgescu, M.G. Current approach to branchial remnants in the neck. *Rom. J. Morphol. Embryol.* **2022**, *63*, 485–490. [CrossRef] [PubMed] [PubMed Central]
6. Wilkins, R.; Zan, E.; Leonardi, O.; Patel, K.N.; Jacobson, A.S.; Jour, G.; Liu, C.Z.; Zhou, F. Case Report: Giant Thyroid Angiolipoma-Challenging Clinical Diagnosis and Novel Genetic Alterations. *Head. Neck Pathol.* **2023**, *17*, 246–252. [CrossRef] [PubMed] [PubMed Central]
7. Tang, T.; Yang, G.; Sun, J.; Chen, X.-L.; Li, W.-N.; Li, Q.; Zhu, J.-J.; Xiong, Y.-F.; Li, J.-D. Giant cervical goiter in Hashimoto's thyroiditis: A case report. *J. Int. Med. Res.* **2022**, *50*, 3000605221096379. [CrossRef] [PubMed] [PubMed Central]
8. De Pasquale, L.; Rabbiosi, D.; Bardazzi, A.; Autelitano, L.; Moro, G.P.; Ghilardi, G. Multidisciplinary approach to follicular thyroid carcinoma with giant mandibular and multiple sites metastases Case report. *Ann. Ital. Chir.* **2014**, *85*, 601–605. [PubMed]
9. Kang, S.; Kim, E.; Lee, S.; Kim, J.K.; Lee, C.R.; Kang, S.W.; Lee, J.; Jeong, J.J.; Nam, K.H.; Chung, W.Y. Do large thyroid nodules (≥4 cm) without suspicious cytology need surgery? *Front. Endocrinol.* **2023**, *14*, 1252503. [CrossRef] [PubMed] [PubMed Central]
10. Campennì, A.; Barbaro, D.; Guzzo, M.; Capoccetti, F.; Giovanella, L. Personalized management of differentiated thyroid cancer in real life—Practical guidance from a multidisciplinary panel of experts. *Endocrine* **2020**, *70*, 280–291. [CrossRef] [PubMed] [PubMed Central]
11. Croce, L.; Ruggeri, R.M.; Cappelli, C.; Virili, C.; Coperchini, F.; Laganà, M.; Costa, P.; Dal Molin, M.; Chytiris, S.; Magri, F.; et al. Cardiovascular and metabolic comorbidities in patients with thyroid nodules: The impact of incidental diagnosis. *J. Endocrinol. Investig.* **2024**, *47*, 827–832. [CrossRef] [PubMed] [PubMed Central]
12. Mazumder, H.; Husain, M.; Hossain, M.F.; Mahmud, S. Prevalence, trend and associated factors of obesity-related cancers among U.S. adults with metabolic syndrome: Evidence from the National Health and Nutrition Examination Survey 2001-2018. *PLoS ONE* **2023**, *18*, e0290994. [CrossRef] [PubMed] [PubMed Central]
13. Marcy, P.Y.; Tassart, M.; Marchand, J.G.; Thariat, J.; Bizeau, A.; Ghanassia, E. Percutaneous Radiofrequency Ablation of Thyroid Carcinomas Ineligible for Surgery, in the Elderly. *Curr. Oncol.* **2023**, *30*, 7439–7449. [CrossRef] [PubMed] [PubMed Central]

14. Ahn, H.Y.; Chae, J.E.; Moon, H.; Noh, J.; Park, Y.J.; Kim, S.G. Trends in the Diagnosis and Treatment of Patients with Medullary Thyroid Carcinoma in Korea. *Endocrinol. Metab.* **2020**, *35*, 811–819. [CrossRef] [PubMed] [PubMed Central]
15. Kefeli, M.; Gucer, H.; Durmuş, E.T.; Atmaca, A.; Colak, R.; Mete, O. Prevalence of Papillary Thyroid Carcinoma is Significantly Higher in Graves Disease with Synchronous Thyroid Nodules. *Turk. Patoloji Derg.* **2024**, *40*, 190–195. [CrossRef] [PubMed]
16. Steponaviciene, R.; Maceika, E.; Kesminiene, A.; Smailyte, G. Recent insights into trends of thyroid cancer incidence in Lithuanian population exposed to Chernobyl fallout early in life. *Ecotoxicol. Environ. Saf.* **2024**, *283*, 116789. [CrossRef] [PubMed]
17. Gong, Y.; Jiang, Q.; Zhai, M.; Tang, T.; Liu, S. Thyroid cancer trends in China and its comparative analysis with G20 countries: Projections for 2020-2040. *J. Glob. Health* **2024**, *14*, 04131. [CrossRef] [PubMed] [PubMed Central]
18. Agilinko, J.; Kueh, T.J.; Smart, L.; Shakeel, M. Primary thyroid squamous cell carcinoma: A challenging management problem. *BMJ Case Rep.* **2021**, *14*, e238560. [CrossRef] [PubMed] [PubMed Central]
19. Birly, A.; Renwick, A.; Patel, P. Recurrent cardiogenic syncope as the first presentation of thyroid carcinoma. *Br. J. Hosp. Med.* **2022**, *83*, 1–3. [CrossRef] [PubMed]
20. Benbakh, M.; Abou-elfadl, M.; Rouadi, S.; Abada, R.L.; Roubal, M.; Mahtar, M. Substernal goiter: Experience with 50 cases. *Eur. Ann. Otorhinolaryngol. Head. Neck Dis.* **2016**, *133*, 19–22. [CrossRef] [PubMed]
21. An, S.Y.; Kim, S.Y.; Oh, D.J.; Min, C.; Sim, S.; Choi, H.G. Obesity is positively related and tobacco smoking and alcohol consumption are negatively related to an increased risk of thyroid cancer. *Sci. Rep.* **2020**, *10*, 19279. [CrossRef] [PubMed] [PubMed Central]
22. Papaleontiou, M.; Norton, E.C.; Reyes-Gastelum, D.; Banerjee, M.; Haymart, M.R. Competing Causes of Death in Older Adults with Thyroid Cancer. *Thyroid* **2021**, *31*, 1359–1365. [CrossRef] [PubMed] [PubMed Central]
23. Du, B.; Wang, F.; Wu, L.; Wang, Z.; Zhang, D.; Huang, Z.; Gao, L.; Li, Y.; Liang, C.; Li, P.; et al. Cause-specific mortality after diagnosis of thyroid cancer: A large population-based study. *Endocrine* **2021**, *72*, 179–189. [CrossRef] [PubMed]
24. Agosto Salgado, S.; Kaye, E.R.; Sargi, Z.; Chung, C.H.; Papaleontiou, M. Management of Advanced Thyroid Cancer: Overview, Advances, and Opportunities. *Am. Soc. Clin. Oncol. Educ. Book* **2023**, *43*, e389708. [CrossRef] [PubMed]
25. Agcaoglu, O.; Sucu, S.; Toprak, S.; Tezelman, S. Techniques for Thyroidectomy and Functional Neck Dissection. *J. Clin. Med.* **2024**, *13*, 1914. [CrossRef]
26. Otsuki, N.; Shimoda, H.; Morita, N.; Furukawa, T.; Teshima, M.; Shinomiya, H.; Nibu, K.I. Salvage surgery for structural local recurrence of papillary thyroid cancer: Recurrence patterns and surgical outcome. *Endocr. J.* **2020**, *67*, 949–956. [CrossRef] [PubMed]
27. Beka, E.; Hanna, H.; Olofsson, P.; Gimm, O. Hemithyroidectomy, does the indication influence the outcome? *Langenbecks Arch. Surg.* **2023**, *409*, 1. [CrossRef] [PubMed] [PubMed Central]
28. Boucek, J.; Zabrodsky, M.; Kuchar, M.; Fanta, O.; Skrivan, J.; Betka, J. A new strategy for the surgical management of RLN infiltrated by well-differentiated thyroid carcinoma. *Biomed. Res. Int.* **2014**, *2014*, 616521. [CrossRef] [PubMed] [PubMed Central]
29. Houten, P.V.; Netea-Maier, R.T.; Smit, J.W. Differentiated thyroid carcinoma: An update. *Best. Pract. Res. Clin. Endocrinol. Metab.* **2023**, *37*, 101687. [CrossRef] [PubMed]
30. Masui, T.; Adachi, S.; Uemura, H.; Kimura, T.; Kitahara, T. Clinical Study on the Risk Factors for the Recurrence of Papillary Thyroid Carcinoma. *ORL J. Otorhinolaryngol. Relat. Spec.* **2023**, *85*, 104–108. [CrossRef] [PubMed]
31. Sugitani, I.; Hasegawa, Y.; Sugasawa, M.; Tori, M.; Higashiyama, T.; Miyazaki, M.; Hosoi, H.; Orita, Y.; Kitano, H. Super-radical surgery for anaplastic thyroid carcinoma: A large cohort study using the Anaplastic Thyroid Carcinoma Research Consortium of Japan database. *Head Neck* **2014**, *36*, 328–333. [CrossRef] [PubMed]
32. Chen, R.; Zhang, K.; Liu, J.; Guo, L.; Liu, K.; Geng, C. Preoperative ultrasound identification and localization of the inferior parathyroid glands in thyroid surgery. *Front. Endocrinol.* **2023**, *14*, 1094379. [CrossRef] [PubMed] [PubMed Central]
33. Adam, M.A.; Thomas, S.; Hyslop, T.; Scheri, R.P.; Roman, S.A.; Sosa, J.A. Exploring the Relationship Between Patient Age and Cancer-Specific Survival in Papillary Thyroid Cancer: Rethinking Current Staging Systems. *J. Clin. Oncol.* **2016**, *34*, 4415–4420. [CrossRef] [PubMed] [PubMed Central]
34. Xing, M. Molecular pathogenesis and mechanisms of thyroid cancer. *Nat. Rev. Cancer* **2013**, *13*, 184–199. [CrossRef] [PubMed] [PubMed Central]
35. Prete, A.; Borges de Souza, P.; Censi, S.; Muzza, M.; Nucci, N.; Sponziello, M. Update on Fundamental Mechanisms of Thyroid Cancer. *Front. Endocrinol.* **2020**, *11*, 102. [CrossRef] [PubMed] [PubMed Central]
36. Zaballos, M.A.; Santisteban, P. Key signaling pathways in thyroid cancer. *J. Endocrinol.* **2017**, *235*, R43–R61. [CrossRef] [PubMed]
37. National Health Commission of the People's Republic of China. National guidelines for diagnosis and treatment of thyroid cancer 2022 in China (English version). *Chin. J. Cancer Res.* **2022**, *34*, 131–150. [CrossRef] [PubMed]

biomedicines

MDPI

Article

The Role of Body Mass Index (BMI) in Differentiated Thyroid Cancer: A Potential Prognostic Factor?

Chiara Mele [1,*,†], Lucrezia De Marchi [2,†], Giulia Marsan [1], Marco Zavattaro [3], Maria Grazia Mauri [3], Paolo Aluffi Valletti [4], Gianluca Aimaretti [1] and Paolo Marzullo [1]

1 Department of Translational Medicine, University of Piemonte Orientale, 28100 Novara, Italy; 20022109@studenti.uniupo.it (G.M.); gianluca.aimaretti@med.uniupo.it (G.A.); paolo.marzullo@med.uniupo.it (P.M.)

2 Department of Endocrinology, UZ Brussel, Laarbeeklaan, 1090 Brussels, Belgium; lucredem@gmail.com

3 Division of Endocrinology, University Hospital "Maggiore della Carità", 28100 Novara, Italy; marco.zavattaro@med.uniupo.it (M.Z.); grazia.mauri@maggioreosp.novara.it (M.G.M.)

4 ENT Division, University of Piemonte Orientale, 28100 Novara, Italy; paolo.aluffi@med.uniupo.it

* Correspondence: chiara.mele1989@gmail.com

† These authors contributed equally to this work.

Abstract: Obesity has been recognized as a potential risk factor for the carcinogenesis of differentiated thyroid cancer (DTC). The aim of this observational study was to investigate the prognostic role of BMI in influencing DTC histopathological aggressiveness and the risk of tumor relapse. We enrolled 257 patients with DTC, consecutively admitted to our Institution between January 2016 and December 2023. The following variables were collected: demographic, anthropometric and clinical parameters, risk factors for DTC, surgical and radioiodine therapy, histopathological features of DTC, and biochemical markers of disease. Tumor recurrence was assessed during short-, medium- and long-term follow-up. According to BMI tertiles (e.g; I: BMI < 23.3 kg/m^2; II: 23.3 $\leq$ BMI < 27.1 kg/m^2; III: BMI $\geq$ 27.1 kg/m^2), the clinical and histopathological characteristics did not differ between groups. The multinomial logistic regression analysis showed that BMI was not associated with clinical and histopathological aggressiveness of DTC, independently from sex, age, and risk factors for DTC onset. Moreover, BMI did not constitute a predictor of tumor recurrence during follow-up. In conclusion, BMI does not represent a predictor of clinical and histopathological aggressiveness of DTC. Since it is not a reliable marker of adiposity, BMI cannot be considered alone in evaluating the potential association between obesity and DTC prognosis.

Keywords: thyroid cancer; body mass index; obesity; tumor aggressiveness; outcome

1. Introduction

Obesity represents a potential risk factor for many types of cancer [1,2], and body mass index (BMI) has been found to be associated with histological and clinical aggressiveness of prostate and breast cancer [3]. Over the last decades, a concomitant increase in the incidence of obesity and differentiated thyroid cancer (DTC) has been documented worldwide [4,5]. While the epidemiological trend of DTC can be partly attributed to a greater diagnostic accuracy [6–8], an increased incidence of larger tumors with aggressive histological features has led some authors to speculate on the increasing exposure to specific risk factors, including radiation, environmental pollutants, and nutritional factors [9–11].

Recently, a slight but significant association was found between the incidence of DTC and the growing prevalence of obesity, suggesting a possible role of obesity in thyroid carcinogenesis [12,13].

Although the mechanisms relating obesity and DTC remain largely unknown, the potential impact of insulin resistance and proinflammatory adipocytokines as risks factors for thyroid tumorigenesis has been postulated [14–16].

Furthermore, several authors have investigated the potential role of obesity as a risk factor for the aggressiveness of thyroid cancer, with conflicting results. Some studies have reported overweight/obesity as a predictor of aggressive histopathological features of DTC (i.e., larger tumor size, multifocality, extrathyroidal invasion, and lymph node metastases) [17–20], while others did not find any relationship between obesity and DTC histopathological aggressiveness [21–24].

Conflicting results have also been published about the risk of DTC relapse in patients with obesity. Some authors observed that patients with obesity have an increased risk of developing locoregional recurrence of papillary thyroid cancer (PTC) during long-term follow-up [25], although most of the studies did not demonstrate a higher risk of tumor relapse in patients with obesity as compared to normal-weight subjects [21,22,24].

Given the lack of univocal results on the relationship between obesity and DTC histology and outcome, the aim of our study was to investigate the potential prognostic role of BMI in influencing DTC histopathological aggressiveness and risk of tumor relapse.

2. Materials and Methods

2.1. Study Design and Population

This observational, retrospective, cohort study included 257 patients with DTC, consecutively admitted to the Endocrinology Unit of the University Hospital "Maggiore della Carità" of Novara, between January 2016 and December 2023. Patients with a history of poorly differentiated, anaplastic, or medullary thyroid carcinomas were excluded.

The study design conformed to the ethical guidelines of the Declaration of Helsinki and was approved by the local Ethical Committee "Comitato Etico Territoriale Interaziendale AOU Maggiore della Carità di Novara". All of the participants signed a written informed consent form.

2.2. Variables, Data, Sources and Measurements

Data were retrieved from electronic hospital records and included the following variables: demographic and anthropometric characteristics, known risk factors for DTC, clinical and family history, surgical approach, histopathological features of DTC, AJCC VIII ed.'s TNM and staging classifications [26], radioiodine (RAI) therapy, and tumor recurrence at 1, 3, and 5 years from diagnosis. Recurrence was defined in accordance with the 2015 ATA dynamic response system [27]. The patients were followed up at regular intervals with periodical biochemical and ultrasonographic evaluations, and timing of follow-up was based on the dynamic risk re-stratification process [27,28]. Thyroglobulin (Tg) levels were considered to evaluate the clinical response when thyroglobulin antibodies (TgAb) were negative. Contrariwise, in the presence of interfering TgAb, their values were considered to define the response to treatment [29].

2.2.1. Body Measurements

All subjects underwent body measurements wearing light underwear, in fasting conditions after voiding, as described previously [15]. Weight and height were measured in the nearest 0.1 kg and 0.1 cm, respectively, using standard methods. BMI was expressed as body mass (kg)/height (m)^2. Overweight was defined as any BMI between 25 and 29.9 kg/m^2 and obesity as any BMI over 30 kg/m^2.

2.2.2. Laboratory Tests

Serum Tg and TgAb were measured with the same methods in all patients at the baseline and during each follow-up visit. Serum Tg levels were determined using an automated chemiluminescence method (LIAISON XL, DiaSorin S.p.A, Saluggia, Italy), with a functional sensitivity of 0.1 ng/mL.

Plasma levels of TgAb were assessed using an automated chemiluminescence assay system (Anti-Tg Ready Pack, Siemens Healthcare Diagnostics). TgAb positivity was defined as serum TgAb levels above 60 IU/mL.

2.2.3. Neck Ultrasound (US)

The US was performed with an Esaote MyLab Twice real-time US system with a linear multifrequency (7–14 MHz) probe. Central and laterocervical lymph node compartments were inspected during each follow-up visit to assess the presence of a locoregional recurrence of the disease. Suspicious lymph nodes were evaluated by using US-guided fine-needle aspiration cytology (FNAC) in association with the Tg measurement in washing fluid.

2.2.4. Surgery

Surgery was performed by the same experienced thyroid surgeon, so that the thyroidectomy and lymph node dissection techniques were consistent across patients. The choice of the type of surgery and lymph node dissection was collegially made by the surgeons and endocrinologists according to ATA guidelines recommendations [27].

2.2.5. Thyroid Histology

Two independent pathologists reviewed the histological slides for the following assessments: tumor size, histological type, foci number, (multi)focality, extrathyroidal extension, vascular invasion, surgical margins, tumor-associated thyroiditis, and presence of locoregional and/or distant metastases, according to the 8th edition of the AJCC TNM Staging System [26].

2.2.6. Radioiodine Therapy (RAI)

RAI was performed after withdrawal of levothyroxine (L-T4) or after recombinant human thyrotropin stimulation (rhTSH). The ^{131}I uptake was measured using a 2-head gamma camera (e.cam Dual-Head 180° Gamma Camera Siemens Medical System, Erlangen, Germany). The choice to perform RAI was made according to the ATA guidelines and recent evidence [27,30,31]

2.3. Statistical Analysis

Values are expressed as mean ± standard deviation (SD) or absolute number and percentage. Data points not normally distributed, obtained by the Shapiro–Wilk test, were log-transformed to improve the symmetry and homoscedasticity of the distribution. The univariate ANOVA for continuous variables and the chi-square tests for categorical variables were used for comparisons between the subgroups of BMI tertiles. Multinomial logistic regression analysis was used to evaluate the association between BMI as a continuous variable and the clinical-histopathological features of DTC, after controlling for age, sex, and risk factors for DTC occurrence.

Univariate logistic regression analysis was conducted to test the potential association between tumor relapse and clinical-histopathological features of DTC. Multivariable logistic regression analysis was performed to identify the independent risk factors of tumor relapse. The regression models included the individual variables considered in the univariate analysis and potential confounders, including sex, age, BMI, histological type, radiation exposure, thyroiditis, and smoking habit. The odds ratio (OR), 95% confidence interval (95% CI), and related significant values obtained from regression are reported. Statistical significance was set at 5%. Statistical analyses were performed using SPSS version 21 (Somers, NY, USA).

3. Results

3.1. Clinical and Histopathological Characteristics

A summary of the clinical and histopathological characteristics of the study population is reported in Table 1. Most patients were female (70.4%, male-to-female ratio 1:2.4), with a mean age at diagnosis of 53.8 ± 15.2 years (range 17–88 years). The majority of patients were Caucasian (93.4%). The mean BMI was 25.9 ± 5.2 kg/m^2, and overweight was found in 87 cases (33.9%) and obesity in 45 cases (17.5%). Smoking habits were documented in 18.7%

of cases. Regarding the risk factors for thyroid cancer, 16 patients (8.5%) were exposed to radiation in the head and neck region, and 55 patients (21.4%) had autoimmune thyroiditis. Overall, 15.9% of patients had a history of cancer in a different site; moreover, the most frequent types were breast cancer in women (29.3%), prostate cancer in men (12.2%), and lymphoma in both sexes (19.5%). A family history of thyroid nodules, autoimmune thyroiditis, and thyroid cancer was found in 11.3%, 4.7%, and 5.4% of cases, respectively. Familiarity for other malignancies was found in 24.5% of patients.

Table 1. Clinical and histopathological characteristics of the population as a whole and subdivided into three groups according to BMI tertiles (1st tertile: BMI < 23.3 kg/m^2; 2nd tertile: $23.3 \leq$ BMI < 27.1 kg/m^2; 3rd tertile: BMI ≥ 27.1 kg/m^2).

Variables	Whole Population (N = 257)	BMI I Tertile (N = 86)	BMI II Tertile (N = 86)	BMI III Tertile (N = 85)	*p*-Value
Sex					
Male	76 (29.6)	16 (18.6)	34 (39.5)	26 (30.6)	0.01
Female	181 (70.4)	70 (81.4)	52 (60.5)	59 (69.4)	
Age at diagnosis	53.8 ± 15.2	49.5 ± 17.0	57.7 ± 14.5	54.1 ± 12.9	0.002
Ethnicity					
Caucasian	240 (93.4)	82 (95.3)	78 (90.7)	80 (94.1)	0.07
Hispanic	9 (3.5)	1 (1.2)	3 (3.5)	5 (5.9)	
Asian	5 (1.9)	3 (3.5)	2 (2.3)	0 (0.0)	
African	3 (1.2)	0 (0.0)	3 (3.5)	0 (0.0)	
Risk factor					
Radiation	16 (6.2)	6 (7.0)	5 (5.8)	5 (5.9)	0.94
Thyroiditis	55 (21.4)	21 (24.4)	15 (17.4)	19 (22.4)	0.52
Smoking	48 (18.7)	17 (19.8)	18 (20.9)	13 (15.3)	0.61
Other tumors	41 (15.9)	15 (17.4)	12 (14.0)	14 (16.5)	0.81
Family history					
Thyroid nodules	29 (11.3)	12 (14.0)	9 (10.5)	8 (9.4)	0.62
Thyroid cancer	14 (5.4)	5 (5.8)	3 (3.5)	6 (7.1)	0.58
Thyroiditis	12 (4.7)	4 (4.7)	3 (3.5)	5 (5.9)	0.76
Other tumors	63 (24.5)	23 (26.7)	19 (22.1)	21 (24.7)	0.78
Surgery					
Lobectomy	15 (5.8)	6 (7.0)	5 (5.8)	4 (4.7)	0.82
Total thyroidectomy	242 (94.2)	80 (93.0)	81 (94.2)	81 (95.3)	
pCND	77 (30.0)	23 (26.7)	30 (34.9)	24 (28.2)	0.46
tCND	96 (37.4)	37 (43.0)	29 (33.7)	30 (35.3)	0.40
LCD	31 (12.1)	14 (16.3)	7 (8.1)	10 (11.8)	0.26
Histotype					
PTC	224 (87.1)	77 (89.5)	74 (86.0)	73 (85.9)	0.96
FTC	22 (8.6)	6 (7.0)	8 (9.3)	8 (9.4)	
Hurtle Cells	11 (4.3)	3 (3.5)	4 (4.7)	4 (4.7)	
PTC variants					
Classical	81 (37.9)	28 (39.4)	31 (43.1)	22 (31.0)	0.67
Follicular	84 (39.2)	25 (35.2)	25 (34.7)	34 (47.9)	
Classical and follicular	28 (13.1)	10 (14.1)	10 (13.9)	8 (11.3)	
Other variants	21 (9.8)	8 (11.3)	6 (8.3)	7 (9.8)	
FTC variants					
Minimally invasive	14 (63.6)	3 (50.0)	5 (62.5)	6 (75.0)	0.63
Invasive	8 (36.4)	3 (50.0)	3 (37.5)	2 (25.0)	
Tumor size (mm)	16.6 ± 13.1	16.1 ± 12.1	17.3 ± 13.5	16.3 ± 14.0	0.82
Bilaterality	66 (25.7)	19 (22.1)	26 (30.2)	21 (24.7)	0.46
Multifocality	94 (36.6)	25 (29.1)	38 (44.2)	31 (36.5)	0.12
Extrathyroidal extension	57 (22.3)	21 (24.4)	19 (22.1)	17 (20.0)	0.78

Table 1. *Cont.*

Variables	Whole Population (N = 257)	BMI I Tertile (N = 86)	BMI II Tertile (N = 86)	BMI III Tertile (N = 85)	*p*-Value
Vascular invasion	43 (16.7)	14 (16.3)	10 (11.6)	19 (22.4)	0.17
Surgical margins					
R0	225 (87.5)	77 (89.5)	74 (86.0)	74 (87.1)	
R1	31 (12.1)	9 (10.5)	11 (12.8)	11 (12.9)	0.68
R2	1 (0.4)	0 (0.0)	1 (1.2)	0 (0.0)	
LND MTS at diagnosis					
Presence of LND MTS	59 (28.9)	22 (29.7)	20 (30.3)	17 (26.6)	0.88
N° of LND MTS	6.3 ± 8.6	7.8 ± 9.0	4.9 ± 8.5	6.1 ± 8.4	0.58
Location of LND MTS					
Central compartment	35 (59.4)	10 (45.5)	17 (85.0)	8 (47.1)	
LC compartment	12 (20.3)	7 (31.8)	1 (5.0)	4 (23.5)	0.06
Both	12 (20.3)	5 (22.7)	2 (10.0)	5 (29.4)	

Data are expressed as mean ± SD or absolute number and percentage. Comparison between groups was performed using univariate ANOVA or χ^2 test. For 3-group comparison analysis, the statistical significance was set at 1% ($p < 0.01$). Abbreviations: pCND, prophylactic central neck dissection; tCND, therapeutic central neck dissection; LCD, laterocervical; PTC, papillary thyroid cancer; FTC, follicular thyroid cancer; LND, lymph nodes; MTS, metastases.

Most of the patients underwent total thyroidectomy (94.2%), with concomitant prophylactic or therapeutic dissection of the central compartment in 30.0% and 37.4% of cases, respectively. In patients with US suspicion of lateral neck lymphadenopathy, a dissection of the lateral neck compartment was also performed (12.1% of cases).

The most frequently found histotype was PTC (87.1%) and the most common variant was the follicular one (39.20%), followed by the classical one (37.9%). The average tumor size was 16.6 ± 13.1 mm, with tumors < 10 mm (microcarcinomas) in 36.2% of cases. Multifocality and bilaterality were detected in 94 (36.6%) and 66 (25.7%) cases, respectively. Extrathyroidal extension was detected in 57 patients (22.3%) and vascular invasion in 43 patients (16.7%).

In more than a quarter of patients (28.9%), lymph node metastases were documented, prevalently in the central compartment (59.4%). The average number of involved lymph nodes was 6.3 ± 8.6.

Based on these histopathological features, and according to the 8th edition of the AJCC TNM Staging System, overall, 65.4% of cases were classified as stage I, followed by stage III (18.3%), stage II (9.3%), and stage IV (7.0%).

Overall, 100 patients (38.9%) underwent radioiodine (RAI) treatment within 6 months after surgery. The average dose of 131I was 81.5 ± 23.2 mCi. The mean stimulated Tg level was 14.5 ± 45.5 ng/mL, and a minority of patients showed TgAb positivity (12.0%). The majority of patients (84.0%) showed whole-body scintigraphy (WBS) uptake in the thyroid bed, while an uptake in the lateral neck compartment or in multiple sites was detected in the 3.0% and 12.0% of cases, respectively (Table 2).

When the population was subgrouped according to BMI tertiles (I tertile: BMI < 23.3 kg/m^2, II tertile: 23.3 ≤ BMI < 27.1 kg/m^2, BMI ≥ 27.1 kg/m^2), no significant differences were found in terms of clinical and histopathological features (Table 1), stage of disease (Figure 1), and dosimetric, laboratory, and WBS characteristics in the context of RAI (Table 2).

A multinomial logistic regression analysis was conducted to evaluate the association between BMI as a continuous variable and the clinical-histopathological characteristics of the tumor (Table 3). BMI was not associated with clinical and histopathological features, independently from potential confounders, including sex, age, and risk factors for DTC.

Table 2. Dosimetric, laboratory, and WBS characteristics of patients who underwent RAI therapy.

Variables	Whole Population (N = 100)	BMI I Tertile (N = 33)	BMI II Tertile (N = 34)	BMI III Tertile (N = 33)	*p*-Value
RAI activity (mCi)	81.5 ± 23.2	84.3 ± 26.2	82.2 ± 20.2	77.9 ± 23.2	0.52
Stimulation regimen					
LT4-withdrawal	82 (82.0)	29 (87.9)	31 (91.2)	22 (66.7)	0.02
rhTSH	18 (18.0)	4 (12.1)	3 (8.8)	11 (33.3)	
Stimulated Tg (ng/dL)	16.7 ± 40.6	26.8 ± 60.2	11.0 ± 23.0	13.6 ± 31.9	0.27
TgAb					
Positive (≥30 IU/mL)	12 (12.0)	4 (12.1)	3 (8.8)	5 (15.2)	0.73
Negative (<30 IU/mL)	88 (88.0)	29 (87.9)	31 (91.2)	28 (84.8)	
WBS uptake					
No uptake	0 (0.0)	0 (0.0)	0 (0.0)	0 (0.0)	
Thyroid bed	84 (84.0)	28 (84.9)	29 (85.3)	27 (81.8)	
Neck LCC	3 (3.0)	0 (0.0)	2 (5.9)	1 (3.0)	0.60
Mediastinum or lungs	0 (0.0)	0 (0.0)	0 (0.0)	0 (0.0)	
Bone	1 (1.0)	1 (3.0)	0 (0.0)	0 (0.0)	

Data are expressed as mean ± SD or absolute number and percentage. Comparison between groups was performed using univariate ANOVA or χ^2 test. For 3-group comparison analysis, the statistical significance was set at 1% ($p < 0.01$). Abbreviations: RAI, radioiodine, LT4, levothyroxine; rhTSH, recombinant human thyrotropin; Tg, Thyroglobulin; TgAb, Thyroglobulin antibodies; LCC, laterocervical compartment; WBS, whole-body scintigraphy.

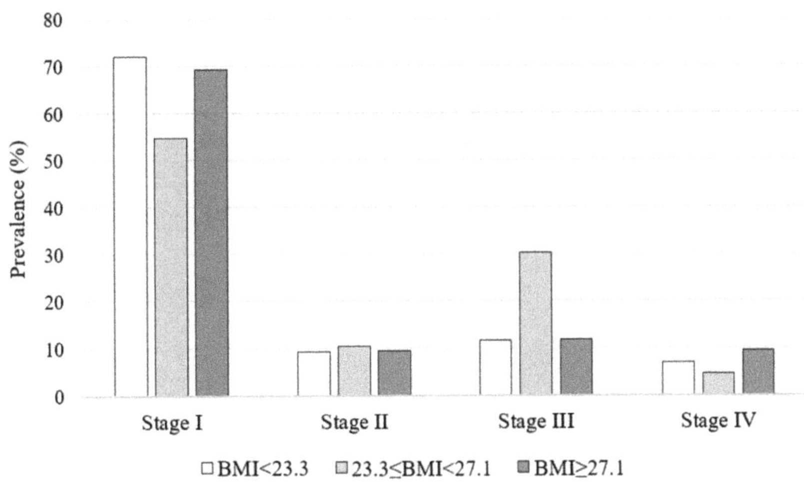

Figure 1. Stage of disease according to BMI tertiles.

Table 3. Multinomial logistic regression analysis to evaluate the association between the BMI as a continuous variable and the histopathological features of the tumor.

Variables	BMI (Continuous Variable)			
	OR (CI 95%)	*p*-Value	OR (CI 95%) (Sex*Age*RFs)	*p*-Value (Sex*Age*RFs)
Histotype				
PTC	Ref	-	Ref	-
FTC	1.01 (0.93–1.10)	0.83	1.01 (0.92–1.11)	0.80
Hurtle Cells	0.99 (0.89–1.12)	0.98	0.99 (0.88–1.13)	0.97

Table 3. *Cont.*

Variables	BMI (Continuous Variable)			
	OR (CI 95%)	*p*-Value	OR (CI 95%) (Sex*Age*RFs)	*p*-Value (Sex*Age*RFs)
PTC variants				
Classical	Ref	-	Ref	-
Follicular	1.06 (0.99–1.13)	0.07	1.07 (1.00–1.14)	0.05
Classical and follicular	1.03 (0.94–1.12)	0.55	1.04 (0.96–1.14)	0.34
Other variants	1.02 (0.90–1.16)	0.77	1.02 (0.88–1.17)	0.82
FTC variants				
Minimally invasive	Ref	-	Ref	-
Invasive	1.02 (0.85–1.22)	0.87	1.03 (0.84–1.25)	0.80
Tumor size				
≤1 cm	Ref	-	Ref	-
>1 cm but ≤2 cm	0.97 (0.92–1.03)	0.35	0.97 (0.92–1.03)	0.34
≥2 cm but ≤4 cm	0.98 (0.92–1.04)	0.48	0.98 (0.92–1.04)	0.50
>4 cm	1.04 (0.95–1.13)	0.44	1.03 (0.94–1.13)	0.56
Bilaterality				
No	Ref	-	Ref	-
Yes	1.02 (0.97–1.07)	0.53	1.02 (0.96–1.07)	0.55
Multifocality				
No	Ref	-	Ref	-
Yes	1.03 (0.98–1.08)	0.29	1.02 (0.97–1.08)	0.34
Extrathyroidal extension				
No	Ref	-	Ref	-
Yes	1.01 (0.95–1.07)	0.87	0.99 (0.94–1.06)	0.91
Vascular invasion				
No	Ref	-	Ref	-
Yes	1.05 (0.99–1.11)	0.14	1.05 (0.99–1.11)	0.12
Surgical margins				
R0	Ref	-	Ref	-
R1	1.03 (0.96–1.10)	0.49	1.02 (0.95–1.09)	0.52
R2	0.97 (0.65–1.17)	0.90	0.99 (0.70–1.43)	0.98
LND MTS at diagnosis				
No	Ref	-	Ref	-
Yes	1.01 (0.96–1.07)	0.65	1.02 (0.96–1.08)	0.62
Location of LND MTS				
Central compartment	Ref	-	Ref	-
LC compartment	1.04 (0.94–1.15)	0.47	1.03 (0.92–1.15)	0.60
Both	0.98 (0.87–1.10)	0.70	0.98 (0.86–1.11)	0.69

Abbreviations: OR, odds ratio; CI, confidence interval; RFs, risk factors; PTC, papillary thyroid cancer; FTC, follicular thyroid cancer; LND, lymph nodes; MTS, metastases; LC, laterocervical.

3.2. Follow-Up

Tumor relapse was observed in 35 patients (15.7%) at one year after diagnosis, in 15 patients (10.5%) at 3 years after diagnosis, and in 12 patients (17.1%) at 5 years after diagnosis. Most of the patients had biochemical evidence of disease (87.1%), whereas, in only eight patients (12.9%), biochemical and instrumental evidence of disease was documented. Of the latter, five patients had local recurrence at the laterocervical lymph nodes, while three patients had lung metastases.

Data on short-term (1 year), medium-term (3 years), and long-term (5 years) follow-up, divided according to tertiles of BMI, are summarized in Table 4. No significant differences in tumor recurrence rates were found between the three groups of BMI tertiles.

Table 4. Short-, medium-, and long-term follow-up in the total population and divided according to BMI tertiles.

Variables	Whole Population	BMI I Tertile	BMI II Tertile	BMI III Tertile	*p* Value
1-year tumor relapse					
No	188 (84.3)	62 (80.5)	65 (90.3)	61 (82.4)	
Biochemical evidence of disease	32 (14.3)	12 (15.6)	7 (9.7)	13 (17.6)	0.10
Biochemical and instrumental evidence of disease	3 (1.4)	3 (3.9)	0 (0.0)	0 (0.0)	
3-year tumor relapse					
No	128 (89.5)	46 (92.0)	39 (90.7)	43 (86.0)	
Biochemical evidence of disease	11 (7.7)	3 (6.0)	3 (7.0)	5 (10.0)	0.90
Biochemical and instrumental evidence of disease	4 (2.8)	1 (2.0)	1 (2.3)	2 (4.0)	
5-year tumor relapse					
No	58 (82.9)	24 (82.8)	15 (83.3)	19 (82.6)	
Biochemical evidence of disease	11 (15.7)	5 (17.2)	2 (11.1)	4 (17.4)	0.52
Biochemical and instrumental evidence of disease	1 (1.4)	0 (0.0)	1 (5.6)	0 (0.0)	

Data are expressed as absolute number and percentage. Comparison between groups was performed using χ^2 test.

3.3. Risk of Tumor Relapse

Univariate logistic regression analysis was conducted to test the potential risk factors of tumor relapse in our population. BMI and risk factors for DTC were not associated with an increased risk of relapse in the short-, medium-, and long-term follow-up. Among the clinical and histopathological features, extrathyroidal extension (OR = 2.29, CI 95% 1.24–4.22, $p = 0.008$), tumoral infiltration of surgical margins (OR = 2.44, CI 95% 1.05–5.69, $p = 0.04$), the presence of lymph node metastases at diagnosis (OR = 4.00, CI 95% 1.65–9.73, $p = 0.002$), and high stimulated Tg levels in the context of RAI (OR = 1.03, CI 95% 1.01–1.05, $p = 0.007$) were identified as risk factors for one-year tumor relapse.

With regard to medium- and long-term follow-up, tumoral infiltration of surgical margins (OR = 4.31, CI 95% 1.44–12.87, $p = 0.009$) and one-year tumor relapse (OR 11.79, CI 95% 3.20–43.48, $p < 0.0001$) represented independent predictors of three-year tumor relapse, while five-year tumor relapse was independently predicted only by one-year tumor relapse (OR = 20.8, CI 95% 3.29–131.91, $p = 0.001$).

Multivariable logistic regression analysis was subsequently conducted to better characterize the associations found with univariate analysis (Table 5). The regression models included the individual variables considered in the univariate analysis to avoid collinearity and potential confounders, including sex, age, BMI, histological type, radiation exposure, thyroiditis, and smoking habit. The analysis confirmed that the variables identified in the univariate analysis represent risk factors for DTC recurrence, regardless of the potential confounders mentioned above.

Table 5. Multivariable logistic regression analysis used to evaluate the risk factors for DTC recurrence in the short-, medium-, and long-term follow-up.

Variables	OR (CI 95%) Model Weighted for Sex, Age, BMI, RFs, and Histological Type	*p*-Value Model Weighted for Sex, Age, BMI, RFs, and Histological Type
1-year follow-up		
Extrathyroidal extension	2.62 (1.36–5.05)	0.004
Infiltration of surgical margins	2.80 (1.17–6.72)	0.02
LND MTS at diagnosis	5.20 (1.95–13.88)	0.001
Stimulated Tg level	1.03 (1.01–1.06)	0.01

Table 5. *Cont.*

Variables	OR (CI 95%) Model Weighted for Sex, Age, BMI, RFs, and Histological Type	*p*-Value Model Weighted for Sex, Age, BMI, RFs, and Histological Type
3-year follow-up		
Infiltration of surgical margins	4.84 (1.52–15.43)	0.008
One-year tumor relapse	14.01 (3.46–56.74)	<0.0001
5-year follow-up		
One-year tumor relapse	32.29 (3.80–274.55)	0.001

Abbreviations: OR, odds ratio; CI, confidence interval; LND, lymph nodes; MTS, metastases; Tg, thyroglobulin.

4. Discussion

The present study investigated the potential association between BMI and aggressiveness of DTC. Our results showed that BMI is not associated with histopathological aggressiveness of DTC, nor with a higher risk of tumor recurrence in the short-, medium-, and long-term follow-up.

Over the last decade, several studies have analyzed the potential relationship between obesity and DTC occurrence. A meta-analysis published in 2021 demonstrated that obesity is associated with a 50% increase in the risk of thyroid cancer (RR = 1.5, CI 95% 1.45–1.55) [32]. In addition, obesity has been claimed to play a role in influencing the histopathological and clinical aggressiveness of DTCs [17,18].

Different pathogenetic mechanisms have been proposed to define the association between obesity and the onset of DTC. An important role in thyroid carcinogenesis could be played by TSH, the levels of which are slightly increased in patients with obesity [33–35]. In this context, while some studies reported an association between higher TSH values and a greater risk of malignancy of thyroid nodules, as well as the aggressiveness of DTC [36,37], others failed to document significant differences in TSH values among DTC patients depending on the presence of obesity, thus downscaling the contribution of circulating TSH on susceptibility to thyroid malignancy in people with obesity [38,39]. Even the excess of adipose tissue seems to promote cancer cell growth and metastasis through a condition of insulin resistance and altered secretion of IGF-1, which have a direct stimulating action on thyrocyte growth [40]. In this setting, the production of adipocytokines by adipose tissue could also be involved in the relationship between obesity and thyroid cancer; moreover, in particular, increased leptin secretion seems to be associated with a poor prognosis and greater tumor aggressiveness [41,42]. On the other hand, adiponectin, which has an insulin-sensitizing and anti-inflammatory action, is reduced in obese subjects and is inversely correlated with BMI [15,43].

On this basis, several studies have evaluated the relationship between obesity and the aggressiveness of thyroid cancer, with controversial results. While some authors found no association between BMI and the histopathological characteristics of thyroid cancer [23,24], others identified a relationship between BMI and some aggressive features of DTC, including tumor size > 1 cm and extrathyroidal extension [19,44].

A recent study by Matrone et al. evaluated 1058 patients with DTC enrolled at the time of first RAI treatment and subgrouped them according to BMI categories (underweight, normal weight, overweight, and obesity) [24]. The authors did not find associations between the clinical-histopathological characteristic of DTC and BMI. However, this study has some limitations, which include the lack of information on risk factors for DTC (e.g., radiation exposure and history of chronic autoimmune thyroiditis) and a family history of thyroid neoplasms. A further limitation is that the authors collected the BMI values at the first RAI treatment, which is commonly performed 3 to 6 months after surgery, a period during which the BMI could be affected by inadequate thyroid compensation.

In the present study, we collected anthropometric and clinical features at the time of DTC diagnosis, in the context of euthyroidism or adequate thyroid compensation, thus avoiding any temporary changes in BMI values. Moreover, we considered potential confounders including family history and the presence of specific risk factors for DTC. No significant associations were observed between BMI and histopathological characteristics of tumor aggressiveness, such as histological type, size, bilaterality, multifocality, extrathyroidal extension, vascular invasion, and the presence of lymph node metastases at diagnosis, after controlling for sex, age at diagnosis, and risk factors for DTC. As opposed to our findings, Kim et al. observed that higher BMI values are associated with PTC size > 1 cm, the presence of extrathyroidal extension, and advanced TNM stage [19]. These results could be explained by the fact that the Asian population, compared to the Caucasian population, has a lower incidence of obesity. In fact, only 4.6% of patients included in the study of Kim et al. were obese, compared to 17.5% in our study and 19.9% in the study by Matrone et al.

A direct association between BMI and extrathyroidal extension was also observed in other studies [19,44], but these included heterogeneous cohorts and a clear prevalence of a single ATA risk class of DTC.

As regards RAI treatment, we did not find any differences in terms of dose of ^{131}I administered, stimulated Tg levels, positivity of TgAb, and WBS results among the three subgroups of BMI tertiles. These results, again, seem to suggest that BMI per se cannot be considered as a marker of DTC aggressiveness.

Finally, we investigated the association between BMI and tumor recurrence in the short-, medium-, and long-term follow-up. In addition, in this case, BMI was not associated with high DTC aggressiveness in terms of biochemical and/or instrumental tumor recurrence. This has been previously reported in other studies [24,45]. In our population, the main predictors for short-term DTC recurrence were extrathyroidal extension, tumoral infiltration of surgical margins, the presence of lymph node metastases at diagnosis, and high stimulated Tg levels in the context of RAI, while medium- and long-term DTC recurrence were independently predicted by one-year tumor relapse.

Our study has several limitations that should be pointed out, as follows: first, the lack of information about the BMI changes that occurred after DTC diagnosis; second, the single-center nature of the study with a limited sample size, especially with regard to follow-up data; and third, the absence of indicators of body composition and fat distribution.

In conclusion, BMI does not represent a predictor of clinical and histopathological aggressiveness of DTC. Since BMI remains an arguable (surrogate) marker of adiposity, it cannot be considered alone in evaluating the potential association between obesity and DTC prognosis. Body composition parameters assessed via bioimpedance or total body DEXA could add key information for evaluating the role of obesity in thyroid cancer aggressiveness.

Author Contributions: Conceptualization, C.M. and L.D.M.; methodology, C.M. and P.M.; formal analysis, C.M. and L.D.M.; investigation, C.M., L.D.M., G.M., M.Z., M.G.M. and P.A.V.; data curation, L.D.M., G.M. and M.Z.; writing—original draft preparation, C.M., L.D.M. and G.M.; writing—review and editing, G.A. and P.M.; supervision, P.A.V., G.A. and P.M. All authors have read and agreed to the published version of the manuscript.

Funding: This research received no external funding.

Institutional Review Board Statement: This study was conducted in accordance with the Declaration of Helsinki and approved by the Institutional Ethics Committee of AOU Maggiore della Carità di Novara (protocol code 804/CE).

Informed Consent Statement: Informed consent was obtained from all subjects involved in this study.

Data Availability Statement: The data presented in this study are available upon request from the corresponding author due to privacy.

Conflicts of Interest: The authors declare no conflicts of interest.

References

1. Wolin, K.Y.; Carson, K.; Colditz, G.A. Obesity and cancer. *Oncologist* **2010**, *15*, 556–565. [CrossRef]

2. Avgerinos, K.I.; Spyrou, N.; Mantzoros, C.S.; Dalamaga, M. Obesity and cancer risk: Emerging biological mechanisms and perspectives. *Metabolism* **2019**, *92*, 121–135. [CrossRef] [PubMed]
3. Lauby-Secretan, B.; Scoccianti, C.; Loomis, D.; Grosse, Y.; Bianchini, F.; Straif, K.; International Agency for Research on Cancer Handbook Working Group. Body Fatness and Cancer—Viewpoint of the IARC Working Group. *N. Engl. J. Med.* **2016**, *375*, 794–798. [CrossRef] [PubMed]
4. Chooi, Y.C.; Ding, C.; Magkos, F. The epidemiology of obesity. *Metabolism* **2019**, *92*, 6–10. [CrossRef] [PubMed]
5. Seib, C.D.; Sosa, J.A. Evolving Understanding of the Epidemiology of Thyroid Cancer. *Endocrinol. Metab. Clin. N. Am.* **2019**, *48*, 23–35. [CrossRef] [PubMed]
6. Kitahara, C.M.; Sosa, J.A. The changing incidence of thyroid cancer. *Nat. Rev. Endocrinol.* **2016**, *12*, 646–653. [CrossRef]
7. Roman, B.R.; Morris, L.G.; Davies, L. The thyroid cancer epidemic, 2017 perspective. *Curr. Opin. Endocrinol. Diabetes Obes.* **2017**, *24*, 332–336. [CrossRef] [PubMed]
8. Fiorentino, V.; Dell'Aquila, M.; Musarra, T.; Martini, M.; Capodimonti, S.; Fadda, G.; Curatolo, M.; Traini, E.; Raffaelli, M.; Lombardi, C.P.; et al. The Role of Cytology in the Diagnosis of Subcentimeter Thyroid Lesions. *Diagnostics* **2021**, *11*, 1043. [CrossRef]
9. Pazaitou-Panayiotou, K.; Iliadou, P.K.; Chrisoulidou, A.; Mitsakis, P.; Doumala, E.; Fotareli, A.; Boudina, M.; Mathiopoulou, L.; Patakiouta, F.; Tziomalos, K. The increase in thyroid cancer incidence is not only due to papillary microcarcinomas: A 40-year study in 1778 patients. *Exp. Clin. Endocrinol. Diabetes* **2013**, *121*, 397–401.
10. Pagano, L.; Mele, C.; Arpaia, D.; Samà, M.T.; Caputo, M.; Ippolito, S.; Peirce, C.; Prodam, F.; Valente, G.; Ciancia, G.; et al. How do etiological factors can explain the different clinical features of patients with differentiated thyroid cancer and their histopathological findings? *Endocrine* **2017**, *56*, 129–137. [CrossRef]
11. Barrea, L.; Gallo, M.; Ruggeri, R.M.; Giacinto, P.D.; Sesti, F.; Prinzi, N.; Adinolfi, V.; Barucca, V.; Renzelli, V.; Muscogiuri, G.; et al. Nutritional status and follicular-derived thyroid cancer: An update. *Crit. Rev. Food Sci. Nutr.* **2021**, *61*, 25–59. [CrossRef] [PubMed]
12. Schmid, D.; Ricci, C.; Behrens, G.; Leitzmann, M.F. Adiposity and risk of thyroid cancer: A systematic review and meta-analysis. *Obes. Rev.* **2015**, *16*, 1042–1054. [CrossRef] [PubMed]
13. Kitahara, C.M.; McCullough, M.L.; Franceschi, S.; Rinaldi, S.; Wolk, A.; Neta, G.; Olov Adami, H.; Anderson, K.; Andreotti, G.; Beane Freeman, L.E.; et al. Anthropometric Factors and Thyroid Cancer Risk by Histological Subtype: Pooled Analysis of 22 Prospective Studies. *Thyroid* **2016**, *26*, 306–318. [CrossRef]
14. Santini, F.; Marzullo, P.; Rotondi, M.; Ceccarini, G.; Pagano, L.; Ippolito, S.; Chiovato, L.; Biondi, B. Mechanisms in endocrinology: The crosstalk between thyroid gland and adipose tissue: Signal integration in health and disease. *Eur. J. Endocrinol.* **2014**, *171*, R137–R152. [CrossRef] [PubMed]
15. Mele, C.; Samà, M.T.; Bisoffi, A.A.; Caputo, M.; Bullara, V.; Mai, S.; Walker, G.E.; Prodam, F.; Marzullo, P.; Aimaretti, G.; et al. Circulating adipokines and metabolic setting in differentiated thyroid cancer. *Endocr. Connect.* **2019**, *8*, 997–1006. [CrossRef] [PubMed]
16. Mele, C.; Caputo, M.; Samà, M.T.; Bullara, V.; Mauri, M.G.; Prodam, F.; Aimaretti, G.; Pagano, L.; Marzullo, P. The role of metabolic setting in predicting the risk of early tumour relapse of differentiated thyroid cancer (DTC). *Eur. J. Clin. Nutr.* **2020**, *74*, 1038–1046. [CrossRef]
17. Dieringer, P.; Klass, E.M.; Caine, B.; Smith-Gagen, J. Associations between body mass and papillary thyroid cancer stage and tumor size: A population-based study. *J. Cancer Res. Clin. Oncol.* **2015**, *141*, 93–98. [CrossRef]
18. Kim, S.H.; Park, H.S.; Kim, K.H.; Yoo, H.; Chae, B.J.; Bae, J.S.; Jung, S.S.; Song, B.J. Correlation between obesity and clinicopathological factors in patients with papillary thyroid cancer. *Surg. Today* **2015**, *45*, 723–729. [CrossRef]
19. Kim, H.J.; Kim, N.K.; Choi, J.H.; Sohn, S.Y.; Kim, S.W.; Jin, S.M.; Jang, H.W.; Suh, S.; Min, Y.K.; Chung, J.H.; et al. Associations between body mass index and clinico-pathological characteristics of papillary thyroid cancer. *Clin. Endocrinol.* **2013**, *78*, 134–140. [CrossRef]
20. Harari, A.; Endo, B.; Nishimoto, S.; Ituarte, P.H.; Yeh, M.W. Risk of advanced papillary thyroid cancer in obese patients. *Arch. Surg.* **2012**, *147*, 805–811. [CrossRef]
21. Paes, J.E.; Hua, K.; Nagy, R.; Kloos, R.T.; Jarjoura, D.; Ringel, M.D. The relationship between body mass index and thyroid cancer pathology features and outcomes: A clinicopathological cohort study. *J. Clin. Endocrinol. Metab.* **2010**, *95*, 4244–4250. [CrossRef] [PubMed]
22. Kwon, H.; Kim, M.; Choi, Y.M.; Jang, E.K.; Jeon, M.J.; Kim, W.G.; Kim, T.Y.; Shong, Y.K.; Song, D.E.; Baek, J.H.; et al. Lack of Associations between Body Mass Index and Clinical Outcomes in Patients with Papillary Thyroid Carcinoma. *Endocrinol. Metab.* **2015**, *30*, 305–311. [CrossRef]
23. Grani, G.; Lamartina, L.; Montesano, T.; Ronga, G.; Maggisano, V.; Falcone, R.; Ramundo, V.; Giacomelli, L.; Durante, C.; Russo, D.; et al. Lack of association between obesity and aggressiveness of differentiated thyroid cancer. *J. Endocrinol. Investig.* **2019**, *42*, 85–90. [CrossRef]
24. Matrone, A.; Ceccarini, G.; Beghini, M.; Ferrari, F.; Gambale, C.; D'Aqui, M.; Piaggi, P.; Torregrossa, L.; Molinaro, E.; Basolo, F.; et al. Potential Impact of BMI on the Aggressiveness of Presentation and Clinical Outcome of Differentiated Thyroid Cancer. *J. Clin. Endocrinol. Metab.* **2020**, *105*, dgz312. [CrossRef]
25. Trésallet, C.; Seman, M.; Tissier, F.; Buffet, C.; Lupinacci, R.M.; Vuarnesson, H.; Leenhardt, L.; Menegaux, F. The incidence of papillary thyroid carcinoma and outcomes in operative patients according to their body mass indices. *Surgery* **2014**, *156*, 1145–1152. [CrossRef] [PubMed]

26. Tuttle, M.; Morris, L.F.; Haugen, B.; Shah, J.; Sosa, J.A.; Rohren, E.; Subramaniam, R.M.; Hunt, J.L.; Perrier, N.D. Thyroid differentiated and anaplastic carcinoma. In *AJCC Cancer Staging Manual*, 8th ed.; Springer International Publishing: New York, NY, USA, 2017; Chapter 73.
27. Haugen, B.R.; Alexander, E.K.; Bible, K.C.; Doherty, G.M.; Mandel, S.J.; Nikiforov, Y.E.; Pacini, F.; Randolph, G.W.; Sawka, A.M.; Schlumberger, M.; et al. 2015 American Thyroid Association Management Guidelines for Adult Patients with Thyroid Nodules and Differentiated Thyroid Cancer: The American Thyroid Association Guidelines Task Force on Thyroid Nodules and Differentiated Thyroid Cancer. *Thyroid* **2016**, *26*, 1–133. [CrossRef]
28. Pacini, F.; Basolo, F.; Bellantone, R.; Boni, G.; Cannizzaro, M.A.; De Palma, M.; Durante, C.; Elisei, R.; Fadda, G.; Frasoldati, A.; et al. Italian consensus on diagnosis and treatment of differentiated thyroid cancer: Joint statements of six Italian societies. *J. Endocrinol. Investig.* **2018**, *41*, 849–876. [CrossRef] [PubMed]
29. Matrone, A.; Latrofa, F.; Torregrossa, L.; Piaggi, P.; Gambale, C.; Faranda, A.; Ricci, D.; Agate, L.; Molinaro, E.; Basolo, F.; et al. Changing Trend of Thyroglobulin Antibodies in Patients with Differentiated Thyroid Cancer Treated with Total Thyroidectomy without 131I Ablation. *Thyroid* **2018**, *28*, 871–879. [CrossRef]
30. Pizzimenti, C.; Fiorentino, V.; Ieni, A.; Rossi, E.D.; Germanà, E.; Giovanella, L.; Lentini, M.; Alessi, Y.; Tuccari, G.; Campennì, A.; et al. BRAF-AXL-PD-L1 Signaling Axis as a Possible Biological Marker for RAI Treatment in the Thyroid Cancer ATA Intermediate Risk Category. *Int. J. Mol. Sci.* **2023**, *24*, 10024. [CrossRef]
31. Rossi, M.; Mele, C.; Rossetto Giaccherino, R.; Meomartino, L.; Brero, D.; Marsan, G.; Aimaretti, G.; Ghigo, E.; Pagano, L. Post-Surgical Indications to Radioiodine Treatment and Potential Risk Factors for Post-Treatment Recurrence in Patients with Intermediate-Risk Differentiated Thyroid Carcinoma. *J. Pers. Med.* **2023**, *13*, 775. [CrossRef]
32. Youssef, M.R.; Reisner, A.S.C.; Attia, A.S.; Hussein, M.H.; Omar, M.; LaRussa, A.; Galvani, C.A.; Aboueisha, M.; Abdelgawad, M.; Toraih, E.A.; et al. Obesity and the prevention of thyroid cancer: Impact of body mass index and weight change on developing thyroid cancer—Pooled results of 24 million cohorts. *Oral. Oncol.* **2021**, *112*, 105085. [CrossRef] [PubMed]
33. Knudsen, N.; Laurberg, P.; Rasmussen, L.B.; Bülow, I.; Perrild, H.; Ovesen, L.; Jørgensen, T. Small differences in thyroid function may be important for body mass index and the occurrence of obesity in the population. *J. Clin. Endocrinol. Metab.* **2005**, *90*, 4019–4024. [CrossRef] [PubMed]
34. Bétry, C.; Challan-Belval, M.A.; Bernard, A.; Charrié, A.; Drai, J.; Laville, M.; Thivolet, C.; Disse, E. Increased TSH in obesity: Evidence for a BMI-independent association with leptin. *Diabetes Metab.* **2015**, *41*, 248–251. [CrossRef] [PubMed]
35. Mele, C.; Mai, S.; Cena, T.; Pagano, L.; Scacchi, M.; Biondi, B.; Aimaretti, G.; Marzullo, P. The pattern of TSH and fT4 levels across different BMI ranges in a large cohort of euthyroid patients with obesity. *Front. Endocrinol.* **2022**, *13*, 1029376. [CrossRef] [PubMed]
36. Fiore, E.; Vitti, P. Serum TSH and risk of papillary thyroid cancer in nodular thyroid disease. *J. Clin. Endocrinol. Metab.* **2012**, *97*, 1134–1145. [CrossRef]
37. McLeod, D.S.; Cooper, D.S.; Ladenson, P.W.; Ain, K.B.; Brierley, J.D.; Fein, H.G.; Haugen, B.R.; Jonklaas, J.; Magner, J.; Ross, D.S.; et al. Prognosis of differentiated thyroid cancer in relation to serum thyrotropin and thyroglobulin antibody status at time of diagnosis. *Thyroid* **2014**, *24*, 35–42. [CrossRef]
38. Han, J.M.; Kim, T.Y.; Jeon, M.J.; Yim, J.H.; Kim, W.G.; Song, D.E.; Hong, S.J.; Bae, S.J.; Kim, H.K.; Shin, M.H.; et al. Obesity is a risk factor for thyroid cancer in a large, ultrasonographically screened population. *Eur. J. Endocrinol.* **2013**, *168*, 879–886. [CrossRef]
39. Fussey, J.M.; Beaumont, R.N.; Wood, A.R.; Vaidya, B.; Smith, J.; Tyrrell, J. Does Obesity Cause Thyroid Cancer? A Mendelian Randomization Study. *J. Clin. Endocrinol. Metab.* **2020**, *105*, e2398–e2407. [CrossRef]
40. Rezzónico, J.N.; Rezzónico, M.; Pusiol, E.; Pitoia, F.; Niepomniszcze, H. Increased prevalence of insulin resistance in patients with differentiated thyroid carcinoma. *Metab. Syndr. Relat. Disord.* **2009**, *7*, 375–380. [CrossRef]
41. Celano, M.; Maggisano, V.; Lepore, S.M.; Sponziello, M.; Pecce, V.; Verrienti, A.; Durante, C.; Maranghi, M.; Lucia, P.; Bulotta, S.; et al. Expression of Leptin Receptor and Effects of Leptin on Papillary Thyroid Carcinoma Cells. *Int. J. Endocrinol.* **2019**, *2019*, 5031696. [CrossRef]
42. Zhang, G.A.; Hou, S.; Han, S.; Zhou, J.; Wang, X.; Cui, W. Clinicopathological implications of leptin and leptin receptor expression in papillary thyroid cancer. *Oncol. Lett.* **2013**, *5*, 797–800. [CrossRef] [PubMed]
43. Mitsiades, N.; Pazaitou-Panayiotou, K.; Aronis, K.N.; Moon, H.S.; Chamberland, J.P.; Liu, X.; Diakopoulos, K.N.; Kyttaris, V.; Panagiotou, V.; Mylvaganam, G.; et al. Circulating adiponectin is inversely associated with risk of thyroid cancer: In vivo and in vitro studies. *J. Clin. Endocrinol. Metab.* **2011**, *96*, E2023–E2028. [CrossRef] [PubMed]
44. Choi, J.S.; Kim, E.K.; Moon, H.J.; Kwak, J.Y. Higher body mass index may be a predictor of extrathyroidal extension in patients with papillary thyroid microcarcinoma. *Endocrine* **2015**, *48*, 264–271. [CrossRef] [PubMed]
45. Gąsior-Perczak, D.; Pałyga, I.; Szymonek, M.; Kowalik, A.; Walczyk, A.; Kopczyński, J.; Lizis-Kolus, K.; Trybek, T.; Mikina, E.; Szyska-Skrobot, D.; et al. The impact of BMI on clinical progress, response to treatment, and disease course in patients with differentiated thyroid cancer. *PLoS ONE* **2018**, *13*, e0204668. [CrossRef]

biomedicines

MDPI

Review

Recent Trends and Potential of Radiotherapy in the Treatment of Anaplastic Thyroid Cancer

Kazumasa Sekihara [1,2], Hidetomo Himuro [3,4], Soji Toda [1,5], Nao Saito [1,2], Ryoichi Hirayama [6], Nobuyasu Suganuma [7], Tetsuro Sasada [3] and Daisuke Hoshino [1,2,*]

1 Cancer Biology Division, Kanagawa Cancer Center Research Institute, Yokohama 2418515, Japan; sekihara.6e20l@kanagawa-pho.jp (K.S.); toda.soj.im@yokohama-cu.ac.jp (S.T.); saito.6d10l@kanagawa-pho.jp (N.S.)
2 Biospecimen Center, Kanagawa Cancer Center, Yokohama 2418515, Japan
3 Division of Cancer Immunotherapy, Kanagawa Cancer Center Research Institute, Yokohama 2418515, Japan; himuro.4l00j@kanagawa-pho.jp (H.H.); sasada.0980e@kanagawa-pho.jp (T.S.)
4 Department of Radiation Oncology, Kanagawa Cancer Center, Yokohama 2418515, Japan
5 Department of Breast and Thyroid Surgery, Yokohama City University Medical Center, Yokohama 2320024, Japan
6 Department of Charged Particle Therapy Research, QST Hospital, National Institutes for Quantum Science and Technology, Chiba 2638555, Japan; hirayama.ryoichi@qst.go.jp
7 Department of Surgery, Yokohama City University, Yokohama 2360004, Japan; suganuma@yokohama-cu.ac.jp
* Correspondence: hoshino.2390e@kanagawa-pho.jp

Abstract: Anaplastic thyroid cancer (ATC) is a rare but highly aggressive malignancy characterized by advanced disease at diagnosis and a poor prognosis. Despite multimodal therapeutic approaches that include surgery, radiotherapy, and chemotherapy, an optimal treatment strategy remains elusive. Current developments in targeted therapies and immunotherapy offer promising avenues for improved outcomes, particularly for *BRAF*-mutant patients. However, challenges remain regarding overcoming drug resistance and developing effective treatments for *BRAF*-wild-type tumors. This comprehensive review examines the clinical and biological features of ATC, outlines the current standards of care, and discusses recent developments with a focus on the evolving role of radiotherapy. Moreover, it emphasizes the necessity of a multidisciplinary approach and highlights the urgent need for further research to better understand ATC pathogenesis and identify new therapeutic targets. Collaborative efforts, including large-scale clinical trials, are essential for translating these findings into improved patient outcomes.

Keywords: anaplastic thyroid cancer (ATC); BRAF; MAPK signaling; PAM signaling; multimodality therapy; radiotherapy; molecular targeted therapy; immune checkpoint inhibitor

1. Introduction

Although anaplastic thyroid cancer (ATC) occurs rarely [1–4], it exhibits an extremely poor prognosis [5–7] and is characterized by the presence of unresectable local extension or distant metastasis at initial diagnosis [8,9]. A radical cure for this malignancy is extremely difficult. To maintain and prolong quality of life (QOL), a multidisciplinary approach combining surgery, radiotherapy, and chemotherapy is currently used, but this approach yields poor results. Recently, clinical trials with kinase inhibitors have been conducted in cases in which specific genetic mutations, such as *BRAF* V600E, have been identified, with the hope of improving the prognosis of ATC. One example of a successful study was the combination of the BRAF inhibitor dabrafenib and the MEK inhibitor trametinib in ATC patients harboring the *BRAF* V600E mutation [10]. Certain reports have suggested the possible beneficial role of immune checkpoint inhibitors [7–9]. However, molecular targeted agents can lead to the emergence of drug resistance during administration, and this is a significant factor that complicates cancer treatment. Additionally, patients who do not possess the target gene mutation are not eligible for these agents. Immunotherapy can cause serious side effects, such as interstitial pneumonia, due to an excessive immune response when T cells in the body are activated.

Here, we summarize the clinical and biological features of ATC and the current standard of care and its problems, and we discuss future prospects for the management of ATC. Several useful review articles exist regarding ATC management [11–15], with emphasis on molecular targeted agents. We would like to distinguish our review from these other manuscripts by highlighting the potential for ATC management in the context of radiotherapy based on the remarkable technological development that has occurred in recent years.

2. The Characteristics of ATC

2.1. Epidemiology and Clinical Presentation

Most thyroid cancers are differentiated thyroid cancers (DTC) originating from follicular cells, such as papillary thyroid cancer (PTC) and follicular thyroid cancer (FTC), generally exhibit a good prognosis [16]. In contrast, ATCs are extremely aggressive and exhibit a poor prognosis. They are considered to be one of the most malignant of all cancer types [17,18] and account for 10–35% of thyroid cancer deaths, despite their low incidence (approximately 1–2% of all thyroid cancers) [2,4,19]. The majority of patients with this disease are older than 60 years of age, and the sex ratio is the lowest compared to other types of thyroid cancer that are more common in women. Patients present with rapidly growing cervical mass and neck pain that develops within weeks, skin erythema, hoarseness, dysphagia, dyspnea, rapid swelling of the cervical lymph nodes, fever, fatigue, and weight loss. Invasion of the gastrointestinal tract is frequently observed. Patients may occasionally develop urgent airway narrowing, such as invasion or compression of the trachea, requires airway clearance to prevent death due to asphyxia. According to the eighth edition of the American Joint Committee on Cancer (AJCC)/Tumor-Node-Metastasis (TMN) cancer staging system [20], the disease is always in an advanced stage (stage IV) and is divided into IVA (localized stage) when the cancer is only within the thyroid gland, IVB (locally advanced stage) when there is gross extra-thyroidal extension or cervical lymph node metastasis, and IVC (metastatic stage) when there is distant metastasis [7,21] (Table 1).

Table 1. Staging and TMN classification of ATC according to the AJCC eighth edition.

Stage	T Category		N Category		M Category	
IVA	T1:	Tumor ≤ 2 cm in greatest dimension limited to the thyroid	N0:	No metastasis to regional nodes	M0:	No distant metastasis
	T2:	Tumor > 2 cm but ≤4 cm in greatest dimension limited to the thyroid				
	T3a:	Tumor > 4 cm limited to the thyroid				
IVB	T1 T2 T3a		N1:	Metastasis to regional nodes	M0	
	T3b:	Gross extrathyroidal extension invading only strap muscles (sternohyoid, sternothyroid, thyrohyoid, or omohyoid muscles) from a tumor of any size	N0–N1		M0	
	T4a:	Gross extrathyroidal extension invading subcutaneous soft tissues, larynx, trachea, esophagus, or recurrent laryngeal nerve from a tumor of any size				

Table 1. *Cont.*

Stage		T Category	N Category		M Category
	T4b:	Gross extrathyroidal extension invading prevertebral fascia or encasing a carotid artery or mediastinal vessels from a tumor of any size			
IVC	T1–T4		N0–N1	M1:	Distant metastasis

Onoda et al. [22] evaluated overall survival (OS) using this system in the national database of the Thyroid Cancer Research Consortium for Japan (ATCCJ) [23], which consisted of 757 patients with ATC. The percentages and median OS for each stage included stage IVA (5.9%, 15.8 months), stage IVB (55.7%, 6.1 months), and stage IVC (38.3%, 2.8 months). Consequently, approximately 90% of patients with ATC exhibited disease progression to surrounding organs or distant metastases at initial diagnosis, and treatment may not have been initiated due to extremely rapid disease progression. Moreover, it is common for patients with ATC to die early after diagnosis if no effective treatment is available. Older patients may not tolerate aggressive radiotherapy or chemotherapy due to impaired immune and/or organ function or complications. Thus, age is a significant prognostic factor for ATC [24]. Additionally, leukocytosis (white blood cell count >10,000/mL), extrathyroidal extension, and distant metastases have been reported as prognostic factors [23,25].

2.2. Genomic Changes

Recently, several analytical studies using next-generation sequencing have been conducted to investigate the genetic alterations in ATC [6,26–33]. According to their findings, the most commonly identified mutations in ATC were *TP53* and *telomerase reverse transcriptase (TERT)* promoter mutations. Although these mutations are observed in DTC and poorly differentiated DTC (PDTC), they are more frequent in ATC than they are in others [6,30]. *TP53* is a well-known tumor suppressor gene involved in a variety of cellular functions, including cell survival, DNA repair, apoptosis, cell cycle checkpoints, and senescence. *TP53* mutations promote cell proliferation and tumor progression through the loss of these functions [34]. This was strongly correlated with the malignant potential of ATC. Landa et al. [30] reported that *TP53* mutations were observed in 8% of PDTC; however, it increased to 73% in ATC. The analyses by Pozdeyev et al. [28] and Xu et al. [6] revealed high frequencies of *TP53* mutations (65% and 63%, respectively). *TERT* promoter mutations (C228T and C250T) are common in ATC. *TERT* is the catalytic subunit of telomerase and is essential for telomerase activity [35]. *TERT* is not expressed in most human somatic cells; however, its expression and transcription are upregulated in many cancers through various mechanisms, including mutations in the core promoter region of the *TERT* gene. Moreover, it elongates telomeres, confers unlimited proliferative capacity to tumor cells, and contributes to tumor progression and aggressiveness [36,37]. Recently, it has been reported that *TERT* interacts with various signaling molecules such as NF-κ B, c-MYC, β-catenin, and TCF-4 to increase cancer malignancy and promote cancer progression [38–41]. Landa et al. reported that *TERT* promoter mutations were observed at a high frequency of 73% in ATCs, compared to 9% in PTCs and 40% in PDTCs [30]. Xu et al. observed this mutation at a high frequency (75%) in ATCs [6].

Two major cascades are responsible for tumorigenesis in ATCs, including the mitogen-activated protein kinase (MAPK) signaling pathway (RAS-RAF-MEK-ERK) and the PI3K-Akt-mTOR (PAM) signaling pathway. As described in Figure 1, both pathways are involved in cell proliferation and survival and essentially start with receptor tyrosine kinase (RTK), which is activated by the binding of ligands such as growth factors such as fibroblast growth factor (FGF) or epidermal growth factor (EGF) to specific receptors. When one of these molecules is continuously activated by a genetic mutation, it consistently activates downstream molecules without signals from the upstream molecules.

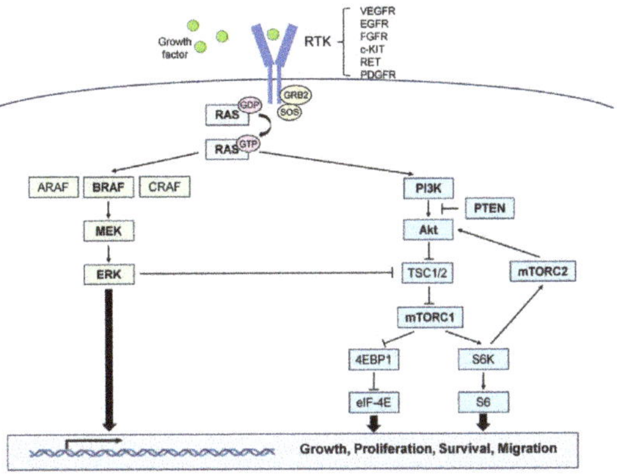

Figure 1. Schematic illustration of the MAPK signaling and PAM signaling pathways in the ATC. Sharp arrows (→) and blunt arrows (⊣) indicate promotion and inhibition, respectively.

The MAPK signaling pathway is involved in various cellular processes such as growth, proliferation, survival (avoidance of apoptosis [42] and induction of autophagy [43]), migration [44], and angiogenesis. The intracellular signaling of the MAPK pathway has been described in detail by Schubert et al. [45] and Cook et al. [46]. Common alterations in the MAPK pathway in ATC include mutations in *BRAF* and *RAS*. *BRAF* mutations are the primary therapeutic targets for this disease. The majority of *BRAF* mutations in ATC are *BRAF V600E* point mutations [29] that play an essential role in the development and progression of tumors [47,48]. This mutation activates BRAF kinase, which phosphorylates multiple targets, including MEK and ERK [49]. The *BRAF V600E* mutation is observed in approximately 20–40% of ATCs [50], and Jannin et al. [12]. reported that the frequency of *BRAF* mutations in ATCs appears to vary in each region. According to recent reports, *BRAF* mutations have been observed in 40–45% of ATC cases in the United States [6,30], 14–37% of cases in Europe [31,33], and 41–48% of cases in East Asia (Japan and Korea) [26,51]. Although the details are unclear, they suggest an association between ethnicity and iodine intake. *BRAF* mutations, the most common mutations originally observed in PTCs, strongly activate the MAPK pathway, ultimately leading to thyroid cell dedifferentiation [52]. Oishi et al. summarized the mutation profiles of PTCs and ATCs and observed that *BRAF* status and *BRAF* genotype matched between PTCs and ATCs in 18 of 21 cases [53]. Yoo et al. [26] and Xu et al. [6] reported similar results. Genomic associations have been demonstrated between PTCs and ATCs, thus suggesting that ATCs are derived from PTCs. *RAS* genes such as *HRAS*, *KRAS*, and *NRAS* have been described. *RAS* mutations are observed at a frequency of 10–50% in ATC, according to next generation sequencer (NGS) analysis data [27,28,54]. Among them, *NRAS* mutations are significantly more common in thyroid cancer [55]. Oishi et al. [53] reported *HRAS* and *KRAS* mutations at 5%, while *NRAS* mutations were detected at 18%. Lai et al. [56] confirmed a high frequency of *NRAS* (30%) compared to that of *HRAS* (0%) and *KRAS* (11%). *RAS* mutations promote the activation of the MAPK and PAM signaling pathways. *KRAS* mutants are major activators of the MAPK pathway, whereas *NRAS* mutants are activators of the PAM pathway [57]. These mutations were frequently detected in FTC [26], thus suggesting that a few ATC may have originated from FTC. Furthermore, certain studies have demonstrated that *eukaryotic translation initiation factor 1A X-linked (EIF1AX)* mutations often occur together with *RAS* mutations in ATCs and that a positive correlation between RAS and EIF1AX proteins results in increased expression of the oncogene *c-MYC* [30,58,59].

The PAM signaling pathway regulates various cellular processes, including metabolism, motility, proliferation, growth, and survival [60]. Intracellular signaling in the PAM pathway has been described in detail by Glaviano et al. [61] and Yang et al. [62]. Hyperactivation of the PAM pathway is observed in many cancers and contributes to accelerated cancer initiation and progression and the development of therapeutic resistance [63,64]. PAM promotes epithelial-mesenchymal transition (EMT) and metastasis [65,66]. Mutations in *PIK3CA*, *PTEN*, and *AKT1* have been identified in the PAM pathway of ATC. *PIK3CA*, which encodes the p110α catalytic subunit, is frequently mutated in various cancers and is known to be associated with cell signaling, proliferation, invasion, and cancer development [67–69]. *PIK3CA* mutations were detected in less than 20% of ATC [29,31]; however, they were more frequent than they were in DTC or PDTC [28,30]. *PTEN* is a representative tumor suppressor gene similar to *TP53* and is frequently mutated in various cancers. PTEN plays a critical role in regulating cell growth, proliferation, survival, migration, and invasion [70]. *PTEN* mutations have been demonstrated to activate the PAM pathway with a loss of function [71,72]. Additionally, loss of PTEN function in combination with alterations in *TP53* has been reported to accelerate tumor progression [73]. *PTEN* mutations in ATCs were less than 20%. Their frequency was higher than that of PTCs and PDTCs and similar to that of FTCs [28,30]. AKT1 regulates key processes such as glucose metabolism, apoptosis, cell proliferation, transcription, and cell migration. However, the *AKT1* gene mutation is rarer than that of *PI3KCA* and *PTEN* in ATC and accounts for less than 10% of mutations in most reports [28,31]. Although genetic mutations in *AKT* are rare, overactivation has been observed in many cancers, including ATC, resulting in tumorigenesis, growth, invasion, and drug resistance [74].

Other mutations were observed in Wnt-β-catenin pathway-related genes (*CTNNB1*, *AXIN1*, and *APC*) [75] and epigenetic-related genes such as SWI/SNF chromatin remodeling complex (*ARID1A*, *SMARCB1*, and *PBRM1*) and histone methyltransferases (*KMT2A*, *KMT2C*, *KMT2D*, and *SETD2*). Moreover, mutations in the *cyclin-dependent kinase inhibitor 2A (CDKN2A)* gene that encodes p16 have been observed in a few ATC cases [28,29]. Furthermore, anaplastic lymphoma kinase (ALK) mutations and fusions that activate both MAPK and PAM pathways have been detected at low rates [28,29]. Similarly, receptor tyrosine kinase (RET) fusions have been observed [76].

Although the details are discussed in Section 3.4, "Targeted Therapy," many drugs specific to these targets are currently under development and in clinical trials. Among these, combination therapy with a BRAF inhibitor and MEK inhibition has exhibited favorable antitumor effects in patients with ATC and the BRAF V600E mutation [10].

3. Treatment of ATC

ATC is difficult to treat as it is aggressive, spreads rapidly within the neck, and possesses the potential to metastasize to distant body sites. After considering the available therapies, comorbidities, and patient wishes, physicians decide whether to provide aggressive treatment or palliative care based on staging and prognosis. In general, radical treatment is difficult to achieve, and multidisciplinary treatment combining surgery, radiotherapy, and chemotherapy is used to prolong life and maintain QOL, except for a few cases (Figure 2). In retrospective studies, patients who received this multimodal therapy exhibited better prognoses than those who did not [17,23,77–79]. Radioactive iodine (RAI) therapy and thyroid-stimulating hormone (TSH) suppression that are commonly used to treat DTC are not effective for ATC [7]. In recent years, targeted therapy has been used with a few successes in cases with specific genetic mutations. Additionally, immune checkpoint inhibitors have been used successfully in a few cases.

In this section, we describe each treatment modality's current status and future perspectives, considering the results of representative recent studies (Table 2) and ongoing clinical trials (Table 3) of multimodal treatments.

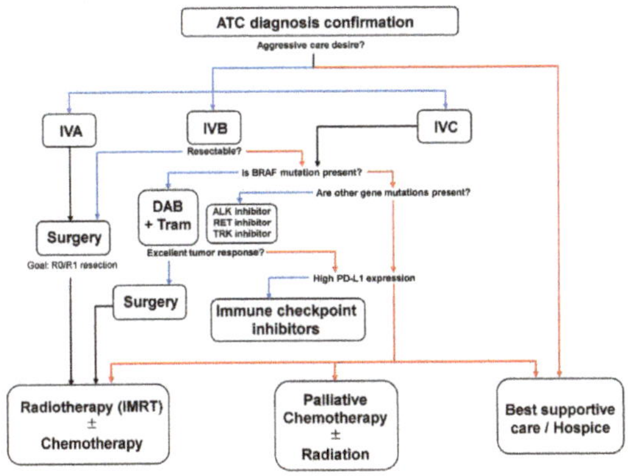

Figure 2. Initial treatment of stages IVA, IVB, and IVC ATC. Taken from [7,12], with a few modifications. For each question, blue arrows indicate "Yes," and red arrows indicate "No." R0: resection for cure or complete remission. R1: complete gross resection; tumor removed grossly but not microscopically.

Table 2. Recent studies with multimodal treatment in ATC.

Treatment	Study	Number of Patients	Number of Patients					Median OS (Months)	ORR (%)	Reference
			Surgery	RT	CTx	MTT	IMM			
RT (66 Gy) + Doxorubicin (10–20 mg/m^2 weekly) or Paclitaxel (80 mg/m^2 weekly)	Retrospective	104 IVA:5 IVB:76 IVC:23	52	101	99	0	0	7	N.D.	Fan et al. (2020) [80]
Doxorubicin + Docetaxel (20 mg/m^2 weekly, each)Carboplatin + Paclitaxel (50 mg/m^2 weekly, each)Doxorubicin only (20 mg/m^2 weekly) Cisplatin only (30 mg/m^2 weekly)	Retrospective	30 IVA:2 IVB:22 IVC:6 ND:5	27	30	30	0	0	21	63	Prasongsook et al. (2017) [81]
Dabrafenib (150 mg twice daily) + Trametinib (2 mg once daily)	Phase 2	36 IV:1 IVC:35	30	30	15	36	4	14.5	56	Subbiah et al. (2022) [10]
Dabrafenib (150 mg twice daily) + Trametinib (2 mg once daily)	Retrospective	16 IVB:4 IVC:12	8	7	9	16	0	9.3	50	Iyer et al. (2018) [82]
Everolimus (10 mg daily)	Phase 2	7 IVC:7	5	4	3	7	0	4.6	14	Hanna et al. (2018) [83]
Lenvatinib (24 mg daily)	Phase 2	17 IV:17	14	9	7	17	0	10.6	24	Takahashi et al.(2019) [84]
Spartalizumab (400 mg every 4 weeks)	Phase 1/2	42 IV:42	28	30	25	4	42	5.9	19	Capdevila et al. (2020) [85]

RT: radiotherapy, CTx: chemotherapy, MTT: molecular targeted therapy, IMM: immunotherapy, OS: overall survival, ORR: overall response rate.

Table 3. Ongoing clinical trials in patients with ATC.

ClinicalTrials.gov Identifier	Intervention/Treatment	Phase	Status
NCT04552769	Abemaciclib	Phase 2	Active, not recruiting
NCT05453799	Vudalimab	Phase 2	Recruiting
NCT04171622	Lenvatinib + Pembrolizumab	Phase 2	Recruiting
NCT03975231	Dabrafenib + Trametinib + IMRT	Phase 1	Recruiting
NCT05119296	Pembrolizumab (Keytruda)	Phase 2	Recruiting
NCT04420754	AIC100 CAR T Cells	Phase 1	Recruiting
NCT03449108	Aldesleukin (IL2) + Autologous Tumor Infiltrating Lymphocytes LN-145 or LN-145-S1	Phase 2	Active, not recruiting
NCT03246958	Nivolumab + Ipilimumab	Phase 2	Active, not recruiting
NCT04675710	Pembrolizumab + Dabrafenib + Trametinib + Surgery + IMRT	Phase 2	Recruiting
NCT03181100	Atezolizumab + Chemotherapy (Cobimetinib, Nab-paclitaxel, Paclitaxel, Vemurafenib)	Phase 2	Active, not recruiting
NCT03085056	Trametinib + Paclitaxel	Early Phase 1	Active, not recruiting
NCT04238624	Dabrafenib + Trametinib	Phase 2	Recruiting

Table 3. *Cont.*

ClinicalTrials.gov Identifier	Intervention/Treatment	Phase	Status
NCT04759911	Selpercatinib + Surgery	Phase 2	Recruiting
NCT06007924	Avutometinib + Defactinib	Phase 2	Recruiting
NCT02041260	Cabozantinib	Phase 2	Unknown
NCT04579757	Surufatinib + Tislelizumab	Phase 1/2	Active, not recruiting
NCT05059470	Pembrolizumab + IMRT	Phase 2	Recruiting

3.1. Surgery

A complete surgical excision followed by adjuvant therapy is the best approach to curing ATC [15]. However, curative resection is currently beneficial in early stage cases (IVA and part of IVB), as it may lead to long-term survival [86], whereas surgery must be carefully approved to maintain QOL in cases where the long-term prognosis is not expected [87]. Specifically, R0/R1 resection can be expected if the tumor does not extend beyond the common carotid artery, whereas tumors that extend beyond the common carotid artery are often inoperable. R0 resection, also known as curative resection, indicates a microscopically margin-negative resection with no residual tumor grossly or microscopically in the primary tumor. R1 resection indicates that all macroscopic lesions are removed, but the microscopic margins are tumor-positive [88,89]. Debulking surgery that minimizes postoperative QOL is considered valuable [90,91]; however, the extent to which it affects prognosis remains unclear. The National Comprehensive Cancer Network recommends total thyroidectomy with therapeutic lymph node dissection (R0/R1) and local radiotherapy if resectable, and tracheostomy with steroids only if more strongly indicated [9,92]; However, as recommended by the American Thyroid Association, it may be practical to perform surgery for local control while taking care not to interfere with other available palliative approaches, including radiation and systemic therapy, and not to compromise QOL [7].

The role of surgery in the treatment of locally advanced and metastatic ATC is currently the subject of considerable debate, with successful cases reported in patients with ATC harboring BRAF V600E mutations who received preoperative dabrafenib plus trametinib and ultimately underwent surgery. Looking to the future, this suggests that the use of surgery may be re-evaluated, even in advanced stages.

3.2. Radiotherapy

Rapid local progression and recurrence of ATC are associated with the aggressive nature of the disease, and local control using surgery or external beam radiotherapy (EBRT) is important. EBRT is a treatment in which X-rays are delivered to the tumor from high-energy radiotherapy equipment located outside of the body. Radiotherapy is recommended, as EBRT is used as a preoperative or postoperative adjuvant therapy and has been demonstrated to improve the median OS in retrospective studies [18,54,93,94]. For example, in a retrospective analysis of 496 patients with ATC, Saeed et al. reported that the survival of 375 patients who received adjuvant EBRT was significantly longer than that of 121 patients who did not receive adjuvant EBRT (12.3 vs. 9.1 months) [95]. The total dose was an important factor in EBRT. Most studies have indicated that OS and local control can be predicted by the total dose [96] that is better managed with irradiation greater than 45 Gy. For example, in a National Cancer Database analysis of 1,288 patients with unresected stage IVB and IVC ATC, Pezzi et al. reported that 1-year OS rates were improved in patients treated with 60–75 Gy compared to those treated with less than 60 Gy (31% vs. 16%) [97]. In a retrospective analysis by Fan et al., delivering 60 Gy or more was significantly associated with a lower risk of local progression and longer OS (10.6 vs. 3.6 months) [80]. Although the conventional irradiation regimen of 2 Gy once daily, as recommended by the American Thyroid Association and National Comprehensive Cancer Network guidelines, has been used as the standard option, hyperfractionated, accelerated, and fractionated irradiation have been studied. Hyperfractionated and accelerated irradiation have been considered to overcome the rapid progression and radioresistance of ATC. While certain reports suggest improved local control [98–100], others conclude that it neither reduces toxicity nor improves outcomes [101,102], ultimately leading to controversy. In contrast, hypofractionated irradiation, which delivers a higher dose in a shorter time, is used to improve quality of life and local control. Several clinical trials have exhibited promising results using hypofractionated RT for the treatment of ATC [103,104]. However, as discussed by Oliinyk et al. [102], limited data are evaluating hypofractionated regimens, and their use in the actual treatment of ATC remains conclusive. Irradiation techniques play an important role. The thyroid gland is located near the spinal cord, and this makes it difficult to avoid the spinal cord and deliver high doses to localized areas of cancer. One technology that makes this possible is intensity-modulated radiation therapy (IMRT). IMRT is a technique that delivers a high dose to the tumor while minimizing the dose to organs at risk (OAR) by varying the intensity of the radiation in the field during treatment, thus allowing precise dose delivery even to tumors with complex shapes. IMRT can precisely deliver radiation to thyroid cancer cells while reducing the radiation dose to the spinal cord [105]. IMRT is recommended as the standard of care for radiation therapy in ATC due to its advantages in reducing local recurrence, toxicity, and treatment complications [7,8]. Recently, volumetric modulated arc therapy has been developed, in which the device is rotated at different speeds and dose rates to modulate intensity, ultimately resulting in shorter treatment times and improved treatment accuracy [106]. Altogether, it is currently accepted that the appropriate treatment is to utilize IMRT to achieve a total dose of 60 Gy or more at 2 Gy per dose. Radiotherapy is often used in combination with chemotherapy, molecular targeted therapy, and immunotherapy to treat ATC. The clinical trials of combination therapies, including radiotherapy, are shown in Table 4.

Table 4. Clinical trials related to radiotherapy in patients with ATC.

ClinicalTrials.gov Identifier	Intervention/Treatment	Phase	Status	Reference
NCT03565536	Sorafenib + Surgery + EBRT	Phase 2	Completed	
NCT05659186	Tislelizumab + Anlotinib + RT	Phase 2	Recruiting	
NCT01236547	IMRT + Paclitaxel + Pazopanib	Phase 2	Completed	Sherman et al. (2023) [107]
NCT03122496	Durvalumab + Tremelimumab +SBRT	Phase 1	Completed	Lee et al. (2022) [108]
NCT03211117	Docetaxel + Doxorubicin + IMRT + Pembrolizumab + Surgery	Phase 2	Completed	
NCT04675710	Pembrolizumab + Dabrafenib + Trametinib + Surgery + IMRT	Phase 2	Recruiting	
NCT03975231	Dabrafenib + Trametinib + IMRT	Phase 1	Recruiting	
NCT00004089	Chemotherapy (Fluorouracil, Hydroxyurea, Paclitaxel) + Surgery + RT	Phase 2	Completed	
NCT00077103	Chemotherapy (Cisplatin, Doxorubicin) + Fosbretabulin + RT	Phase 1/2	Terminated	
NCT05059470	Pembrolizumab + IMRT	Phase 2	Recruiting	

RT: radiotherapy, SBRT: stereotactic body radiotherapy.

However, photon beam radiotherapy exhibits limitations regarding delivering a radical dose to the tumor site while accounting for damage to the OAR. From a future perspective, one way to overcome this problem is to use particle beam radiotherapy such as proton beam radiotherapy (PBRT) and carbon ion radiotherapy (CIRT). Particle beams enter the body with low energy when they enter the surface, transfer most of their energy to a certain depth that is called the Bragg peak, and then decay rapidly. These physical characteristics allow particle beams to deliver higher doses to cancers while protecting the OAR compared to radiation therapy using photon beams. The relative biological effectiveness (RBE) of a proton beam is 1.1- to 1.2-fold higher than that of X-rays [109], whereas that of carbon ion beams is 2- to 3-fold higher than that of X-rays [110]. As higher RBE values indicate greater cell-killing capacity, particle beams are more effective for cancer treatment than X-rays [111]. The only actual application of particle therapy for ATC was reported by Youssef et al. [112]. Patients with ATC with recurrence after thyroidectomy and radioiodine therapy were treated with two cycles of intensity-modulated PBRT (IMPT) with QUAD shot radiation (3.7 Gy delivered in four fractions twice daily at least 6 h apart for 2 consecutive days, repeated every 4 weeks, and with concurrent chemotherapy with doxorubicin and dacarbazine). At the last follow-up at 12 months, the disease had not progressed locally or systemically, thus indicating that PBRT was effective for treating ATC. Carbon ion beams are even more biologically effective than proton beams and thus exert more promising therapeutic effects. Recently, intensity-modulated CIRT (IMCT) was developed using pencil beam scanning technology, in which the total dose is made uniform by the sum of the individual beams, but the intensity of each beam is different as in IMRT [113]. IMCT can further reduce the dose of irradiation to neighboring OARs compared to that of conventional CIRT. Although not included in ATC, there have been several reports detailing the results of IMCT in head and neck cancer that indicate a favorable therapeutic effect and a low incidence of acute and late toxicity [114,115]. Multi-ion radiotherapy (MIRT) is currently under development. Moreover, it combines ion beams with different linear energy transfers (LETs) of noncarbon ions with carbon ion beams, such as higher LET beams (e.g., oxygen and neon ions) targeting areas of resistance and lower LET beams (e.g., helium ions) for the boundary with normal tissue near the tumor. This approach offers a promising new treatment option for patients with complex cancers [116]. Additionally, the higher LET beams used in MIRT are more effective against radioresistant hypoxic cells than are carbon ions, thus potentially leading to earlier tumor reoxygenation [117–119].

3.3. Chemotherapy

Anthracyclines such as doxorubicin, platinum-based drugs such as cisplatin and carboplatin, and taxanes such as paclitaxel and docetaxel are the main chemotherapeutic drugs used for ATC [81]. However, the effects of these agents on ATCs are moderate and transient and are often disappointing. These guidelines recommend the rapid use of paclitaxel + carboplatin, docetaxel + doxorubicin, paclitaxel alone, or docetaxel alone when there are no therapeutic targets without molecular abnormalities or when targeted therapies are not available [7,8]. They can be used as bridging chemotherapeutic agents before the use of molecularly targeted agents [82]. Among these, taxanes have been reported to be effective for the treatment of ATC. For example, Higashiyama et al. treated stage IVB and IVC patients with ATC and weekly PTX induction chemotherapy and observed complete (CR) and partial response (PR) in 8% and 23% of patients, respectively [120]. They reported that the OS rate of paclitaxel-treated patients with stage IVB disease was better than that of patients who did not receive chemotherapy or those who received drugs other than paclitaxel. However, it is challenging to treat ATC with anticancer drugs alone.

Therefore, a future strategy is to use them in combination with other modalities. For example, taxanes increase the percentage of radiosensitive G2/M phase cells; as a result, their combination with radiotherapy may be effective. A report evaluated the use of docetaxel in combination with radiotherapy in patients with ATC and observed that 67% of patients achieved CR and the remaining 33% achieved PR, although the number of patients was small [121]. They reported that 83% of patients were alive at a median follow-up of 21.5 months. These findings suggest that a combination of taxane-based chemotherapy and radiotherapy may be effective for patients with ATC.

3.4. Targeted Therapy

Recently, genome sequencing analysis revealed molecules that are frequently mutated in ATCs and are involved in tumor progression and malignant transformation. Therapeutic agents targeting these molecules have been investigated. These agents target receptor tyrosine kinases (RTK) and downstream molecules of the MAPK and PAM signaling pathways.

3.4.1. Inhibitors of MAPK Pathway

Inhibitors of the MAPK pathway are potential agents for cancer therapy, and many compounds have been identified in clinical and preclinical trials. Several RAF and MEK inhibitors have been approved; however, no ERK inhibitors have yet been approved.

Dabrafenib is a BRAFV600E kinase inhibitor, and trametinib is an MEK inhibitor. Their combination therapy has been approved by the U.S. Food and Drug Administration (FDA) for the treatment of patients with ATC and BRAF V600E mutations. This is due to resistance to BRAF inhibitors that develops within months of BRAF blockade alone [122]. Several mechanisms have been proposed to induce this resistance, including the expression of splicing variants of the BRAF gene [123], inhibition of the negative feedback mechanism in the MAPK pathway [124], and activation of integrin/FAK signaling [125]. In vitro studies revealed that dabrafenib and trametinib inhibit ATC cell proliferation [126]. Subbiah et al. reported that in a phase II study evaluating the efficacy of dabrafenib plus trametinib in 36 patients with ATC, the CR and PR were 8% and 47%, respectively, and the median OS was 14.5 months [10]. In a recently reported UK clinical trial, CR and PR were achieved in 12% and 71% of patients with ATC, respectively, with a median OS of 6.9 months [127].

Another combination of BRAF and MEK inhibitors includes encorafenib (BRAF inhibitor) and binimetinib (MEK inhibitor). In a phase II study of 22 patients with thyroid cancer, including five patients with ATC and BRAF mutation-positive ATC with local invasion or distant metastasis, that evaluated the efficacy of the combination of encorafenib and binimetinib, the overall response rate (ORR) was 80% (CR, one case; PR, three cases) [128].

Vemurafenib is a selective BRAF inhibitor approved by the FDA for the treatment of patients with metastatic melanoma harboring the BRAF V600E mutation [129]. Zhang et al. reported that vemurafenib inhibits tumor growth in an in vivo xenograft mouse model using an ATC cell line [130]. A clinical trial evaluating the efficacy of vemurafenib in patients with cancer due to the BRAF V600E mutation, including seven patients with ATC, indicated that the percentages of patients with cancer achieving CR and PR were 14% and 14%, respectively [131]. Clinical trials are currently evaluating the efficacy of combining vemurafenib with cobimetinib, a MEK inhibitor, in BRAF-positive thyroid cancers, including ATC.

Other drugs, such as PLX8394 (BRAF inhibitor) and selumetinib (MEK inhibitor), have been investigated for the treatment of thyroid cancer [132]. Additionally, the ERK inhibitor DEL-22379 has been reported to decrease cell viability and inhibit the metastasis of ATC cells with BRAF mutations in vitro and in vivo [133].

3.4.2. Inhibitors of PAM Pathway

Molecules involved in this signaling pathway have received considerable attention in recent years, and many drugs targeting them have been studied and evaluated in animals and humans.

Everolimus inhibits the mTOR complex 1 (mTORC1). Owonikoko et al. reported that everolimus is effective against ATC cells both in vitro and in vivo [134]. However, the results of clinical trials investigating the efficacy of everolimus have been disappointing [83,135,136]. mTOR exists in two functionally and structurally distinct complexes, mTOR complex 1 (mTORC1) and mTORC2. Inhibition of mTORC1 inhibits ribosome biogenesis and suppresses cell proliferation, whereas inhibition of mTORC2 activates AKT and promotes cell growth [137]. This may have been due to the limited efficacy of everolimus.

In contrast, ATP-competitive dual mTORC1/2 inhibitors such as MLN0128 [138], AZD2014 [139,140], and AZD8055 [141] have been developed that can efficiently block the PAM pathway without causing negative feedback induction of mTORC2. Among these compounds, a phase II clinical trial is currently underway to evaluate the efficacy of MLN0128 for the treatment of metastatic ATC.

Other compounds, including CUDC-907 (PI3K and HDAC inhibitor) [142], copanlisib (PI3K inhibitor) [143], and buparlisib (PI3K inhibitor) [144], have been studied in the context of thyroid cancer.

3.4.3. RTK Inhibitors

RTKs are transmembrane glycoproteins on the cell surface that regulate cell proliferation, differentiation, and survival by activating several important intracellular signaling pathways, such as the MAPK and PAM pathways. RTKs include vascular endothelial growth factor receptor (VEGFR), epidermal growth factor receptor (EGFR), fibroblast growth factor receptor (FGFR), cluster of differentiation 117 (c-KIT), rearranged during transfection (RET), and platelet-derived growth factor receptor (PDGFR). Overexpression and activation of mutations in cancer cells have been reported, and drugs targeting them have been developed.

Lenvatinib is an inhibitor of VEGFR, FGFR, c-kit, RET, and PDGFR, and it is approved by the FDA and the European Medicines Agency for the treatment of iodine-131 (I-131) refractory DTC [145]. Ferrari et al. reported that lenvatinib suppresses the proliferative capacity of ATC cells in vitro and in vivo [146]. In a clinical trial of patients with ATC, Takahashi et al. reported a median OS of 10.4 months and an ORR of 24% in the lenvatinib group [84]. Reports have suggested that lenvatinib provides clinical benefits to patients with advanced ATC [147,148]. Although a high response rate can be expected, there is a risk of a shortened prognosis in patients with tracheal or carotid artery invasion due to fistula formation. Furthermore, lenvatinib alone is not an effective treatment for ATC [149] and has been disappointing in terms of prolonging the survival of unresectable ATC [150].

Similar to lenvatinib, single-agent multi-kinase inhibitors (MKIs), including sorafenib, gefitinib, imatinib, sunitinib, and pazopanib, have exhibited efficacy in vitro and in vivo [151–157] but have not exhibited promising results in clinical trials [107,158–163]. These MKIs are not effective when prescribed alone for the treatment of ATC but may be potentially useful in combination with other targeted therapies. Furthermore, the therapeutic effects of TRK or RET inhibitors are expected to be effective when mutations or fusions of TRK or RET are observed.

Targeted drugs have been developed against various target molecules, and a few of them, such as dabrafenib plus trametinib and encorafenib plus binimetinib, have demonstrated therapeutic efficacy. However, the emergence of drug resistance within a few months after a successful response has become a problem. Overcoming drug-resistant cancer is a major challenge in the development of molecularly targeted cancer therapies. Currently, there are no concrete, effective means to solve this problem.

Future prospects include elucidating the mechanisms of drug resistance at the basic research level and, in clinical practice, identifying effective therapeutic agents by studying the mutations that occur when drug resistance develops through genetic testing.

3.5. *Immunotherapy*

Tumor cells grow and metastasize through various mechanisms to escape recognition and attack by the immune system. Tumor-induced immunosuppression occurs in two ways. The first occurs through the induction of immunosuppressive cells that accumulate around the tumor and secrete immunosuppressive factors. Another mechanism involves the expression of immunosuppressive molecules and their receptors, such as programmed death ligand/programmed death-1 (PD-L1/PD-1), galectin-9/TIM-3, LAG-3, and CTLA-4. These are known as immune checkpoints that inhibit the activation of effector T lymphocytes, ultimately leading to the immune escape of the tumor. A recent trend in immunotherapy is the inhibition of these immune checkpoints and the restoration of immune function.

PD-L1 expressed on tumor cells binds to PD-1 on T cells and suppresses the proliferation and function of T cells, thereby weakening their immune response to tumor cells. PD-L1 expression in cancer cells may be primarily expressed or induced in the cancer microenvironment by the stimulation of inflammatory cytokines produced by tumor-infiltrating lymphocytes (TILs) and tumor-associated macrophages (TAMs) surrounding tumor cells [164]. PD-L1 is highly expressed in ATC [85,165,166], and Cantara et al. reported that immunohistochemistry using two PD-L1 antibodies exhibited high positivity rates of 65% and 90%, respectively [167]. Therefore, anti-PD-L1 and anti-PD-1 antibodies may be effective therapies for ATC. In contrast, CTLA-4 expressed on T cells binds to B7 molecules (CD80 and CD86) on antigen-presenting cells and inhibits T cell activation. CTLA-4 is expressed in regulatory T cells (Tregs). When Tregs bind to antigen-presenting cells, T cells cannot bind to antigen-presenting cells and cannot be activated. Therefore, anti-CTLA-4 antibodies are expected to be used for cancer therapy.

There are reports of the use of the anti-PD-1 antibodies spartalizumab and pembrolizumab and the anti-PD-L1 antibody atezolizumab in the treatment of ATC. In a phase II study by Capdevila et al. involving 42 patients with ATC treated with spartalizumab intravenously at a dose of 400 mg every 4 weeks, the ORR was 19% (CR, 7%; PR, 12%), and it was 29% in patients with PD-L1 expression and even higher in patients with high PD-L1 expression. The median OS was 5.9 months, with 40% of patients surviving for 1 year [85]. In a retrospective study, Iyer et al. demonstrated the efficacy of pembrolizumab in combination with lenvatinib, trametinib, or a combination of dabrafenib and trametinib in patients with ATC [168]. Moreover, there were no CRs, but 42% of patients achieved OR. The median OS after the addition of pembrolizumab was 6.93 months. Wang et al. investigated six patients with ATC and BRAF V600E mutation who underwent complete surgical resection and received dabrafenib plus trametinib with or without pembrolizumab [169]. No local recurrence was detected in any patient. Four patients with pembrolizumab achieved CR within the observation period (7.8–26.0 months), while two patients without pembrolizumab died due to distant metastasis. These results suggest that the combination of dabrafenib and trametinib with ICI would be more effective for patients with ATC and the BRAF V600E mutation. A phase 2 pilot study is ongoing to evaluate the efficacy of dabrafenib and trametinib in combination with cemiplimab, an anti-PD-1 antibody, in the context of ATC treatment. Moreover, reports suggest that a combination of lenvatinib and pembrolizumab may be effective for treating ATC [170]. A study evaluating the efficacy of lenvatinib in combination with nivolumab is ongoing in Japan (jRCT2080224758), and results are expected in the near future. While immunotherapy is successful in a few cases, it can cause side effects. Immune checkpoint inhibitors reactivate immune cells that have been suppressed by cancer cells. These side effects are known as immune-related adverse events (irAEs) and have been reported to include interstitial pneumonia, colitis, type 1 diabetes, endocrine disorders such as thyroid dysfunction, liver and kidney dysfunction, skin disorders, myasthenia gravis, myositis, and uveitis [171,172]. Chronic side effects have been reported, such as those that persist for more than three months after the end of treatment with immune checkpoint inhibitors [173].

The irAEs are becoming very complicated due to the combination of immunotherapy and other therapies. In the future, it is necessary to move toward establishing and managing a safety management system across medical departments and professions in collaboration with multiple professions to address these issues.

3.6. Others

Recently, it has been increasingly recognized that microbiota, including those in the gut and oral cavity, influence the pathogenesis, prognosis, and treatment response of various diseases, including cancer [174]. Several studies have reported a relationship between thyroid cancer and the microbiota. Research on the relationship between oral bacteria has reported that an increase in the genera *Alloprevotella*, *Anaeroglobus*, and *Acinetobacter*, unclassified *Bacteroidales*, and unclassified *Cyanobacteriales* was observed in the saliva of patients with thyroid cancer [175,176]. Moreover, studies exist on the relationship between gut microbiota and thyroid cancer. The relative abundances of *Neisseria* and *Streptococcus* were significantly higher in the gut flora of patients with thyroid cancer than those in healthy controls [177]. A study examining patients with PTC revealed that the abundance of *Firmicutes* was higher in the fecal flora than it was in healthy participants [178].

Previously, the thyroid gland was believed to be a sterile organ; however, recent technological advances have revealed that it is colonized by microorganisms. Microorganisms exist in thyroid cancer tissues, and a relationship between bacterial flora and disease status has been reported. One study has demonstrated a correlation between *Sphingomonas* abundance within the tumor microenvironment and lymph node metastasis [179]. A study examining patients with PTC revealed a high abundance of *Proteobacteria* in the tumors. Additionally, tumor bacterial diversity increased in patients with a higher T stage [178]. Regarding the therapeutic response to postoperative I-131 treatment for PTC, low levels of the genera Dorea and Bifidobacterium were associated with a poor prognosis [180]. However, there have been no reports investigating the relationship between ATC and the bacterial flora. Treatment methods for ATC, such as radiotherapy, chemotherapy, and immunotherapy, are associated with bacterial flora [181]. Therefore, in the future, microflora will attract attention as a target for new treatment strategies for ATC, and further research and development are expected [182].

3.7. Best Supportive Care

Although promising therapies have been developed for the treatment of ATC in recent years, it remains a difficult-to-cure cancer with a high mortality rate. The patient wishes to be fully considered when deciding whether to pursue aggressive treatment, including palliative care for pain and dyspnea and hospice care [183].

4. Conclusions

Although the treatment of ATC is evolving and diversifying, the optimal treatment has not yet been identified, ultimately resulting in a poor prognosis. The rapid progression of ATC necessitates immediate diagnosis and treatment. A multidisciplinary care team, including endocrinologists, oncologic surgeons, medical oncologists, radiation oncologists, radiologists, and palliative care staff, must be formed to determine the treatment plan and provide appropriate care as soon as possible while considering patient wishes. Recent studies have demonstrated that BRAF-mutant ATCs exhibit dramatically improved prognosis. However, the problem of drug resistance and treatment strategies for wild-type BRAF remain underexplored. A better understanding of the molecular biology of ATCs is expected to lead to the development of novel targeted therapies. Although radiotherapy remains the mainstay of ATC treatment, recent technological developments such as intensity-modulated irradiation and particle therapy are remarkable. The successful use of combinations of these novel drugs and therapies may lead to the development of treatment strategies to improve the ATC prognosis. Further clinical trials using many patients are required.

Author Contributions: Conceptualization, K.S. and D.H.; methodology, K.S. and D.H.; data curation, K.S., H.H. and D.H.; writing—original draft preparation, K.S., H.H. and D.H.; writing—review and editing, K.S., H.H., S.T., N.S. (Nao Saito), R.H., N.S. (Nobuyasu Suganuma), T.S. and D.H. All authors have read and agreed to the published version of the manuscript.

Funding: This research received no external funding.

Conflicts of Interest: The authors declare no conflict of interest.

References

1. Siegel, R.L.; Miller, K.D.; Fuchs, H.E.; Jemal, A. Cancer statistics, 2022. *CA Cancer J. Clin.* **2022**, *72*, 7–33. [CrossRef] [PubMed]
2. Janz, T.A.; Neskey, D.M.; Nguyen, S.A.; Lentsch, E.J. Is the incidence of anaplastic thyroid cancer increasing: A population based epidemiology study. *World J. Otorhinolaryngol. Head Neck Surg.* **2019**, *5*, 34–40. [CrossRef] [PubMed]
3. Casali, P.G.; Trama, A. Rationale of the rare cancer list: A consensus paper from the Joint Action on Rare Cancers (JARC) of the European Union (EU). *ESMO Open* **2020**, *5*, e000666. [CrossRef] [PubMed]

4. Pereira, M.; Williams, V.L.; Hallanger Johnson, J.; Valderrabano, P. Thyroid Cancer Incidence Trends in the United States: Association with Changes in Professional Guideline Recommendations. *Thyroid* **2020**, *30*, 1132–1140. [CrossRef] [PubMed]
5. Takahashi, S.; Tahara, M.; Ito, K.; Tori, M.; Kiyota, N.; Yoshida, K.; Sakata, Y.; Yoshida, A. Safety and Effectiveness of Lenvatinib in 594 Patients with Unresectable Thyroid Cancer in an All-Case Post-Marketing Observational Study in Japan. *Adv. Ther.* **2020**, *37*, 3850–3862. [CrossRef] [PubMed]
6. Xu, B.; Fuchs, T.; Dogan, S.; Landa, I.; Katabi, N.; Fagin, J.A.; Tuttle, R.M.; Sherman, E.; Gill, A.J.; Ghossein, R. Dissecting Anaplastic Thyroid Carcinoma: A Comprehensive Clinical, Histologic, Immunophenotypic, and Molecular Study of 360 Cases. *Thyroid* **2020**, *30*, 1505–1517. [CrossRef] [PubMed]
7. Bible, K.C.; Kebebew, E.; Brierley, J.; Brito, J.P.; Cabanillas, M.E.; Clark, T.J., Jr.; Di Cristofano, A.; Foote, R.; Giordano, T.; Kasperbauer, J.; et al. 2021 American Thyroid Association Guidelines for Management of Patients with Anaplastic Thyroid Cancer. *Thyroid* **2021**, *31*, 337–386. [CrossRef] [PubMed]
8. Filetti, S.; Durante, C.; Hartl, D.; Leboulleux, S.; Locati, L.D.; Newbold, K.; Papotti, M.G.; Berruti, A. Thyroid cancer: ESMO Clinical Practice Guidelines for diagnosis, treatment and follow-up†. *Ann. Oncol.* **2019**, *30*, 1856–1883. [CrossRef] [PubMed]
9. Haddad, R.I.; Bischoff, L.; Ball, D.; Bernet, V.; Blomain, E.; Busaidy, N.L.; Campbell, M.; Dickson, P.; Duh, Q.Y.; Ehya, H.; et al. Thyroid Carcinoma, Version 2.2022, NCCN Clinical Practice Guidelines in Oncology. *J. Natl. Compr. Cancer Netw.* **2022**, *20*, 925–951. [CrossRef]
10. Subbiah, V.; Kreitman, R.J.; Wainberg, Z.A.; Cho, J.Y.; Schellens, J.H.M.; Soria, J.C.; Wen, P.Y.; Zielinski, C.C.; Cabanillas, M.E.; Boran, A.; et al. Dabrafenib plus trametinib in patients with BRAF V600E-mutant anaplastic thyroid cancer: Updated analysis from the phase II ROAR basket study. *Ann. Oncol.* **2022**, *33*, 406–415. [CrossRef]
11. De Leo, S.; Trevisan, M.; Fugazzola, L. Recent advances in the management of anaplastic thyroid cancer. *Thyroid Res.* **2020**, *13*, 17. [CrossRef]
12. Jannin, A.; Escande, A.; Al Ghuzlan, A.; Blanchard, P.; Hartl, D.; Chevalier, B.; Deschamps, F.; Lamartina, L.; Lacroix, L.; Dupuy, C.; et al. Anaplastic Thyroid Carcinoma: An Update. *Cancers* **2022**, *14*, 1061. [CrossRef]
13. Abe, I.; Lam, A.K. Anaplastic Thyroid Carcinoma: Current Issues in Genomics and Therapeutics. *Curr. Oncol. Rep.* **2021**, *23*, 31. [CrossRef] [PubMed]
14. Chiacchio, S.; Lorenzoni, A.; Boni, G.; Rubello, D.; Elisei, R.; Mariani, G. Anaplastic thyroid cancer: Prevalence, diagnosis and treatment. *Minerva Endocrinol.* **2008**, *33*, 341–357. [PubMed]
15. Califano, I.; Smulever, A.; Jerkovich, F.; Pitoia, F. Advances in the management of anaplastic thyroid carcinoma: Transforming a life-threatening condition into a potentially treatable disease. *Rev. Endocr. Metab. Disord.* **2024**, *25*, 123–147. [CrossRef]
16. Shaha, A.R. Implications of prognostic factors and risk groups in the management of differentiated thyroid cancer. *Laryngoscope* **2004**, *114*, 393–402. [CrossRef] [PubMed]
17. Maniakas, A.; Dadu, R.; Busaidy, N.L.; Wang, J.R.; Ferrarotto, R.; Lu, C.; Williams, M.D.; Gunn, G.B.; Hofmann, M.C.; Cote, G.; et al. Evaluation of Overall Survival in Patients With Anaplastic Thyroid Carcinoma, 2000–2019. *JAMA Oncol.* **2020**, *6*, 1397–1404. [CrossRef]
18. Song, T.; Chen, L.; Zhang, H.; Lu, Y.; Yu, K.; Zhan, W.; Fang, M. Multimodal treatment based on thyroidectomy improves survival in patients with metastatic anaplastic thyroid carcinoma: A SEER analysis from 1998 to 2015. *Gland Surg.* **2020**, *9*, 1205–1213. [CrossRef]
19. de Ridder, M.; Nieveen van Dijkum, E.; Engelsman, A.; Kapiteijn, E.; Klümpen, H.J.; Rasch, C.R.N. Anaplastic thyroid carcinoma: A nationwide cohort study on incidence, treatment and survival in the Netherlands over 3 decades. *Eur. J. Endocrinol.* **2020**, *183*, 203–209. [CrossRef]
20. Tuttle, R.M.; Haugen, B.; Perrier, N.D. Updated American Joint Committee on Cancer/Tumor-Node-Metastasis Staging System for Differentiated and Anaplastic Thyroid Cancer (Eighth Edition): What Changed and Why? *Thyroid* **2017**, *27*, 751–756. [CrossRef]
21. Molinaro, E.; Romei, C.; Biagini, A.; Sabini, E.; Agate, L.; Mazzeo, S.; Materazzi, G.; Sellari-Franceschini, S.; Ribechini, A.; Torregrossa, L.; et al. Anaplastic thyroid carcinoma: From clinicopathology to genetics and advanced therapies. *Nat. Rev. Endocrinol.* **2017**, *13*, 644–660. [CrossRef]
22. Onoda, N.; Sugitani, I.; Ito, K.I.; Suzuki, A.; Higashiyama, T.; Fukumori, T.; Suganuma, N.; Masudo, K.; Nakayama, H.; Uno, A.; et al. Evaluation of the 8th Edition TNM Classification for Anaplastic Thyroid Carcinoma. *Cancers* **2020**, *12*, 552. [CrossRef]
23. Sugitani, I.; Miyauchi, A.; Sugino, K.; Okamoto, T.; Yoshida, A.; Suzuki, S. Prognostic factors and treatment outcomes for anaplastic thyroid carcinoma: ATC Research Consortium of Japan cohort study of 677 patients. *World J. Surg.* **2012**, *36*, 1247–1254. [CrossRef] [PubMed]
24. Haymart, M.R.; Banerjee, M.; Yin, H.; Worden, F.; Griggs, J.J. Marginal treatment benefit in anaplastic thyroid cancer. *Cancer* **2013**, *119*, 3133–3139. [CrossRef] [PubMed]
25. Akaishi, J.; Sugino, K.; Kitagawa, W.; Nagahama, M.; Kameyama, K.; Shimizu, K.; Ito, K.; Ito, K. Prognostic factors and treatment outcomes of 100 cases of anaplastic thyroid carcinoma. *Thyroid* **2011**, *21*, 1183–1189. [CrossRef]
26. Yoo, S.K.; Song, Y.S.; Lee, E.K.; Hwang, J.; Kim, H.H.; Jung, G.; Kim, Y.A.; Kim, S.J.; Cho, S.W.; Won, J.K.; et al. Integrative analysis of genomic and transcriptomic characteristics associated with progression of aggressive thyroid cancer. *Nat. Commun.* **2019**, *10*, 2764. [CrossRef] [PubMed]
27. Ravi, N.; Yang, M.; Gretarsson, S.; Jansson, C.; Mylona, N.; Sydow, S.R.; Woodward, E.L.; Ekblad, L.; Wennerberg, J.; Paulsson, K. Identification of Targetable Lesions in Anaplastic Thyroid Cancer by Genome Profiling. *Cancers* **2019**, *11*, 402. [CrossRef]

28. Pozdeyev, N.; Gay, L.M.; Sokol, E.S.; Hartmaier, R.; Deaver, K.E.; Davis, S.; French, J.D.; Borre, P.V.; LaBarbera, D.V.; Tan, A.C.; et al. Genetic Analysis of 779 Advanced Differentiated and Anaplastic Thyroid Cancers. *Clin. Cancer Res.* **2018**, *24*, 3059–3068. [CrossRef]
29. Khan, S.A.; Ci, B.; Xie, Y.; Gerber, D.E.; Beg, M.S.; Sherman, S.I.; Cabanillas, M.E.; Busaidy, N.L.; Burtness, B.A.; Heilmann, A.M.; et al. Unique mutation patterns in anaplastic thyroid cancer identified by comprehensive genomic profiling. *Head Neck* **2019**, *41*, 1928–1934. [CrossRef]
30. Landa, I.; Ibrahimpasic, T.; Boucai, L.; Sinha, R.; Knauf, J.A.; Shah, R.H.; Dogan, S.; Ricarte-Filho, J.C.; Krishnamoorthy, G.P.; Xu, B.; et al. Genomic and transcriptomic hallmarks of poorly differentiated and anaplastic thyroid cancers. *J. Clin. Investig.* **2016**, *126*, 1052–1066. [CrossRef]
31. Bonhomme, B.; Godbert, Y.; Perot, G.; Al Ghuzlan, A.; Bardet, S.; Belleannée, G.; Crinière, L.; Do Cao, C.; Fouilloux, G.; Guyetant, S.; et al. Molecular Pathology of Anaplastic Thyroid Carcinomas: A Retrospective Study of 144 Cases. *Thyroid* **2017**, *27*, 682–692. [CrossRef] [PubMed]
32. Duan, H.; Li, Y.; Hu, P.; Gao, J.; Ying, J.; Xu, W.; Zhao, D.; Wang, Z.; Ye, J.; Lizaso, A.; et al. Mutational profiling of poorly differentiated and anaplastic thyroid carcinoma by the use of targeted next-generation sequencing. *Histopathology* **2019**, *75*, 890–899. [CrossRef] [PubMed]
33. Romei, C.; Tacito, A.; Molinaro, E.; Piaggi, P.; Cappagli, V.; Pieruzzi, L.; Matrone, A.; Viola, D.; Agate, L.; Torregrossa, L.; et al. Clinical, pathological and genetic features of anaplastic and poorly differentiated thyroid cancer: A single institute experience. *Oncol. Lett.* **2018**, *15*, 9174–9182. [CrossRef] [PubMed]
34. Marei, H.E.; Althani, A.; Afifi, N.; Hasan, A.; Caceci, T.; Pozzoli, G.; Morrione, A.; Giordano, A.; Cenciarelli, C. p53 signaling in cancer progression and therapy. *Cancer Cell Int.* **2021**, *21*, 703. [CrossRef] [PubMed]
35. McKelvey, B.A.; Umbricht, C.B.; Zeiger, M.A. Telomerase Reverse Transcriptase (TERT) Regulation in Thyroid Cancer: A Review. *Front. Endocrinol.* **2020**, *11*, 485. [CrossRef] [PubMed]
36. Panebianco, F.; Nikitski, A.V.; Nikiforova, M.N.; Nikiforov, Y.E. Spectrum of TERT promoter mutations and mechanisms of activation in thyroid cancer. *Cancer Med.* **2019**, *8*, 5831–5839. [CrossRef] [PubMed]
37. Matsuse, M.; Mitsutake, N. TERT promoter mutations in thyroid cancer. *Endocr. J.* **2023**, *70*, 1035–1049. [CrossRef] [PubMed]
38. Akıncılar, S.C.; Chua, J.Y.H.; Ng, Q.F.; Chan, C.H.T.; Eslami, S.Z.; Chen, K.; Low, J.L.; Arumugam, S.; Aswad, L.; Chua, C.; et al. Identification of mechanism of cancer-cell-specific reactivation of hTERT offers therapeutic opportunities for blocking telomerase specifically in human colorectal cancer. *Nucleic Acids Res.* **2023**, *51*, 1–16. [CrossRef] [PubMed]
39. Low, K.C.; Tergaonkar, V. Telomerase: Central regulator of all of the hallmarks of cancer. *Trends Biochem. Sci.* **2013**, *38*, 426–434. [CrossRef]
40. Chen, S.; Yang, L.; Dong, H.; Guo, H. Human telomerase reverse transcriptase recruits the β-catenin/TCF-4 complex to transactivate chemokine (C-C motif) ligand 2 expression in colorectal cancer. *Biomed. Pharmacother.* **2019**, *112*, 108700. [CrossRef]
41. Kumar, N.; Sethi, G. Telomerase and hallmarks of cancer: An intricate interplay governing cancer cell evolution. *Cancer Lett.* **2023**, *578*, 216459. [CrossRef] [PubMed]
42. Lavoie, H.; Gagnon, J.; Therrien, M. ERK signalling: A master regulator of cell behaviour, life and fate. *Nat. Rev. Mol. Cell Biol.* **2020**, *21*, 607–632. [CrossRef] [PubMed]
43. Luo, W.; Sun, R.; Chen, X.; Li, J.; Jiang, J.; He, Y.; Shi, S.; Wen, H. ERK Activation-Mediated Autophagy Induction Resists Licochalcone A-Induced Anticancer Activities in Lung Cancer Cells in vitro. *OncoTargets Ther.* **2020**, *13*, 13437–13450. [CrossRef] [PubMed]
44. Samson, S.C.; Khan, A.M.; Mendoza, M.C. ERK signaling for cell migration and invasion. *Front. Mol. Biosci.* **2022**, *9*, 998475. [CrossRef] [PubMed]
45. Schubert, L.; Mariko, M.L.; Clerc, J.; Huillard, O.; Groussin, L. MAPK Pathway Inhibitors in Thyroid Cancer: Preclinical and Clinical Data. *Cancers* **2023**, *15*, 710. [CrossRef] [PubMed]
46. Cook, F.A.; Cook, S.J. Inhibition of RAF dimers: It takes two to tango. *Biochem. Soc. Trans.* **2021**, *49*, 237–251. [CrossRef] [PubMed]
47. Rosove, M.H.; Peddi, P.F.; Glaspy, J.A. BRAF V600E inhibition in anaplastic thyroid cancer. *N. Engl. J. Med.* **2013**, *368*, 684–685. [CrossRef] [PubMed]
48. Rushton, S.; Burghel, G.; Wallace, A.; Nonaka, D. Immunohistochemical detection of BRAF V600E mutation status in anaplastic thyroid carcinoma. *Histopathology* **2016**, *69*, 524–526. [CrossRef]
49. Perri, F.; Pezzullo, L.; Chiofalo, M.G.; Lastoria, S.; Di Gennaro, F.; Scarpati, G.D.; Caponigro, F. Targeted therapy: A new hope for thyroid carcinomas. *Crit. Rev. Oncol./Hematol.* **2015**, *94*, 55–63. [CrossRef]
50. Hlozek, J.; Pekova, B.; Rotnágl, J.; Holý, R.; Astl, J. Genetic Changes in Thyroid Cancers and the Importance of Their Preoperative Detection in Relation to the General Treatment and Determination of the Extent of Surgical Intervention-A Review. *Biomedicines* **2022**, *10*, 1515. [CrossRef]
51. Yamazaki, H.; Kunisaki, C.; Sugimori, M.; Rino, Y.; Saito, A. Genetic landscape of 482 thyroid carcinomas: Analysis with the national datacenter for cancer genomic medicine in Japan. *Endocrine* **2024**, *in press*. [CrossRef] [PubMed]
52. Rusinek, D.; Chmielik, E.; Krajewska, J.; Jarzab, M.; Oczko-Wojciechowska, M.; Czarniecka, A.; Jarzab, B. Current Advances in Thyroid Cancer Management. Are We Ready for the Epidemic Rise of Diagnoses? *Int. J. Mol. Sci.* **2017**, *18*, 1817. [CrossRef] [PubMed]

53. Oishi, N.; Kondo, T.; Ebina, A.; Sato, Y.; Akaishi, J.; Hino, R.; Yamamoto, N.; Mochizuki, K.; Nakazawa, T.; Yokomichi, H.; et al. Molecular alterations of coexisting thyroid papillary carcinoma and anaplastic carcinoma: Identification of TERT mutation as an independent risk factor for transformation. *Mod. Pathol.* **2017**, *30*, 1527–1537. [CrossRef] [PubMed]
54. Ferrari, S.M.; Elia, G.; Ragusa, F.; Ruffilli, I.; La Motta, C.; Paparo, S.R.; Patrizio, A.; Vita, R.; Benvenga, S.; Materazzi, G.; et al. Novel treatments for anaplastic thyroid carcinoma. *Gland. Surg.* **2020**, *9*, S28–S42. [CrossRef] [PubMed]
55. Gilani, S.M.; Abi-Raad, R.; Garritano, J.; Cai, G.; Prasad, M.L.; Adeniran, A.J. RAS mutation and associated risk of malignancy in the thyroid gland: An FNA study with cytology-histology correlation. *Cancer Cytopathol.* **2022**, *130*, 284–293. [CrossRef] [PubMed]
56. Lai, W.A.; Liu, C.Y.; Lin, S.Y.; Chen, C.C.; Hang, J.F. Characterization of Driver Mutations in Anaplastic Thyroid Carcinoma Identifies RAS and PIK3CA Mutations as Negative Survival Predictors. *Cancers* **2020**, *12*, 1973. [CrossRef] [PubMed]
57. Haigis, K.M.; Kendall, K.R.; Wang, Y.; Cheung, A.; Haigis, M.C.; Glickman, J.N.; Niwa-Kawakita, M.; Sweet-Cordero, A.; Sebolt-Leopold, J.; Shannon, K.M.; et al. Differential effects of oncogenic K-Ras and N-Ras on proliferation, differentiation and tumor progression in the colon. *Nat. Genet.* **2008**, *40*, 600–608. [CrossRef] [PubMed]
58. Kunstman, J.W.; Juhlin, C.C.; Goh, G.; Brown, T.C.; Stenman, A.; Healy, J.M.; Rubinstein, J.C.; Choi, M.; Kiss, N.; Nelson-Williams, C.; et al. Characterization of the mutational landscape of anaplastic thyroid cancer via whole-exome sequencing. *Hum. Mol. Genet.* **2015**, *24*, 2318–2329. [CrossRef] [PubMed]
59. Krishnamoorthy, G.P.; Davidson, N.R.; Leach, S.D.; Zhao, Z.; Lowe, S.W.; Lee, G.; Landa, I.; Nagarajah, J.; Saqcena, M.; Singh, K.; et al. EIF1AX and RAS Mutations Cooperate to Drive Thyroid Tumorigenesis through ATF4 and c-MYC. *Cancer Discov.* **2019**, *9*, 264–281. [CrossRef]
60. Janku, F.; Yap, T.A.; Meric-Bernstam, F. Targeting the PI3K pathway in cancer: Are we making headway? *Nat. Rev. Clin. Oncol.* **2018**, *15*, 273–291. [CrossRef]
61. Glaviano, A.; Foo, A.S.C.; Lam, H.Y.; Yap, K.C.H.; Jacot, W.; Jones, R.H.; Eng, H.; Nair, M.G.; Makvandi, P.; Geoerger, B.; et al. PI3K/AKT/mTOR signaling transduction pathway and targeted therapies in cancer. *Mol. Cancer* **2023**, *22*, 138. [CrossRef] [PubMed]
62. Yang, J.; Nie, J.; Ma, X.; Wei, Y.; Peng, Y.; Wei, X. Targeting PI3K in cancer: Mechanisms and advances in clinical trials. *Mol. Cancer* **2019**, *18*, 26. [CrossRef] [PubMed]
63. Martini, M.; De Santis, M.C.; Braccini, L.; Gulluni, F.; Hirsch, E. PI3K/AKT signaling pathway and cancer: An updated review. *Ann. Med.* **2014**, *46*, 372–383. [CrossRef] [PubMed]
64. Mayer, I.A.; Arteaga, C.L. The PI3K/AKT Pathway as a Target for Cancer Treatment. *Annu. Rev. Med.* **2016**, *67*, 11–28. [CrossRef] [PubMed]
65. Deng, J.; Bai, X.; Feng, X.; Ni, J.; Beretov, J.; Graham, P.; Li, Y. Inhibition of PI3K/Akt/mTOR signaling pathway alleviates ovarian cancer chemoresistance through reversing epithelial-mesenchymal transition and decreasing cancer stem cell marker expression. *BMC Cancer* **2019**, *19*, 618. [CrossRef] [PubMed]
66. Peng, Y.; Wang, Y.; Zhou, C.; Mei, W.; Zeng, C. PI3K/Akt/mTOR Pathway and Its Role in Cancer Therapeutics: Are We Making Headway? *Front. Oncol.* **2022**, *12*, 819128. [CrossRef]
67. Samuels, Y.; Diaz, L.A., Jr.; Schmidt-Kittler, O.; Cummins, J.M.; Delong, L.; Cheong, I.; Rago, C.; Huso, D.L.; Lengauer, C.; Kinzler, K.W.; et al. Mutant PIK3CA promotes cell growth and invasion of human cancer cells. *Cancer Cell* **2005**, *7*, 561–573. [CrossRef]
68. Thorpe, L.M.; Yuzugullu, H.; Zhao, J.J. PI3K in cancer: Divergent roles of isoforms, modes of activation and therapeutic targeting. *Nat. Rev. Cancer* **2015**, *15*, 7–24. [CrossRef]
69. Pinto, N.; Ruicci, K.M.; Khan, M.I.; Shaikh, M.H.; Zeng, Y.F.P.; Yoo, J.; Fung, K.; MacNeil, S.D.; Mendez, A.; Mymryk, J.S.; et al. Introduction and expression of PIK3CA(E545K) in a papillary thyroid cancer BRAF(V600E) cell line leads to a dedifferentiated aggressive phenotype. *J. Otolaryngol. Head Neck Surg.* **2022**, *51*, 7. [CrossRef]
70. Worby, C.A.; Dixon, J.E. PTEN. *Annu. Rev. Biochem.* **2014**, *83*, 641–669. [CrossRef]
71. Hashemi, M.; Taheriazam, A.; Daneii, P.; Hassanpour, A.; Kakavand, A.; Rezaei, S.; Hejazi, E.S.; Aboutalebi, M.; Gholamrezaie, H.; Saebfar, H.; et al. Targeting PI3K/Akt signaling in prostate cancer therapy. *J. Cell Commun. Signal.* **2023**, *17*, 423–443. [CrossRef] [PubMed]
72. Paskeh, M.D.A.; Ghadyani, F.; Hashemi, M.; Abbaspour, A.; Zabolian, A.; Javanshir, S.; Razzazan, M.; Mirzaei, S.; Entezari, M.; Goharrizi, M.; et al. Biological impact and therapeutic perspective of targeting PI3K/Akt signaling in hepatocellular carcinoma: Promises and Challenges. *Pharmacol. Res.* **2023**, *187*, 106553. [CrossRef] [PubMed]
73. Puzio-Kuter, A.M.; Castillo-Martin, M.; Kinkade, C.W.; Wang, X.; Shen, T.H.; Matos, T.; Shen, M.M.; Cordon-Cardo, C.; Abate-Shen, C. Inactivation of p53 and Pten promotes invasive bladder cancer. *Genes Dev.* **2009**, *23*, 675–680. [CrossRef] [PubMed]
74. Jin, Z.; Cheng, X.; Feng, H.; Kuang, J.; Yang, W.; Peng, C.; Shen, B.; Qiu, W. Apatinib Inhibits Angiogenesis Via Suppressing Akt/GSK3β/ANG Signaling Pathway in Anaplastic Thyroid Cancer. *Cell. Physiol. Biochem.* **2017**, *44*, 1471–1484. [CrossRef] [PubMed]
75. Prete, A.; Matrone, A.; Gambale, C.; Torregrossa, L.; Minaldi, E.; Romei, C.; Ciampi, R.; Molinaro, E.; Elisei, R. Poorly Differentiated and Anaplastic Thyroid Cancer: Insights into Genomics, Microenvironment and New Drugs. *Cancers* **2021**, *13*, 3200. [CrossRef] [PubMed]
76. Toda, S.; Hiroshima, Y.; Iwasaki, H.; Masudo, K. Genomic landscape and clinical features of advanced thyroid carcinoma: A national database study in Japan. *J. Clin. Endocrinol. Metab.* **2024**, dgae271. [CrossRef] [PubMed]

77. Lee, H.; Kim, S.Y.; Kim, S.M.; Chang, H.J.; Lee, Y.S.; Park, C.S.; Chang, H.S. Long-term survival of patients with anaplastic thyroid cancer after multimodal treatment. *Transl. Cancer Res.* **2020**, *9*, 5430–5436. [CrossRef]
78. Guo, H.; Lin, H. The value of multimodal treatment in anaplastic thyroid cancer patients with distant metastasis. *BMC Surg.* **2024**, *24*, 79. [CrossRef] [PubMed]
79. Hvilsom, G.B.; Londero, S.C.; Hahn, C.H.; Schytte, S.; Pedersen, H.B.; Christiansen, P.; Kiss, K.; Larsen, S.R.; Jespersen, M.L.; Lelkaitis, G.; et al. Anaplastic thyroid carcinoma in Denmark 1996-2012: A national prospective study of 219 patients. *Cancer Epidemiol.* **2018**, *53*, 65–71. [CrossRef]
80. Fan, D.; Ma, J.; Bell, A.C.; Groen, A.H.; Olsen, K.S.; Lok, B.H.; Leeman, J.E.; Anderson, E.; Riaz, N.; McBride, S.; et al. Outcomes of multimodal therapy in a large series of patients with anaplastic thyroid cancer. *Cancer* **2020**, *126*, 444–452. [CrossRef]
81. Prasongsook, N.; Kumar, A.; Chintakuntlawar, A.V.; Foote, R.L.; Kasperbauer, J.; Molina, J.; Garces, Y.; Ma, D.; Wittich, M.A.N.; Rubin, J.; et al. Survival in Response to Multimodal Therapy in Anaplastic Thyroid Cancer. *J. Clin. Endocrinol. Metab.* **2017**, *102*, 4506–4514. [CrossRef] [PubMed]
82. Iyer, P.C.; Dadu, R.; Ferrarotto, R.; Busaidy, N.L.; Habra, M.A.; Zafereo, M.; Gross, N.; Hess, K.R.; Gule-Monroe, M.; Williams, M.D.; et al. Real-World Experience with Targeted Therapy for the Treatment of Anaplastic Thyroid Carcinoma. *Thyroid* **2018**, *28*, 79–87. [CrossRef] [PubMed]
83. Hanna, G.J.; Busaidy, N.L.; Chau, N.G.; Wirth, L.J.; Barletta, J.A.; Calles, A.; Haddad, R.I.; Kraft, S.; Cabanillas, M.E.; Rabinowits, G.; et al. Genomic Correlates of Response to Everolimus in Aggressive Radioiodine-refractory Thyroid Cancer: A Phase II Study. *Clin. Cancer Res.* **2018**, *24*, 1546–1553. [CrossRef]
84. Takahashi, S.; Kiyota, N.; Yamazaki, T.; Chayahara, N.; Nakano, K.; Inagaki, L.; Toda, K.; Enokida, T.; Minami, H.; Imamura, Y.; et al. A Phase II study of the safety and efficacy of lenvatinib in patients with advanced thyroid cancer. *Future Oncol.* **2019**, *15*, 717–726. [CrossRef] [PubMed]
85. Capdevila, J.; Wirth, L.J.; Ernst, T.; Ponce Aix, S.; Lin, C.C.; Ramlau, R.; Butler, M.O.; Delord, J.P.; Gelderblom, H.; Ascierto, P.A.; et al. PD-1 Blockade in Anaplastic Thyroid Carcinoma. *J. Clin. Oncol.* **2020**, *38*, 2620–2627. [CrossRef]
86. Moreno, F.; Reyes, C.; Pineda, C.A.; Castellanos, G.; Cálix, F.; Calderón, J.; Vasquez-Bonilla, W.O. Anaplastic thyroid carcinoma with unusual long-term survival: A case report. *J. Med. Case Rep.* **2022**, *16*, 39. [CrossRef]
87. Sugitani, I.; Hasegawa, Y.; Sugasawa, M.; Tori, M.; Higashiyama, T.; Miyazaki, M.; Hosoi, H.; Orita, Y.; Kitano, H. Super-radical surgery for anaplastic thyroid carcinoma: A large cohort study using the Anaplastic Thyroid Carcinoma Research Consortium of Japan database. *Head Neck* **2014**, *36*, 328–333. [CrossRef]
88. Hermanek, P.; Wittekind, C. Residual tumor (R) classification and prognosis. *Semin. Surg. Oncol.* **1994**, *10*, 12–20. [CrossRef]
89. Wittekind, C.; Compton, C.; Quirke, P.; Nagtegaal, I.; Merkel, S.; Hermanek, P.; Sobin, L.H. A uniform residual tumor (R) classification: Integration of the R classification and the circumferential margin status. *Cancer* **2009**, *115*, 3483–3488. [CrossRef]
90. Pierie, J.P.; Muzikansky, A.; Gaz, R.D.; Faquin, W.C.; Ott, M.J. The effect of surgery and radiotherapy on outcome of anaplastic thyroid carcinoma. *Ann. Surg. Oncol.* **2002**, *9*, 57–64. [CrossRef]
91. Chang, H.S.; Nam, K.H.; Chung, W.Y.; Park, C.S. Anaplastic thyroid carcinoma: A therapeutic dilemma. *Yonsei Med. J.* **2005**, *46*, 759–764. [CrossRef] [PubMed]
92. Oliinyk, D.; Augustin, T.; Rauch, J.; Koehler, V.F.; Belka, C.; Spitzweg, C.; Käsmann, L. Role of surgery to the primary tumor in metastatic anaplastic thyroid carcinoma: Pooled analysis and SEER-based study. *J. Cancer Res. Clin. Oncol.* **2023**, *149*, 3527–3547. [CrossRef] [PubMed]
93. Huang, N.S.; Shi, X.; Lei, B.W.; Wei, W.J.; Lu, Z.W.; Yu, P.C.; Wang, Y.; Ji, Q.H.; Wang, Y.L. An Update of the Appropriate Treatment Strategies in Anaplastic Thyroid Cancer: A Population-Based Study of 735 Patients. *Int. J. Endocrinol.* **2019**, *2019*, 8428547. [CrossRef] [PubMed]
94. Jacob, J.; Vordermark, D.; Lorenz, K.; Medenwald, D. Prognostic factors in radiotherapy of anaplastic thyroid carcinoma: A single center study over 31 years. *Radiat. Oncol.* **2023**, *18*, 71. [CrossRef] [PubMed]
95. Saeed, N.A.; Kelly, J.R.; Deshpande, H.A.; Bhatia, A.K.; Burtness, B.A.; Judson, B.L.; Mehra, S.; Edwards, H.A.; Yarbrough, W.G.; Peter, P.R.; et al. Adjuvant external beam radiotherapy for surgically resected, nonmetastatic anaplastic thyroid cancer. *Head Neck* **2020**, *42*, 1031–1044. [CrossRef]
96. Nachalon, Y.; Stern-Shavit, S.; Bachar, G.; Shvero, J.; Limon, D.; Popovtzer, A. Aggressive Palliation and Survival in Anaplastic Thyroid Carcinoma. *JAMA Otolaryngol. Head Neck Surg.* **2015**, *141*, 1128–1132. [CrossRef] [PubMed]
97. Pezzi, T.A.; Mohamed, A.S.R.; Sheu, T.; Blanchard, P.; Sandulache, V.C.; Lai, S.Y.; Cabanillas, M.E.; Williams, M.D.; Pezzi, C.M.; Lu, C.; et al. Radiation therapy dose is associated with improved survival for unresected anaplastic thyroid carcinoma: Outcomes from the National Cancer Data Base. *Cancer* **2017**, *123*, 1653–1661. [CrossRef] [PubMed]
98. Tennvall, J.; Lundell, G.; Wahlberg, P.; Bergenfelz, A.; Grimelius, L.; Akerman, M.; Hjelm Skog, A.L.; Wallin, G. Anaplastic thyroid carcinoma: Three protocols combining doxorubicin, hyperfractionated radiotherapy and surgery. *Br. J. Cancer* **2002**, *86*, 1848–1853. [CrossRef]
99. De Crevoisier, R.; Baudin, E.; Bachelot, A.; Leboulleux, S.; Travagli, J.P.; Caillou, B.; Schlumberger, M. Combined treatment of anaplastic thyroid carcinoma with surgery, chemotherapy, and hyperfractionated accelerated external radiotherapy. *Int. J. Radiat. Oncol. Biol. Phys.* **2004**, *60*, 1137–1143. [CrossRef]
100. Wang, Y.; Tsang, R.; Asa, S.; Dickson, B.; Arenovich, T.; Brierley, J. Clinical outcome of anaplastic thyroid carcinoma treated with radiotherapy of once- and twice-daily fractionation regimens. *Cancer* **2006**, *107*, 1786–1792. [CrossRef]

101. Dandekar, P.; Harmer, C.; Barbachano, Y.; Rhys-Evans, P.; Harrington, K.; Nutting, C.; Newbold, K. Hyperfractionated Accelerated Radiotherapy (HART) for anaplastic thyroid carcinoma: Toxicity and survival analysis. *Int. J. Radiat. Oncol. Biol. Phys.* **2009**, *74*, 518–521. [CrossRef]
102. Oliinyk, D.; Augustin, T.; Koehler, V.F.; Rauch, J.; Belka, C.; Spitzweg, C.; Käsmann, L. Hypofractionated Radiotherapy for Anaplastic Thyroid Cancer: Systematic Review and Pooled Analysis. *Cancers* **2020**, *12*, 2506. [CrossRef] [PubMed]
103. Stavas, M.J.; Shinohara, E.T.; Attia, A.; Ning, M.S.; Friedman, J.M.; Cmelak, A.J. Short course high dose radiotherapy in the treatment of anaplastic thyroid carcinoma. *J. Thyroid Res.* **2014**, *2014*, 764281. [CrossRef]
104. Takahashi, N.; Matsushita, H.; Umezawa, R.; Yamamoto, T.; Ishikawa, Y.; Katagiri, Y.; Tasaka, S.; Takeda, K.; Fukui, K.; Kadoya, N.; et al. Hypofractionated Radiotherapy for Anaplastic Thyroid Carcinoma: 15 Years of Experience in a Single Institution. *Eur. Thyroid J.* **2019**, *8*, 24–30. [CrossRef]
105. Nutting, C.M.; Convery, D.J.; Cosgrove, V.P.; Rowbottom, C.; Vini, L.; Harmer, C.; Dearnaley, D.P.; Webb, S. Improvements in target coverage and reduced spinal cord irradiation using intensity-modulated radiotherapy (IMRT) in patients with carcinoma of the thyroid gland. *Radiother. Oncol.* **2001**, *60*, 173–180. [CrossRef]
106. Verbakel, W.F.; Cuijpers, J.P.; Hoffmans, D.; Bieker, M.; Slotman, B.J.; Senan, S. Volumetric intensity-modulated arc therapy vs. conventional IMRT in head-and-neck cancer: A comparative planning and dosimetric study. *Int. J. Radiat. Oncol. Biol. Phys.* **2009**, *74*, 252–259. [CrossRef]
107. Sherman, E.J.; Harris, J.; Bible, K.C.; Xia, P.; Ghossein, R.A.; Chung, C.H.; Riaz, N.; Gunn, G.B.; Foote, R.L.; Yom, S.S.; et al. Radiotherapy and paclitaxel plus pazopanib or placebo in anaplastic thyroid cancer (NRG/RTOG 0912): A randomised, double-blind, placebo-controlled, multicentre, phase 2 trial. *Lancet Oncol.* **2023**, *24*, 175–186. [CrossRef] [PubMed]
108. Lee, N.Y.; Riaz, N.; Wu, V.; Brinkman, T.; Tsai, C.J.; Zhi, W.; Fetten, J.; Ho, A.; Wong, R.J.; Ghossein, R.; et al. A Pilot Study of Durvalumab (MEDI4736) with Tremelimumab in Combination with Image-Guided Stereotactic Body Radiotherapy in the Treatment of Metastatic Anaplastic Thyroid Cancer. *Thyroid* **2022**, *32*, 799–806. [CrossRef] [PubMed]
109. Paganetti, H.; Niemierko, A.; Ancukiewicz, M.; Gerweck, L.E.; Goitein, M.; Loeffler, J.S.; Suit, H.D. Relative biological effectiveness (RBE) values for proton beam therapy. *Int. J. Radiat. Oncol. Biol. Phys.* **2002**, *53*, 407–421. [CrossRef]
110. Matsumoto, Y.; Fukumitsu, N.; Ishikawa, H.; Nakai, K.; Sakurai, H. A Critical Review of Radiation Therapy: From Particle Beam Therapy (Proton, Carbon, and BNCT) to Beyond. *J. Pers. Med.* **2021**, *11*, 825. [CrossRef]
111. Sekihara, K.; Himuro, H.; Saito, N.; Ota, Y.; Kouro, T.; Kusano, Y.; Minohara, S.; Hirayama, R.; Katoh, H.; Sasada, T.; et al. Evaluation of X-ray and carbon-ion beam irradiation with chemotherapy for the treatment of cervical adenocarcinoma cells in 2D and 3D cultures. *Cancer Cell Int.* **2022**, *22*, 391. [CrossRef]
112. Youssef, I.; Yoon, J.; Mohamed, N.; Zakeri, K.; Press, R.H.; Yu, Y.; Kang, J.J.; Wong, R.J.; Tuttle, R.M.; Shaha, A.; et al. Outcomes and Toxicities of Nonmedullary Thyroid Tumors Treated with Proton Beam Radiation Therapy. *Int. J. Part. Ther.* **2022**, *9*, 20–30. [CrossRef]
113. Mohamad, O.; Makishima, H.; Kamada, T. Evolution of Carbon Ion Radiotherapy at the National Institute of Radiological Sciences in Japan. *Cancers* **2018**, *10*, 66. [CrossRef] [PubMed]
114. Mattke, M.; Vogt, K.; Bougatf, N.; Welzel, T.; Oelmann-Avendano, J.; Hauswald, H.; Jensen, A.; Ellerbrock, M.; Jäkel, O.; Haberer, T.; et al. High control rates of proton- and carbon-ion-beam treatment with intensity-modulated active raster scanning in 101 patients with skull base chondrosarcoma at the Heidelberg Ion Beam Therapy Center. *Cancer* **2018**, *124*, 2036–2044. [CrossRef]
115. Huang, Q.; Hu, W.; Hu, J.; Gao, J.; Yang, J.; Qiu, X.; Kong, L.; Lu, J.J. Intensity-modulated proton and carbon-ion radiation therapy in the management of major salivary gland carcinomas. *Ann. Transl. Med.* **2022**, *10*, 1195. [CrossRef] [PubMed]
116. Ebner, D.K.; Frank, S.J.; Inaniwa, T.; Yamada, S.; Shirai, T. The Emerging Potential of Multi-Ion Radiotherapy. *Front. Oncol.* **2021**, *11*, 624786. [CrossRef]
117. Hirayama, R.; Uzawa, A.; Obara, M.; Takase, N.; Koda, K.; Ozaki, M.; Noguchi, M.; Matsumoto, Y.; Li, H.; Yamashita, K.; et al. Determination of the relative biological effectiveness and oxygen enhancement ratio for micronuclei formation using high-LET radiation in solid tumor cells: An in vitro and in vivo study. *Mutat. Res./Genet. Toxicol. Environ. Mutagen.* **2015**, *793*, 41–47. [CrossRef]
118. Ito, A.; Kitabatake, S.; Furuichi, W.; Takase, N.; Nakahara, T.; Akiyama, T.; Yoshida, S.; Kusano, Y.; Furusawa, Y.; Hirayama, R. LET Dependence of 8-Hydroxy-2′-deoxyguanosine (8-OHdG) Generation in Mammalian Cells under Air-Saturated and Hypoxic Conditions: A Possible Experimental Approach to the Mechanism of the Decreasing Oxygen Effect in the High-LET Region. *Radiat. Res.* **2024**, *201*, 189–196. [CrossRef] [PubMed]
119. Imaizumi, A.; Hirayama, R.; Ikoma, Y.; Nitta, N.; Obata, T.; Hasegawa, S. Neon ion ($^{20}Ne^{10+}$) charged particle beams manipulate rapid tumor reoxygenation in syngeneic mouse models. *Cancer Sci.* **2024**, *115*, 227–236. [CrossRef]
120. Higashiyama, T.; Ito, Y.; Hirokawa, M.; Fukushima, M.; Uruno, T.; Miya, A.; Matsuzuka, F.; Miyauchi, A. Induction chemotherapy with weekly paclitaxel administration for anaplastic thyroid carcinoma. *Thyroid* **2010**, *20*, 7–14. [CrossRef]
121. Troch, M.; Koperek, O.; Scheuba, C.; Dieckmann, K.; Hoffmann, M.; Niederle, B.; Raderer, M. High efficacy of concomitant treatment of undifferentiated (anaplastic) thyroid cancer with radiation and docetaxel. *J. Clin. Endocrinol. Metab.* **2010**, *95*, E54–E57. [CrossRef] [PubMed]
122. Hanrahan, A.J.; Chen, Z.; Rosen, N.; Solit, D.B. BRAF—A tumour-agnostic drug target with lineage-specific dependencies. *Nat. Rev. Clin. Oncol.* **2024**, *21*, 224–247. [CrossRef] [PubMed]

123. Poulikakos, P.I.; Persaud, Y.; Janakiraman, M.; Kong, X.; Ng, C.; Moriceau, G.; Shi, H.; Atefi, M.; Titz, B.; Gabay, M.T.; et al. RAF inhibitor resistance is mediated by dimerization of aberrantly spliced BRAF(V600E). *Nature* **2011**, *480*, 387–390. [CrossRef] [PubMed]
124. Lito, P.; Pratilas, C.A.; Joseph, E.W.; Tadi, M.; Halilovic, E.; Zubrowski, M.; Huang, A.; Wong, W.L.; Callahan, M.K.; Merghoub, T.; et al. Relief of profound feedback inhibition of mitogenic signaling by RAF inhibitors attenuates their activity in BRAFV600E melanomas. *Cancer Cell* **2012**, *22*, 668–682. [CrossRef] [PubMed]
125. Hirata, E.; Girotti, M.R.; Viros, A.; Hooper, S.; Spencer-Dene, B.; Matsuda, M.; Larkin, J.; Marais, R.; Sahai, E. Intravital imaging reveals how BRAF inhibition generates drug-tolerant microenvironments with high integrin β1/FAK signaling. *Cancer Cell* **2015**, *27*, 574–588. [CrossRef] [PubMed]
126. Kurata, K.; Onoda, N.; Noda, S.; Kashiwagi, S.; Asano, Y.; Hirakawa, K.; Ohira, M. Growth arrest by activated BRAF and MEK inhibition in human anaplastic thyroid cancer cells. *Int. J. Oncol.* **2016**, *49*, 2303–2308. [CrossRef]
127. Lorimer, C.; Cheng, L.; Chandler, R.; Garcez, K.; Gill, V.; Graham, K.; Grant, W.; Sardo Infirri, S.; Wadsley, J.; Wall, L.; et al. Dabrafenib and Trametinib Therapy for Advanced Anaplastic Thyroid Cancer—Real-World Outcomes From UK Centres. *Clin. Oncol.* **2023**, *35*, e60–e66. [CrossRef] [PubMed]
128. Tahara, M.; Kiyota, N.; Imai, H.; Takahashi, S.; Nishiyama, A.; Tamura, S.; Shimizu, Y.; Kadowaki, S.; Ito, K.I.; Toyoshima, M.; et al. A Phase 2 Study of Encorafenib in Combination with Binimetinib in Patients with Metastatic BRAF-Mutated Thyroid Cancer in Japan. *Thyroid* **2024**, *34*, 467–476. [CrossRef] [PubMed]
129. Kim, G.; McKee, A.E.; Ning, Y.M.; Hazarika, M.; Theoret, M.; Johnson, J.R.; Xu, Q.C.; Tang, S.; Sridhara, R.; Jiang, X.; et al. FDA approval summary: Vemurafenib for treatment of unresectable or metastatic melanoma with the BRAFV600E mutation. *Clin. Cancer Res.* **2014**, *20*, 4994–5000. [CrossRef]
130. Zhang, L.; Gaskins, K.; Yu, Z.; Xiong, Y.; Merino, M.J.; Kebebew, E. An in vivo mouse model of metastatic human thyroid cancer. *Thyroid* **2014**, *24*, 695–704. [CrossRef]
131. Hyman, D.M.; Puzanov, I.; Subbiah, V.; Faris, J.E.; Chau, I.; Blay, J.Y.; Wolf, J.; Raje, N.S.; Diamond, E.L.; Hollebecque, A.; et al. Vemurafenib in Multiple Nonmelanoma Cancers with BRAF V600 Mutations. *N. Engl. J. Med.* **2015**, *373*, 726–736. [CrossRef] [PubMed]
132. Li, Q.; Li, Z.; Luo, T.; Shi, H. Targeting the PI3K/AKT/mTOR and RAF/MEK/ERK pathways for cancer therapy. *Mol. Biomed.* **2022**, *3*, 47. [CrossRef]
133. Zaballos, M.A.; Acuña-Ruiz, A.; Morante, M.; Riesco-Eizaguirre, G.; Crespo, P.; Santisteban, P. Inhibiting ERK dimerization ameliorates BRAF-driven anaplastic thyroid cancer. *Cell. Mol. Life Sci.* **2022**, *79*, 504. [CrossRef] [PubMed]
134. Owonikoko, T.K.; Zhang, G.; Lallani, S.B.; Chen, Z.; Martinson, D.E.; Khuri, F.R.; Lonial, S.; Marcus, A.; Sun, S.Y. Evaluation of preclinical efficacy of everolimus and pasireotide in thyroid cancer cell lines and xenograft models. *PLoS ONE* **2019**, *14*, e0206309. [CrossRef]
135. Lim, S.M.; Chang, H.; Yoon, M.J.; Hong, Y.K.; Kim, H.; Chung, W.Y.; Park, C.S.; Nam, K.H.; Kang, S.W.; Kim, M.K.; et al. A multicenter, phase II trial of everolimus in locally advanced or metastatic thyroid cancer of all histologic subtypes. *Ann. Oncol.* **2013**, *24*, 3089–3094. [CrossRef]
136. Schneider, T.C.; de Wit, D.; Links, T.P.; van Erp, N.P.; van der Hoeven, J.J.; Gelderblom, H.; Roozen, I.C.; Bos, M.; Corver, W.E.; van Wezel, T.; et al. Everolimus in Patients With Advanced Follicular-Derived Thyroid Cancer: Results of a Phase II Clinical Trial. *J. Clin. Endocrinol. Metab.* **2017**, *102*, 698–707. [CrossRef] [PubMed]
137. Shimobayashi, M.; Hall, M.N. Making new contacts: The mTOR network in metabolism and signalling crosstalk. *Nat. Rev. Mol. Cell Biol.* **2014**, *15*, 155–162. [CrossRef] [PubMed]
138. Gökmen-Polar, Y.; Liu, Y.; Toroni, R.A.; Sanders, K.L.; Mehta, R.; Badve, S.; Rommel, C.; Sledge, G.W., Jr. Investigational drug MLN0128, a novel TORC1/2 inhibitor, demonstrates potent oral antitumor activity in human breast cancer xenograft models. *Breast Cancer Res. Treat.* **2012**, *136*, 673–682. [CrossRef]
139. Harada, M.; Benito, J.; Yamamoto, S.; Kaur, S.; Arslan, D.; Ramirez, S.; Jacamo, R.; Platanias, L.; Matsushita, H.; Fujimura, T.; et al. The novel combination of dual mTOR inhibitor AZD2014 and pan-PIM inhibitor AZD1208 inhibits growth in acute myeloid leukemia via HSF pathway suppression. *Oncotarget* **2015**, *6*, 37930–37947. [CrossRef]
140. Sekihara, K.; Saitoh, K.; Han, L.; Ciurea, S.; Yamamoto, S.; Kikkawa, M.; Kazuno, S.; Taka, H.; Kaga, N.; Arai, H.; et al. Targeting mantle cell lymphoma metabolism and survival through simultaneous blockade of mTOR and nuclear transporter exportin-1. *Oncotarget* **2017**, *8*, 34552–34564. [CrossRef]
141. Jordan, N.J.; Dutkowski, C.M.; Barrow, D.; Mottram, H.J.; Hutcheson, I.R.; Nicholson, R.I.; Guichard, S.M.; Gee, J.M. Impact of dual mTORC1/2 mTOR kinase inhibitor AZD8055 on acquired endocrine resistance in breast cancer in vitro. *Breast Cancer Res.* **2014**, *16*, R12. [CrossRef]
142. Kotian, S.; Zhang, L.; Boufraqech, M.; Gaskins, K.; Gara, S.K.; Quezado, M.; Nilubol, N.; Kebebew, E. Dual Inhibition of HDAC and Tyrosine Kinase Signaling Pathways with CUDC-907 Inhibits Thyroid Cancer Growth and Metastases. *Clin. Cancer Res.* **2017**, *23*, 5044–5054. [CrossRef]
143. Hescheler, D.A.; Hartmann, M.J.M.; Riemann, B.; Michel, M.; Bruns, C.J.; Alakus, H.; Chiapponi, C. Anaplastic thyroid cancer: Genome-based search for new targeted therapy options. *Endocr. Connect.* **2022**, *11*, e210624. [CrossRef] [PubMed]
144. Massacesi, C.; Di Tomaso, E.; Urban, P.; Germa, C.; Quadt, C.; Trandafir, L.; Aimone, P.; Fretault, N.; Dharan, B.; Tavorath, R.; et al. PI3K inhibitors as new cancer therapeutics: Implications for clinical trial design. *OncoTargets Ther.* **2016**, *9*, 203–210. [CrossRef]

145. Lorusso, L.; Newbold, K. Lenvatinib: A new option for the treatment of advanced iodine refractory differentiated thyroid cancer? *Future Oncol.* **2015**, *11*, 1719–1727. [CrossRef] [PubMed]
146. Ferrari, S.M.; Bocci, G.; Di Desidero, T.; Elia, G.; Ruffilli, I.; Ragusa, F.; Orlandi, P.; Paparo, S.R.; Patrizio, A.; Piaggi, S.; et al. Lenvatinib exhibits antineoplastic activity in anaplastic thyroid cancer in vitro and in vivo. *Oncol. Rep.* **2018**, *39*, 2225–2234. [CrossRef]
147. Koyama, S.; Miyake, N.; Fujiwara, K.; Morisaki, T.; Fukuhara, T.; Kitano, H.; Takeuchi, H. Lenvatinib for Anaplastic Thyroid Cancer and Lenvatinib-Induced Thyroid Dysfunction. *Eur. Thyroid J.* **2018**, *7*, 139–144. [CrossRef] [PubMed]
148. Iñiguez-Ariza, N.M.; Ryder, M.M.; Hilger, C.R.; Bible, K.C. Salvage Lenvatinib Therapy in Metastatic Anaplastic Thyroid Cancer. *Thyroid* **2017**, *27*, 923–927. [CrossRef]
149. Wirth, L.J.; Brose, M.S.; Sherman, E.J.; Licitra, L.; Schlumberger, M.; Sherman, S.I.; Bible, K.C.; Robinson, B.; Rodien, P.; Godbert, Y.; et al. Open-Label, Single-Arm, Multicenter, Phase II Trial of Lenvatinib for the Treatment of Patients With Anaplastic Thyroid Cancer. *J. Clin. Oncol.* **2021**, *39*, 2359–2366. [CrossRef]
150. Higashiyama, T.; Sugino, K.; Hara, H.; Ito, K.I.; Nakashima, N.; Onoda, N.; Tori, M.; Katoh, H.; Kiyota, N.; Ota, I.; et al. Phase II study of the efficacy and safety of lenvatinib for anaplastic thyroid cancer (HOPE). *Eur. J. Cancer* **2022**, *173*, 210–218. [CrossRef]
151. Ishihara, S.; Onoda, N.; Noda, S.; Asano, Y.; Tauchi, Y.; Morisaki, T.; Kashiwagi, S.; Takashima, T.; Ohira, M. Sorafenib inhibits vascular endothelial cell proliferation stimulated by anaplastic thyroid cancer cells regardless of BRAF mutation status. *Int. J. Oncol.* **2019**, *55*, 1069–1076. [CrossRef] [PubMed]
152. Kim, S.; Yazici, Y.D.; Calzada, G.; Wang, Z.Y.; Younes, M.N.; Jasser, S.A.; El-Naggar, A.K.; Myers, J.N. Sorafenib inhibits the angiogenesis and growth of orthotopic anaplastic thyroid carcinoma xenografts in nude mice. *Mol. Cancer Ther.* **2007**, *6*, 1785–1792. [CrossRef] [PubMed]
153. Schiff, B.A.; McMurphy, A.B.; Jasser, S.A.; Younes, M.N.; Doan, D.; Yigitbasi, O.G.; Kim, S.; Zhou, G.; Mandal, M.; Bekele, B.N.; et al. Epidermal growth factor receptor (EGFR) is overexpressed in anaplastic thyroid cancer, and the EGFR inhibitor gefitinib inhibits the growth of anaplastic thyroid cancer. *Clin. Cancer Res.* **2004**, *10*, 8594–8602. [CrossRef] [PubMed]
154. Nobuhara, Y.; Onoda, N.; Yamashita, Y.; Yamasaki, M.; Ogisawa, K.; Takashima, T.; Ishikawa, T.; Hirakawa, K. Efficacy of epidermal growth factor receptor-targeted molecular therapy in anaplastic thyroid cancer cell lines. *Br. J. Cancer* **2005**, *92*, 1110–1116. [CrossRef] [PubMed]
155. Podtcheko, A.; Ohtsuru, A.; Tsuda, S.; Namba, H.; Saenko, V.; Nakashima, M.; Mitsutake, N.; Kanda, S.; Kurebayashi, J.; Yamashita, S. The selective tyrosine kinase inhibitor, STI571, inhibits growth of anaplastic thyroid cancer cells. *J. Clin. Endocrinol. Metab.* **2003**, *88*, 1889–1896. [CrossRef] [PubMed]
156. Di Desidero, T.; Fioravanti, A.; Orlandi, P.; Canu, B.; Giannini, R.; Borrelli, N.; Man, S.; Xu, P.; Fontanini, G.; Basolo, F.; et al. Antiproliferative and proapoptotic activity of sunitinib on endothelial and anaplastic thyroid cancer cells via inhibition of Akt and ERK1/2 phosphorylation and by down-regulation of cyclin-D1. *J. Clin. Endocrinol. Metab.* **2013**, *98*, E1465–E1473. [CrossRef] [PubMed]
157. Di Desidero, T.; Orlandi, P.; Gentile, D.; Bocci, G. Effects of Pazopanib Monotherapy vs. Pazopanib and Topotecan Combination on Anaplastic Thyroid Cancer Cells. *Front. Oncol.* **2019**, *9*, 1202. [CrossRef]
158. Savvides, P.; Nagaiah, G.; Lavertu, P.; Fu, P.; Wright, J.J.; Chapman, R.; Wasman, J.; Dowlati, A.; Remick, S.C. Phase II trial of sorafenib in patients with advanced anaplastic carcinoma of the thyroid. *Thyroid* **2013**, *23*, 600–604. [CrossRef] [PubMed]
159. Ito, Y.; Onoda, N.; Ito, K.I.; Sugitani, I.; Takahashi, S.; Yamaguchi, I.; Kabu, K.; Tsukada, K. Sorafenib in Japanese Patients with Locally Advanced or Metastatic Medullary Thyroid Carcinoma and Anaplastic Thyroid Carcinoma. *Thyroid* **2017**, *27*, 1142–1148. [CrossRef]
160. Pennell, N.A.; Daniels, G.H.; Haddad, R.I.; Ross, D.S.; Evans, T.; Wirth, L.J.; Fidias, P.H.; Temel, J.S.; Gurubhagavatula, S.; Heist, R.S.; et al. A phase II study of gefitinib in patients with advanced thyroid cancer. *Thyroid* **2008**, *18*, 317–323. [CrossRef]
161. Ha, H.T.; Lee, J.S.; Urba, S.; Koenig, R.J.; Sisson, J.; Giordano, T.; Worden, F.P. A phase II study of imatinib in patients with advanced anaplastic thyroid cancer. *Thyroid* **2010**, *20*, 975–980. [CrossRef] [PubMed]
162. Ravaud, A.; de la Fouchardière, C.; Caron, P.; Doussau, A.; Do Cao, C.; Asselineau, J.; Rodien, P.; Pouessel, D.; Nicolli-Sire, P.; Klein, M.; et al. A multicenter phase II study of sunitinib in patients with locally advanced or metastatic differentiated, anaplastic or medullary thyroid carcinomas: Mature data from the THYSU study. *Eur. J. Cancer* **2017**, *76*, 110–117. [CrossRef] [PubMed]
163. Bible, K.C.; Suman, V.J.; Menefee, M.E.; Smallridge, R.C.; Molina, J.R.; Maples, W.J.; Karlin, N.J.; Traynor, A.M.; Kumar, P.; Goh, B.C.; et al. A multiinstitutional phase 2 trial of pazopanib monotherapy in advanced anaplastic thyroid cancer. *J. Clin. Endocrinol. Metab.* **2012**, *97*, 3179–3184. [CrossRef] [PubMed]
164. Jiang, X.; Wang, J.; Deng, X.; Xiong, F.; Ge, J.; Xiang, B.; Wu, X.; Ma, J.; Zhou, M.; Li, X.; et al. Role of the tumor microenvironment in PD-L1/PD-1-mediated tumor immune escape. *Mol. Cancer* **2019**, *18*, 10. [CrossRef] [PubMed]
165. Adam, P.; Kircher, S.; Sbiera, I.; Koehler, V.F.; Berg, E.; Knösel, T.; Sandner, B.; Fenske, W.K.; Bläker, H.; Smaxwil, C.; et al. FGF-Receptors and PD-L1 in Anaplastic and Poorly Differentiated Thyroid Cancer: Evaluation of the Preclinical Rationale. *Front. Endocrinol.* **2021**, *12*, 712107. [CrossRef] [PubMed]
166. Chintakuntlawar, A.V.; Rumilla, K.M.; Smith, C.Y.; Jenkins, S.M.; Foote, R.L.; Kasperbauer, J.L.; Morris, J.C.; Ryder, M.; Alsidawi, S.; Hilger, C.; et al. Expression of PD-1 and PD-L1 in Anaplastic Thyroid Cancer Patients Treated With Multimodal Therapy: Results From a Retrospective Study. *J. Clin. Endocrinol. Metab.* **2017**, *102*, 1943–1950. [CrossRef] [PubMed]

167. Cantara, S.; Bertelli, E.; Occhini, R.; Regoli, M.; Brilli, L.; Pacini, F.; Castagna, M.G.; Toti, P. Blockade of the programmed death ligand 1 (PD-L1) as potential therapy for anaplastic thyroid cancer. *Endocrine* **2019**, *64*, 122–129. [CrossRef] [PubMed]
168. Iyer, P.C.; Dadu, R.; Gule-Monroe, M.; Busaidy, N.L.; Ferrarotto, R.; Habra, M.A.; Zafereo, M.; Williams, M.D.; Gunn, G.B.; Grosu, H.; et al. Salvage pembrolizumab added to kinase inhibitor therapy for the treatment of anaplastic thyroid carcinoma. *J. Immunother. Cancer* **2018**, *6*, 68. [CrossRef] [PubMed]
169. Wang, J.R.; Zafereo, M.E.; Dadu, R.; Ferrarotto, R.; Busaidy, N.L.; Lu, C.; Ahmed, S.; Gule-Monroe, M.K.; Williams, M.D.; Sturgis, E.M.; et al. Complete Surgical Resection Following Neoadjuvant Dabrafenib Plus Trametinib in BRAF(V600E)-Mutated Anaplastic Thyroid Carcinoma. *Thyroid* **2019**, *29*, 1036–1043. [CrossRef]
170. Boudin, L.; Morvan, J.B.; Thariat, J.; Métivier, D.; Marcy, P.Y.; Delarbre, D. Rationale Efficacy and Safety Evidence of Lenvatinib and Pembrolizumab Association in Anaplastic Thyroid Carcinoma. *Curr. Oncol.* **2022**, *29*, 7718–7731. [CrossRef]
171. Kang, Y.K.; Boku, N.; Satoh, T.; Ryu, M.H.; Chao, Y.; Kato, K.; Chung, H.C.; Chen, J.S.; Muro, K.; Kang, W.K.; et al. Nivolumab in patients with advanced gastric or gastro-oesophageal junction cancer refractory to, or intolerant of, at least two previous chemotherapy regimens (ONO-4538-12, ATTRACTION-2): A randomised, double-blind, placebo-controlled, phase 3 trial. *Lancet* **2017**, *390*, 2461–2471. [CrossRef] [PubMed]
172. Michot, J.M.; Bigenwald, C.; Champiat, S.; Collins, M.; Carbonnel, F.; Postel-Vinay, S.; Berdelou, A.; Varga, A.; Bahleda, R.; Hollebecque, A.; et al. Immune-related adverse events with immune checkpoint blockade: A comprehensive review. *Eur. J. Cancer* **2016**, *54*, 139–148. [CrossRef] [PubMed]
173. Patrinely, J.R., Jr.; Johnson, R.; Lawless, A.R.; Bhave, P.; Sawyers, A.; Dimitrova, M.; Yeoh, H.L.; Palmeri, M.; Ye, F.; Fan, R.; et al. Chronic Immune-Related Adverse Events Following Adjuvant Anti-PD-1 Therapy for High-risk Resected Melanoma. *JAMA Oncol.* **2021**, *7*, 744–748. [CrossRef] [PubMed]
174. Park, E.M.; Chelvanambi, M.; Bhutiani, N.; Kroemer, G.; Zitvogel, L.; Wargo, J.A. Targeting the gut and tumor microbiota in cancer. *Nat. Med.* **2022**, *28*, 690–703. [CrossRef] [PubMed]
175. Jiao, J.; Zheng, Y.; Zhang, Q.; Xia, D.; Zhang, L.; Ma, N. Saliva microbiome changes in thyroid cancer and thyroid nodules patients. *Front. Cell. Infect. Microbiol.* **2022**, *12*, 989188. [CrossRef] [PubMed]
176. Kun, Y.; Xiaodong, W.; Haijun, W.; Xiazi, N.; Dai, Q. Exploring the oral-gut microbiota during thyroid cancer: Factors affecting the thyroid functions and cancer development. *Food Sci. Nutr.* **2023**, *11*, 5657–5674. [CrossRef] [PubMed]
177. Zhang, J.; Zhang, F.; Zhao, C.; Xu, Q.; Liang, C.; Yang, Y.; Wang, H.; Shang, Y.; Wang, Y.; Mu, X.; et al. Dysbiosis of the gut microbiome is associated with thyroid cancer and thyroid nodules and correlated with clinical index of thyroid function. *Endocrine* **2019**, *64*, 564–574. [CrossRef] [PubMed]
178. Liu, C.J.; Chen, S.Q.; Zhang, S.Y.; Wang, J.L.; Tang, X.D.; Yang, K.X.; Li, X.R. The comparison of microbial communities in thyroid tissues from thyroid carcinoma patients. *J. Microbiol.* **2021**, *59*, 988–1001. [CrossRef]
179. Dai, D.; Yang, Y.; Yang, Y.; Dang, T.; Xiao, J.; Wang, W.; Teng, L.; Xu, J.; Ye, J.; Jiang, H. Alterations of thyroid microbiota across different thyroid microhabitats in patients with thyroid carcinoma. *J. Transl. Med.* **2021**, *19*, 488. [CrossRef]
180. Zheng, L.; Zhang, L.; Tang, L.; Huang, D.; Pan, D.; Guo, W.; He, S.; Huang, Y.; Chen, Y.; Xiao, X.; et al. Gut microbiota is associated with response to (131)I therapy in patients with papillary thyroid carcinoma. *Eur. J. Nucl. Med. Mol. Imaging* **2023**, *50*, 1453–1465. [CrossRef]
181. Zhao, L.Y.; Mei, J.X.; Yu, G.; Lei, L.; Zhang, W.H.; Liu, K.; Chen, X.L.; Kołat, D.; Yang, K.; Hu, J.K. Role of the gut microbiota in anticancer therapy: From molecular mechanisms to clinical applications. *Signal Transduct. Target. Ther.* **2023**, *8*, 201. [CrossRef] [PubMed]
182. Liu, Q.; Sun, W.; Zhang, H. Interaction of Gut Microbiota with Endocrine Homeostasis and Thyroid Cancer. *Cancers* **2022**, *14*, 2656. [CrossRef] [PubMed]
183. Moyer, K.F.; Marcadis, A.R.; Shaha, A.R. Airway management, symptom relief and best supportive care in anaplastic thyroid cancer. *Curr. Opin. Otolaryngol. Head Neck Surg.* **2020**, *28*, 74–78. [CrossRef] [PubMed]

biomedicines

MDPI

Review

Molecular Pathology of Thyroid Tumors: Essential Points to Comprehend Regarding the Latest WHO Classification

Tomohiro Chiba [1,2]

[1] Department of Cytology, Cancer Institute Hospital, Japanese Foundation for Cancer Research, 3-8-31 Ariake, Koto-ku, Tokyo 135-8550, Japan; tomohiro.chiba@jfcr.or.jp; Tel.: +81-3-3520-0111; Fax: +81-3-3570-0558

[2] Department of Pathology, Cancer Institute Hospital, Japanese Foundation for Cancer Research, 3-8-31 Ariake, Koto-ku, Tokyo 135-8550, Japan

Abstract: In 2022, the new WHO Classification of Endocrine and Neuroendocrine Tumors, Fifth Edition (beta version) (WHO 5th), was published. Large-scale genomic analyses such as The Cancer Genome Atlas (TCGA) have revealed the importance of understanding the molecular genetics of thyroid tumors. Consequently, the WHO 5th was fundamentally revised, resulting in a systematic classification based on the cell of origin of tumors and their clinical risk. This paper outlines the following critical points of the WHO 5th. 1. Genetic mutations in follicular cell-derived neoplasms (FDNs) highlight the role of mutations in the MAP kinase pathway, including *RET*, *RAS*, and *BRAF*, as drivers of carcinogenesis. Differentiated thyroid cancers such as follicular thyroid carcinoma (FTC) and papillary thyroid carcinoma (PTC) have specific genetic alterations that correlate with morphological classifications: *RAS*-like tumors (RLTs) and *BRAF* p.V600E-like tumors (BLTs), respectively. 2. The framework for benign lesions has been revised. The WHO 5th introduces a new category: "developmental abnormalities". Benign FDNs comprise "thyroid follicular nodular disease", follicular thyroid adenoma (FTA), FTA with papillary architecture, and oncocytic adenoma (OA). "Hürthle cell adenoma/carcinoma" is renamed oncocytic adenoma/carcinoma of the thyroid (OA/OCA), which can be distinguished from FTA/FTC by its unique genetic background. 3. Low-risk tumors include NIFTP, TT-UMP, and HTT, and they have an extremely low malignant potential or an uncertain malignant potential. 4. PTC histological variants are reclassified as "subtypes" in the WHO 5th. 5. The concept of high-grade carcinomas is introduced, encompassing poorly differentiated thyroid carcinoma (PDTC), differentiated high-grade thyroid carcinoma (DHGTC), and high-grade medullary thyroid carcinoma (MTC). 6. Squamous cell carcinoma is included in anaplastic thyroid carcinoma (ATC) in the WHO 5th due to their shared genetic and prognostic features. 7. Other miscellaneous tumors are categorized as salivary-gland-type carcinomas of the thyroid, thyroid tumors of uncertain histogenesis, thymic tumors within the thyroid, and embryonal thyroid neoplasms. The WHO 5th thus emphasizes the importance of classifying tumors based on both genetic abnormalities and histomorphology. This approach aids in achieving accurate pathological diagnosis and facilitates the early selection of appropriate treatment options, including molecular targeted therapies.

Keywords: thyroid cancer; genomic alterations; pathological diagnosis; WHO classification

1. Introduction

Thyroid cancer diagnoses, particularly in women, are on the rise. Improved detection methods have likely contributed to this trend, although environmental factors are also under investigation. Despite the increase in diagnoses, mortality rates remain low. Thyroid tumors are classified by listing the major histologic types: follicular thyroid adenoma (FTA), a benign tumor; papillary thyroid carcinoma (PTC); follicular thyroid carcinoma (FTC); anaplastic thyroid carcinoma (ATC); and medullary thyroid carcinoma (MTC) [1,2]. The results of large-scale genome analyses, including TCGA (The Cancer Genome Atlas), have accumulated. The fourth edition of the WHO Classification of Endocrine Tumors

(WHO 4th), published in 2017, included information on the driver genes associated with thyroid cancer [2]. WHO released a beta version of the new classification of endocrine and neuroendocrine tumors (WHO 5th) in 2022 [3,4]. Continuing the trend of the WHO 4th and taking tumor-specific molecular genetic information into account, the WHO 5th has been fundamentally revised. It now includes a systematic classification based on the cell of origin and the clinical risk (Table 1). The main categories are follicular cell-derived neoplasms (FDNs) and parafollicular cell (C cell)-derived tumors, with FDNs further divided into three classes: benign, low-risk, and malignant (Table 1). The only C cell-derived tumor is the malignant MTC, which encompasses low-grade and high-grade subcategories. Other tumors are also re-classified as salivary-gland-type carcinomas of the thyroid, thyroid tumors of uncertain histogenesis, thymic tumors within the thyroid, and embryonal thyroid neoplasms. This paper outlines critical points that enable us to better understand the WHO 5th.

Table 1. Summary of the WHO classification, 5th edition (beta, 2022).

WHO 4th Edition	WHO 5th Edition
Follicular thyroid adenoma (FTA) Hyalinizing trabecular tumour (HTT) Other encapsulated follicular-patterned thyroid tumours Follicular tumour of uncertain malignant potential (FT-UMP), Well-differentiated tumour of uncertain malignant potential (WDT-UMP), Non-invasive follicular thyroid neoplasm with papillary-like nuclear features (NIFTP) Papillary thyroid carcinoma (PTC) Follicular thyroid carcinoma (FTC), NOS Hürthle cell tumours Hürthle cell adenoma, Hürthle cell carcinoma Poorly differentiated thyroid carcinoma (PDTC) Anaplastic thyroid carcinoma (ATC) Squamous cell carcinoma (SCC) Medullary thyroid carcinoma (MTC) Mixed medullary and follicular thyroid carcinoma Mucoepidermoid carcinoma (MEC) Sclerosing mucoepidermoid carcinoma with eosinophilia (SMECE) Mucinous carcinoma Ectopic thymoma Spindle epithelial tumor with thymus-like elements (SETTLE) Intrathyroidal thymic carcinoma (ITC)	1. Developmental abnormalities 2. Follicular cell-derived neoplasms 2.1 Benign tumours: Thyroid follicular nodular disease (TFND), FTA, Oncocytic adenoma (OA) 2.2 Low-risk neoplasm: NIFTP, Thyroid tumor UMP (TT-UMP), HTT 2.3 Malignant neoplasms: FTC, Invasive encapsulated follicular variant of papillary thyroid carcinoma (IEFVPTC), PTC, Oncocytic carcinoma (OCA), Differentiated high-grade thyroid carcinoma (DHGTC)/PDTC, ATC 3. Thyroid C-cell derived carcinoma MTC: low-grade, high-grade 4. Mixed medullary and follicular cell-derived carcinomas 5. Salivary gland-type carcinomas of the thyroid MEC, Secretory carcinoma 6. Thyroid tumours of uncertain histogenesis SMECE, Cribriform morular carcinoma 7. Thymic tumours within the thyroid Thymoma, SETTLE, ITC 8. Embryonal thyroid neoplasms Thyroblastoma

2. Essential Points to Comprehend the Latest WHO Classification

2.1. Genetic Mutations in Follicular Cell-Derived Tumors (FDNs)

In FDNs, genetic abnormalities in the MAP kinase pathway, starting from receptor-type tyrosine kinases such as *RET*, *RAS*, and *BRAF*, are the drivers of carcinogenesis [2–5]. In differentiated thyroid cancers such as PTC and FTC, a limited number of mutations such as *BRAF* p.V600E, *RET* translocations (*CCDC6::RET*, *NCOA4::RET*, etc.), *H/K/NRAS* mutations such as *NRAS* p.Q61R, and *PAX8::PPARG* translocation are often found, and these are mutually exclusive (Figure 1).

BRAF p.V600E mutation, along with *RET* and *NTRK* rearrangements, have been identified as primary genetic aberrations in PTC [2–4]. Notably, *BRAF* p.V600E exhibits a high specificity for PTC. Their detection, even in minute quantities within fine-needle aspiration cytology specimens, plays a pivotal role in diagnosing PTC [6]. Additionally, *RAS* point mutations have been documented in follicular PTC and FTC. It is worth noting that *RAS* mutations have also been observed in FTA and benign thyroid nodules. Furthermore, nodules harboring *RAS* mutations have been associated with accelerated growth rates [7].

Unlike the well-known *BRAF* p.V600E mutation, other alterations in the *BRAF* gene, such as p.K601 mutations and gene rearrangements, have been detected in FTC as well as benign follicular tumors [2–4].

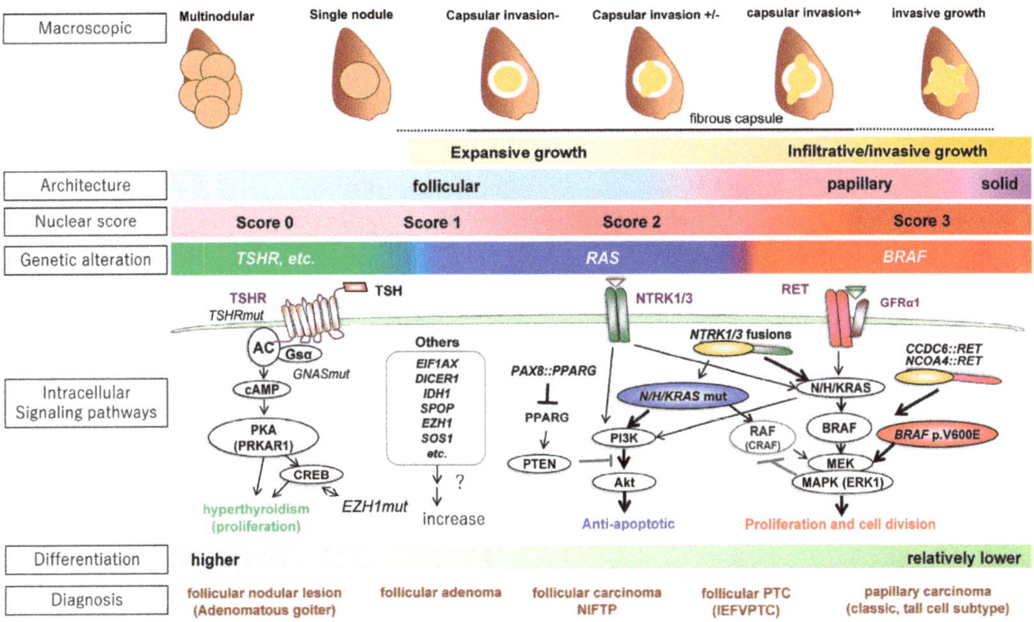

Figure 1. Morphology, genetic abnormalities, and intracellular signaling pathways of differentiated thyroid tumors. The three most important gross characteristics of thyroid tumors are (i) single or multiple nodules, (ii) capsule formation, and (iii) the presence or absence of invasive growth. A lesion with a single nodule and a thick fibrous capsule indicates a neoplastic lesion that has expansively grown over time. Multinodular lesions are more likely to be non-neoplastic. Lesions with irregular margins are suspected of infiltrative growth and may be malignant. The most important histological findings are the histological architecture (follicular, papillary, or solid) and papillary carcinoma (PTC)-like nuclear features ("nuclear score": nuclear enlargement, glassy chromatin, and irregular nuclear shape [nuclear grooves and pseudo-inclusions]), with one point given for each [Total 0–3 points]). Regarding genetic mutations, well-differentiated tumors such as thyroid follicular nodular disease (or functional nodules) show abnormalities in the TSHR to GNAS/cAMP/PKA pathway. Differentiated tumors can be classified into *RAS*-like tumors (RLTs) and *BRAF* p.V600E-like tumors (BLTs). Many of the driver gene mutations in differentiated thyroid cancer contribute to the activation of the MAPK and PI3K/Akt pathways downstream of tyrosine kinase receptors such as RET and NTRKs. RLTs activate the MAPK and PI3K pathways, and CRAF induces negative feedback to inhibit MAPK. As a result, the anti-apoptotic effect via the PI3K pathway is predominant in RLTs. BLTs activate the MAPK pathway, which is highly proliferative. In well-differentiated thyroid tumors such as thyroid follicular nodular disease (or functional nodule), activation of the TSH receptor-mediated cAMP pathway is predominant; this promotes hormonal functions, such as iodine metabolism and the expression of hormone-related genes.

The findings from a comprehensive thyroid cancer genome analysis [8] have demonstrated a strong correlation between driver gene types and morphological classifications. Through genetic alteration pattern analysis, the TCGA study introduced the BRAF-RAS score, delineating two distinct subgroups within PTC: *BRAF* p.V600E-like tumors (BLTs) and *RAS*-like tumors (RLTs). Moreover, compiled evidence from several next-generation sequence (NGS) analyses have demonstrated that this dichotomous classification is not only applicable to PTC, but also extends to FTA and FTC, with BLTs displaying a classic PTC morphology and RLTs encompassing FTA, FTC, and follicular PTC [Korea].

The driver gene mutations of the typical FTC are *RAS* mutations or *PAX8::PPARG* translocation (PAX8::PPARG fusion protein), and FTC grows expansively with a retained follicular structure and forms a fibrous capsule (Figure 1). FTC expresses iodine metabolism-related and hormone-related genes, showing thyroidal differentiation. Such tumors are called "RAS-like tumors (RLTs)" with regard to the genetic mutations.

On the other hand, the typical PTC has *BRAF* p.V600E mutations and *RET* fusion genes and grows invasively with a papillary structure and characteristic nuclear atypia (e.g., ground glass-like chromatin, nuclear grooves, and intranuclear cytoplasmic inclusions). Such tumors are referred to as "*BRAF* p.V600E-like tumors (BLTs)". BLTs have a lower iodine metabolic capacity and lower hormone differentiation compared to RLTs. The *BRAF* p.K601E mutation is found in RLTs. Some tumors are difficult to classify as BLTs or RLTs (non-*BRAF*/non-*RAS* tumors: NBNRs).

2.2. Revision of the Framework for Benign Lesions

The fourth edition of WHO (WHO 4th) listed only FTA and Hürthle cell adenoma as benign lesions. The WHO 5th adopted a new category, namely "developmental abnormalities", to include pathologies such as thyroglossal duct cysts; it also added "thyroid follicular nodular disease (TFND [or multinodular goiter: MNG])", which often exhibits clonality [3–5], to the benign FDN classification (Table 1).

While most FTAs are RLTs, TFND has a cluster of genetic abnormalities in the thyroid-stimulating hormone receptor (TSHR) and its downstream pathway consisting of Gsα-adenylyl cyclase-protein kinase A (PKA). The most frequent mutation in TFND is the *TSHR* mutation (~70%). Other driver genes in TFND include *GNAS*, *EZH1*, *ZNF148*, and *SPOP* [9,10]. Carney complex (CNC) is an autosomal dominant tumor predisposition syndrome that affects endocrine glands, including the thyroid [3]. Up to 60% of CNC patients develop thyroid nodules. CNC is associated with pathological variations in *PRKAR1A* downstream of cAMP. DICER1 syndrome, caused by pathogenic variants in *DICER1*, is another autosomal dominant tumor predisposition syndrome that affects multiple organs, including the thyroid [3]. The most common manifestation is benign thyroid nodules (MNG), which occur in approximately 75% of females and 10–20% of males with *DICER1* pathogenic variants by the age of 40.

FTA with papillary architecture (FTAPA) is a benign non-invasive encapsulated FDN characterized by an intrafollicular papillary architecture; this lacks PTC-like nuclear features and is often associated with hyperthyroidism. Like TFND, mutations in *TSHR*, *GNAS*, *PRKAR1A*, and *EZH1* are common.

Hürthle cell adenoma (formerly called follicular adenoma, oxyphilic cell variant) is renamed oncocytic adenoma of the thyroid (OA) in the WHO 5th. Accordingly, the malignant counterpart of OA is renamed oncocytic carcinoma of the thyroid (OCA). The name "Hürthle cell tumor" is no longer used because it is inappropriate. OA/OCA were distinguished from FTA/FTC by their characteristic morphology, as well as their unique genetic background [11,12]. OA/OCA have a high frequency of gene mutations in the mitochondrial biosynthesis system, such as *ESRRA* and *PPARGC1A*, and have characteristic genetic abnormalities such as a near-haploid (or monoploid) karyotype. OA/OCA, on the other hand, have a low frequency of *RAS* mutations and *PAX8::PPARG* translocations, which are the major driver mutations of FN. Oxyphilic PTC, which generally has *BRAF* p.V600E-like genetic backgrounds, is not included in OCA.

The criteria for differentiating OA from OCA are the same as those for follicular tumors: the presence of capsular invasion and vascular invasion. Like the subclassification of FTC, OCA is subdivided into three subtypes: minimally invasive, encapsulated angioinvasive, and widely invasive OCA.

2.3. Low-Risk Tumors

"Low-risk tumors" in FDNs are a morphological and clinical intermediate between benign and malignant tumors. Low-risk tumors have the potential to metastasize but do so infrequently. Low-risk tumors comprise non-invasive follicular thyroid neoplasms with papillary-like nuclear features (NIFTPs), thyroid tumors of uncertain malignant potential (TT-UMPs), and hyalinizing trabecular tumors (HTTs).

NIFTPs are encapsulated FDNs with a follicular growth pattern and PTC-like nuclear features, lacking capsular and/or vascular invasion (Figure 2A–C). NIFTPs were previously diagnosed as an encapsulated follicular variant PTC and renamed due to their favorable prognosis [13]. The exclusion criteria for NIFTPs are (i) psammoma bodies, (ii) a mitotic count of >3/2 mm^2, (iii) tumor necrosis, and (iv) the presence of genetic alterations including *BRAF* p.V600E, *RET* rearrangement, and *TERT* promoter mutation. In WHO 5th, NIFTPs now incorporate tumors smaller than 1 cm and oncocytic tumors, which were previously excluded.

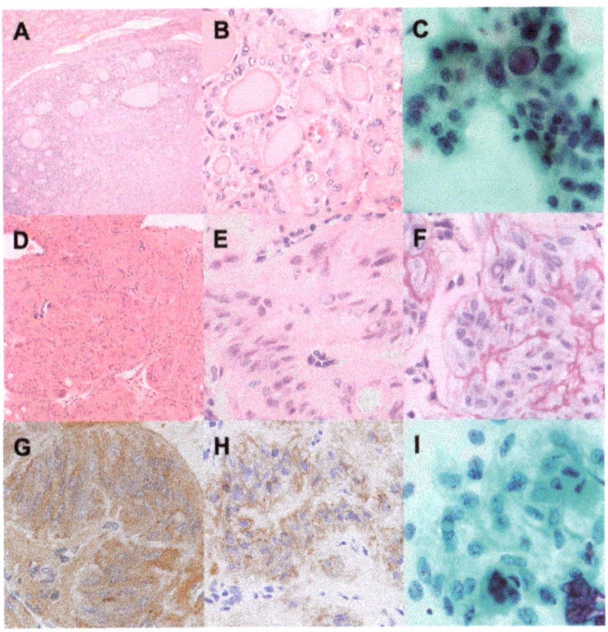

Figure 2. Low-risk neoplasms of the thyroid. (**A–C**): Non-invasive follicular thyroid neoplasm with papillary-like nuclear features (NIFTP). HE staining images of NIFTP at a low (**A**) and high magnification (**B**). Papanicolaou staining image of an NIFTP fine-needle aspiration specimen (**C**). (**D–I**): Hyalinizing trabecular tumor (HTT). HE staining images of HTT at a low (**A**) and high magnification (**B**). PAS staining image of HTT (**F**). Immunohistochemical staining with the MIB1 antibody revealed cytoplasmic (**G**) and cell membranous (**H**) immunoreactivity. Papanicolaou staining image of an HTT fine-needle aspiration specimen (**I**).

TT-UMPs are defined as tumors of "questionable" capsular or vascular invasion; those without PTC-like nuclear atypia are follicular tumors of uncertain malignant potential (FT-UMPs), and those with PTC-like nuclear atypia are well-differentiated tumors of uncertain malignant potential (WDT-UMPs). These diagnostic terms should be carefully used after a thorough pathological investigation of the specimen. Driver gene mutations in TT-UMPs are diverse. While RAS-like mutations are the most common type, mutations in *EIF1AX* and *TSHR*, as well as *PAX8::PPARG* rearrangements, can also be detected.

HTTs were first reported by Carney et al. in 1987 as benign tumors (hyalinizing trabecular "adenoma") and were later renamed after findings that were suggestive of malignancy, such as lymph node metastasis, were presented [14,15]. The presence of PTC-like nuclear atypia and the cell membrane staining of Ki-67 (MIB1), but not the nucleus, are key diagnostic features of HTTs (Figure 2D–I). HTTs commonly exhibit the translocations of *PAX8::GLIS3* (93%) or *PAX8::GLIS1* (7%) [16]. Neither *RAS* nor *BRAF* mutations have been detected in HTTs.

2.4. Subtypes of PTC

PTC subtypes have been described as "variants", but to distinguish them from genetic variants, the term "subtype" is adopted in the WHO 5th (Table 2). The previous "cribriform morular variant PTC" is considered as "cribriform morular carcinoma" in tumors of uncertain histogenesis because they are associated with the constitutive activation of the WNT/β-catenin pathway, which can occur with familial adenomatous polyposis or sporadically. Among the follicular PTCs, those with wide invasive growth remain in the PTC subtype as infiltrative follicular PTC (ifPTC), while the invasive encapsulated follicular variant of papillary thyroid carcinoma (IEFVPTC) has become a unique classification. This is because the genetic background classifies most ifPTCs as BLTs and most IEFVPTCs as RLTs.

Table 2. Papillary thyroid carcinoma (PTC) subtypes (WHO 5th edition, 2022).

PTC Subtypes	Propotion Required for Diagnosis	Major Genetic Abnormalities	Prognosis
Classic PTC	-	*BRAF* p.V600E, *CCDC6::RET*, *NCOA4::RET*	-
Infiltrative follicular PTC	≥90%	*BRAF* p.V600E, *NRAS*, *RET* fusions, *NTRK* and *ALK* fusions	favorable
Tall cell PTC	≥30%	*BRAF* p.V600E, miR-21, *TERT* promoter, *TP53*	high risk
Columnar cell PTC	Not available (NA)	*BRAF* p.V600E, *BRAF* fusions, *CDKN2A* loss, gain of ch.1	high risk
Hobnail PTC	≥30%	*BRAF* p.V600E, *TERT* promoter, *TP53*, *PIK3CA*	high risk
Solid/trabecular PTC	>50	*CCDC6::RET*, *NCOA4::RET*, *ETV6::NTRK3*, *BRAF* p.V600E (rare)	Slightly higher risk
Diffuse sclerosing PTC	100%	*NCOA4::RET*, *BRAF* p.V600E(20%), *ALK* fusions (10%)	Slightly higher risk
PTC with fibromatosis/fasciitis like/desmoid-type stroma	-	*CTNNB1* mutations, *BRAF* p.V600E (frequent)	unknown
Oncocytic PTC	NA (>75%?)	*BRAF* p.V600E, *GRIM-19*, *RET* fusions	Equivalent to classic
Warthin-like PTC	NA	BRAF p.V600E	unknown

The subtypes with a poor prognosis include tall-cell PTC (tcPTC), hobnail PTC (hPTC), and columnar cell PTC (ccPTC). These predominantly comprise *BRAF* p.V600E mutations and often meet the diagnostic criteria for high-grade differentiated carcinomas, as described below. Solid/trabecular PTC (stPTC) also constitutes a slightly higher risk and has a higher frequency of *RET* rearrangements. tcPTC and hPTC are diagnosed when they represent more than 30% of all tumors, and stPTC when it represents more than half of all tumors. CDX2 is often immunohistochemically positive in ccPTC. The risk of diffuse sclerosing PTC is controversial, but it might constitute a higher risk [17].

2.5. High-Grade Thyroid Carcinomas

It has been repeatedly reported that some differentiated follicular cell-derived carcinoma cases, including FTC, PTC, and oncocytic carcinoma (OCA), and some MTC cases have a poor prognosis [3–5]. The WHO 5th introduced the concept of high-grade carcinomas, encompassing high-grade follicular cell-derived non-anaplastic thyroid carcinoma and high-grade MTC. The former category includes PDTC and a newly proposed histological classification termed "differentiated high-grade thyroid carcinoma (DHGTC)" (Table 3).

Table 3. Diagnostic criteria for high-grade follicular cell-derived non-anaplastic thyroid carcinoma and high-grade medullary carcinoma.

	Poorly Differentiated Carcinoma (PDTC)	**Differentiated High-grade Thyroid Carcinoma (DHGTC)**	**Medullary Carcinoma (MTC), High-Grade**
Cell-of-origin	Follicular cell	Follicular cell	C cell
Growth pattern	Solid/trabecular/insular	Papillary, follicular, (solid)	Any
Nuclear findings	No PTC-like nuclear atypia	Any	Any
Other conditions	(At least one of the following features is satisfied)		
	1. Mitosis ($\geq$3/2 mm^2) 2. Tumor necrosis 3. Convoluted nuclei	1. Mitosis ($\geq$5/2 mm^2) 2. Tumor necrosis	1. Mitosis ($\geq$5/2 mm^2) 2. MIB1 labeling idex $\geq$5% 3. Tumor necrosis
Anaplastic features	None	None	None

Poorly differentiated thyroid carcinoma (PDTC) has clinicopathological characteristics that are intermediate between well-differentiated follicular cell-derived carcinoma with excellent prognosis and anaplastic thyroid carcinoma (ATC). PDTC is diagnosed based on the Turin consensus criteria [18]: (i) the presence of a solid/trabecular/insular growth pattern, (ii) an absence of the conventional nuclear features of papillary carcinoma, and (iii) the presence of at least one of the following: convoluted nuclei, increased mitotic counts ($\geq$3 per 2 mm^2), and tumor necrosis.

In well-differentiated follicular cell-derived carcinomas, there are high-risk cases comparable to PDTC [19]. These cases are named "DHGTC" in the WHO 5th and can be morphologically differentiated by increased mitotic counts ($\geq$5 fissions/2 mm^2) or/and tumor necrosis in authentic differentiated thyroid carcinomas including FTC, PTC, and OCA (Figure 3).

In PDTC and DHGTC, *RAS* and *BRAF* mutations are detected at a frequency similar to that in well-differentiated carcinomas. The *TP53*, *CDKN2A*, *PIK3CA*, and *AKT1* mutations are high-risk mutations related to a poor prognosis and malignant transformation. *TERT* promoter mutations (C228T and C250T) are also high-risk genetic alterations. Several studies have suggested the prognostic importance of the co-existence of *BRAF* p.V600E and *TERT* promoter mutations in differentiated thyroid cancer [20,21]. This combination of *BRAF* p.V600E and *TERT* promoter mutations is called a "genetic duet". Recent studies have further recognized the importance of the regulatory single-nucleotide polymorphism (rSNP) rs2853669 in the *TERT* promoter as an additional predictor of risk for PTC [22,23].

The concept of high-grade carcinoma was also introduced for MTC, a calcitonin-producing C cell-derived carcinoma. MTC exhibits neuroendocrine differentiation and is a primary neuroendocrine tumor/carcinoma (NET/NEC) of the thyroid gland. Like NET/NEC in other organs, the prognosis for MTC varies significantly from case to case. The proliferative activities of the tumor can stratify the long-term risk of MTC [24,25]. The WHO 5th recommended a two-tier risk assessment system based on the tumor's proliferative activity and necrosis [4]: (i) mitotic counts, $\geq$5 cells/2 mm^2; (ii) Ki67 labeling index, $\geq$5%; and (iii) presence of tumor necrosis (Table 3).

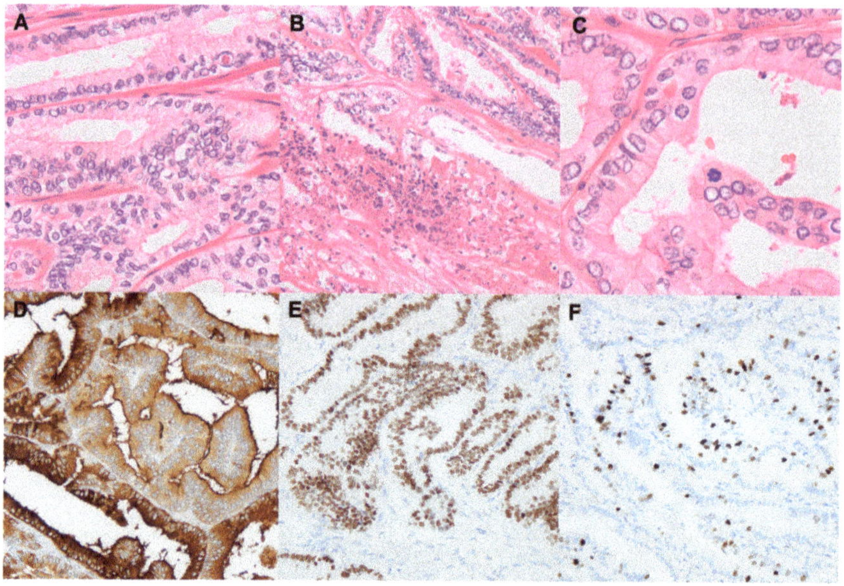

Figure 3. Differentiated high-grade thyroid carcinoma (DHGTC). HE staining images of a DHGTC case (**A–C**). This case is a tall-cell papillary thyroid carcinoma (PTC) (**A**) that meets the criteria of DHGTC. It shows tumor necrosis (**B**) and mitosis (**C**). Immunohistochemistry of Thyroglobulin (**D**) and TTF1 (**E**). The Ki-67 (MIB1) labeling index is about 15% (**F**).

Most cases of hereditary MTC and about half of sporadic MTC cases have *RET* mutations. The second most frequent mutations in sporadic MTC are *RAS* mutations. The clinical risk varies depending on the type of *RET* mutation, with the frequent *RET* p.M918T mutation being that with the highest risk [3–5].

2.6. Changes in the Definition of Anaplastic Thyroid Carcinoma (ATC)

Squamous cell carcinoma (SCC) without a well-differentiated thyroid carcinoma component has been considered a unique histologic type. The WHO 5th edition has incorporated SCC into ATC because SCC of the thyroid generally shows *BRAF* p.V600E mutations (87%) and is immunohistologically positive for the follicular cell markers PAX8 (91%) and TTF1 (38%) [3–5]. SCC of the thyroid also exhibits a poor prognosis comparable to that of other ATCs. The squamous metaplasia of follicular cells and the squamous differentiation of PTC should not be mistaken for ATC. The direct invasion of primary SCC of the head and neck region should also be excluded.

2.7. Miscellaneous Thyroid Tumors

Miscellaneous tumors were classified into four categories based on their cellular origin or differentiation: (i) salivary-gland-type carcinomas of the thyroid, (ii) thymic tumors within the thyroid, (iii) thyroid tumors of uncertain histogenesis, and (iv) embryonal thyroid neoplasms (Table 1).

Salivary-gland-type tumors include mucoepidermoid carcinoma of the thyroid (MEC) and secretory carcinoma of the salivary gland type (SC). MEC consists predominantly of epidermoid cells mixed with a smaller number of mucocytes. Two theories exist regarding the origin of MEC: one posits derivation from ectopic salivary glands, while the other suggests derivation from a solid cell nest within the thyroid gland. In some MEC cases, the *CRTC1::MAML2* fusion gene, characteristic of salivary gland MEC, is detected. SC cases commonly involve the *ETV6::NTRK3* fusion gene.

Intrathyroid thymic tumors include thymoma, intrathyroidal thymic carcinoma (ITC), and spindle cell tumor with thymus-like differentiation (SETTLE). The WHO 4th has remained the same for these classifications.

Sclerosing mucoepidermoid carcinoma with eosinophilia (SMECE) and cribriform morular thyroid carcinoma (CMTC) were classified as tumors of uncertain histogenesis. SMECE was considered a subtype of MEC, but became an independent histologic type due to the absence of the *MAML2* fusion gene and the presence of Hashimoto's disease in the background. CMTC, which was a subtype of PTC in the WHO 4th, is related to familial adenomatous polyposis (FAP) and genetic abnormalities in the β-catenin system such as *APC*. CMTC became independent because it does not show apparent follicular cell differentiation, namely the lack of thyroglobulin production.

Thyroblastoma has been introduced in a new category of embryonal thyroid neoplasms. Thyroblastoma is a highly aggressive tumor, consisting of primitive thyroid-like follicular cells, a primitive small cell component, and mesenchymal stroma. Most thyroblastoma cases have been classified as malignant thyroid teratoma or carcinosarcoma. *DICER1* somatic mutations are common.

It is noteworthy that lymphomas and mesenchymal tumors have been removed from the specific classification of thyroid tumors because they are now grouped together with other endocrine organs.

3. Diagnostic Procedure According to WHO 5th

The WHO 5th simplified the diagnosis of thyroid cancer by dividing it into three steps, as illustrated in Figure 4. The first step involves considering the cell of origin or the cellular differentiation of the tumor cells. The second steps involves an assessment of gene mutations, while the third entails a detailed examination of various histomorphological features, such as capsular/vascular invasion, mitosis, and tumor necrosis.

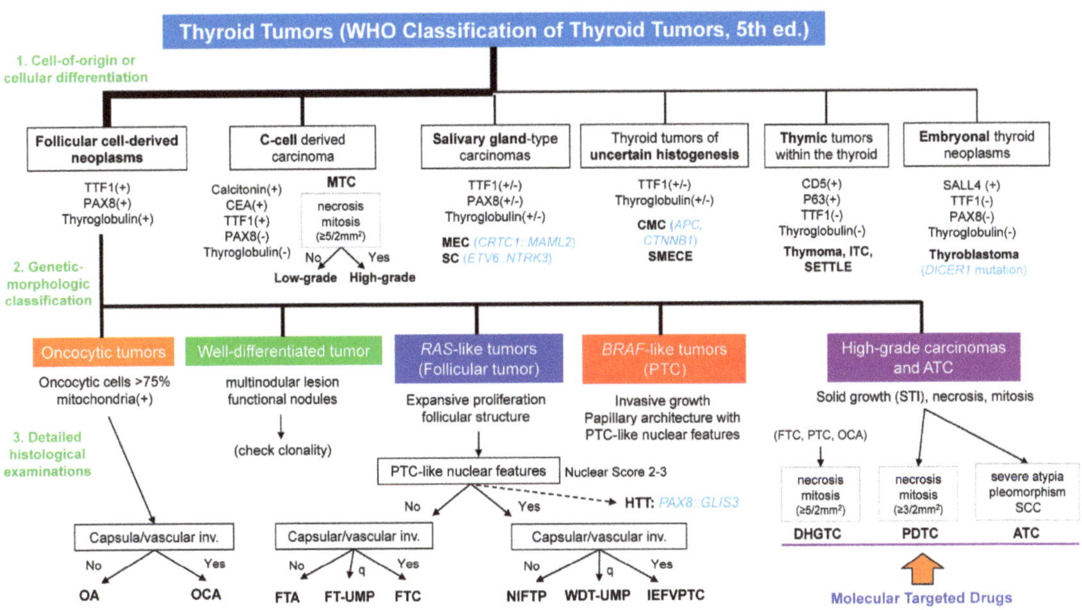

Figure 4. Algorithm for diagnosis of thyroid tumors (WHO 5th edition). The WHO 5th simplified the diagnosis of thyroid cancer by dividing it into three steps: (i) a consideration of the origin or cellular

differentiation of the tumor cells, (ii) an assessment of the gene mutations, and (iii) a detailed examination of various histomorphological features, including capsular/vascular invasion, mitosis, and tumor necrosis. The cell of origin or cellular differentiation can be examined using immunohistological markers such as TTF1, PAX8, and calcitonin. The most frequent follicular cell-derived neoplasms are classified into five categories according to genetic mutations, which are closely related to tumor morphology. Oncocytic tumors and *RAS*-like tumors (RLTs) are commonly encapsulated and are further classified morphologically by the presence or absence of capsular/vascular invasion. Tumors with "Questionable (q)" invasion are diagnosed as FT-UMP or WDT-UMP. In RLTs, papillary-like nuclear features are also important. *BRAF* p.V600E-like tumors (BLTs) commonly show infiltrative growth with apparent PTC-like nuclear features and papillary structures. Tumors with predominantly solid growth are likely classified as high-grade carcinomas or anaplastic thyroid carcinomas (ATCs). Mitotic counts and tumor necrosis are critical in the diagnosis of high-grade carcinomas.

Following the diagnostic algorithm enables the efficient differential diagnosis of thyroid tumors. In facilities with access to genetic analysis, a preliminary diagnosis can be made without relying solely on histomorphological analyses. Conversely, in settings where genetic analysis is not available, it is still possible to narrow down the types of driver genes to some extent through histomorphological analyses. The 5th edition of the WHO aims to minimize interdiagnostic variability and promote more accurate and timely diagnoses.

3.1. Consideration of the Cell-of-Origin or Cellular Differentiation

Thyroid tumor diagnosis primarily relies on determining the cell of origin or tumor differentiation, which is evaluated through histomorphological observation and differentiation markers. For follicular cell differentiation, immunohistological markers such as TTF1, PAX8, and Thyroglobulin are utilized. Additional differentiation markers include calcitonin for C cell differentiation, CD5 for thymus-like differentiation, and SALL4 for embryonal features (Figure 4). Gene expression analysis is also capable of identifying cell differentiation, with current NGS-based thyroid cancer comprehensive panel tests utilizing gene expression patterns for this purpose. Additionally, these tests can directly detect unique driver gene mutations that are closely associated with diagnosis, including *APC*, *CRTC1::MAML2*, and *ETV6::NTRK3*.

3.2. Genetic-Morphologic Classification of the FDNs into Subcategories

FDNs, the most frequent thyroid tumors, are generally classified into five types according to their genetic alterations: (i) oncocytic tumors, (ii) well-differentiated tumors such as TFND, (iii) RLTs, (iv) BLTs, and (v) high-grade carcinomas and ATC. This classification can be performed by gene expression analysis. This classification can be readily achieved using NGS-based genetic analysis. However, the strong correlation between driver genes and morphological features in thyroid cancer allows for a morphological observation-based classification as well. Immunostaining for mitochondria aids in differentiating oncocytic tumors. The diagnosis of oncocytic tumors requires the presence of oncocytes in more than 75% of tumors.

PDTC and ATC typically display solid growth patterns, whereas DHGTC can manifest various growth patterns. DHGTC is diagnosed in FTC, PTC, and OCA based on the presence of increased mitotic figures and/or tumor necrosis. It should be noted that tumors showing solid growth patterns with PTC-like nuclear features are diagnosed as the PTC subtype "stPTC".

3.3. Detailed Histological Examination for the Diagnosis

Further detailed histomorphological evaluation is necessary to confirm the diagnosis of FDNs. Oncocytic tumors and RLTs typically present as encapsulated nodular lesions. The evaluation of capsular and vascular invasion is crucial in determining their benign or malignant status. In RLTs, the diagnosis is determined by assessing the presence or absence of PTC-like nuclear features (nuclear score 2–3 for presence, nuclear score 0–1 for absence) and capsular and vascular invasion. A diagnosis of FTA is established when there are no PTC-like nuclear features and no capsular or vascular invasion. Conversely, a diagnosis of FTC is made when there are no PTC-like nuclear features, but capsular or vascular invasion is present. This indicates that the presence of a *RAS* mutation alone is insufficient to determine malignancy. When PTC-like nuclear features are present without capsular or vascular invasion, the tumor is classified as a NIFTP; meanwhile, if PTC-like nuclear features are present with capsular or vascular invasion, the tumor is categorized as IEFVPTC. When the capsular or vascular invasion is "questionable", the diagnostic term "uncertain malignant potential (UMP)" is used. If the tumor shows PTC-like nuclear features, the diagnosis is well-differentiated tumor-UMP (WDT-UMP); otherwise, it is follicular tumor-UMP (FT-UMP).

High-grade carcinoma and ATC are associated with high-risk gene mutations such as *TERT* promoter mutations, *TP53* mutations, and *CDKN2A/2B* loss, which can be detected through genetic analysis. Tumors harboring these high-risk mutations exhibit morphological features such as brisk mitotic activity and tumor necrosis. These characteristics are utilized to identify high-grade carcinomas morphologically. The diagnosis of high-grade carcinomas is crucial for the early initiation of molecular targeted therapy because a variety of drugs such as Selpercatinib, Entrectinib, Dabrafenib, and Trametinib are currently available for radioactive iodine-resistant thyroid carcinomas.

4. Conclusions

In the WHO 5th edition, the classification was revamped to a systematic approach based on the cell of origin, clinical risk, and genetic alterations. In follicular cell-derived tumors, there exists a close relationship between driver genes and morphological features, enabling the estimation of driver genes to some extent through morphological observation. Conversely, if the driver gene can be identified via genetic testing, it can provide additional confirmation for histological diagnosis. This classification system facilitates the standardization of pathological diagnosis for thyroid tumors, enabling early intervention for high-grade tumors. Understanding genetic alterations has become essential not only in the pathological diagnosis of thyroid tumors, but also in the selection of treatment options.

Funding: This work was supported by JSPS KAKENHI, Grant-in-Aid for Scientific Research (C), Grant Number JP23K06456.

Acknowledgments: The author thanks the members of the Department of Cytology and the Department of Pathology, the Cancer Institute Hospital of JFCR, for their essential assistance.

Conflicts of Interest: The author declares no conflicts of interest.

References

1. Kamma, H.; Kameyama, K.; Kondo, T.; Imamura, Y.; Nakashima, M.; Chiba, T.; Hirokawa, M. Pathological diagnosis of general rules for the description of thyroid cancer by Japanese Society of Thyroid Pathology and Japan Association of Endocrine Surgery. *Endocr. J.* **2022**, *69*, 139–154. [CrossRef]
2. Lloyd, R.V.; Osamura, R.Y.; Klöppel, G.; Rosai, J. *WHO Classification of Tumours of Endocrine Organs*, 4th ed.; IARC: Lyon, France, 2017.
3. Asa, S.L.; Baloch, Z.W.; de Krijger, R.R.; Erickson, L.A.; Ghossein, R.A.; Hyrcza, M.D.; Klimstra, D.S.; Mete, O.; Nosé, V.; Osamura, R.Y.; et al. *WHO Classification of Tumours of Endocrine Organs [Internet]*, 5th ed.; IARC: Lyon, France, 2022.
4. Baloch, Z.W.; Asa, S.L.; Barletta, J.A.; Ghossein, R.A.; Juhlin, C.C.; Jung, C.K.; LiVolsi, V.A.; Papotti, M.G.; Sobrinho-Simões, M.; Tallini, G.; et al. Overview of the 2022 WHO Classification of Thyroid Neoplasms. *Endocr. Pathol.* **2022**, *33*, 27–63. [CrossRef] [PubMed]
5. Nikiforov, Y.E.; Biddinger, P.W.; Thompson, L.D.R. *Diagnostic Pathology and Molecular Genetics of the Thyroid*, 3rd ed.; Wolters Kluwer: Alphen aan den Rijn, The Netherlands, 2020; pp. 347–387.
6. Marotta, V.; Sapio, M.R.; Guerra, A.; Vitale, M. BRAF mutation in cytology samples as a diagnostic tool for papillary thyroid carcinoma. *Expert. Opin. Med. Diag* **2011**, *5*, 277–290. [CrossRef] [PubMed]
7. Puzziello, A.; Guerra, A.; Murino, A.; Izzo, G.; Carrano, M.; Angrisani, E.; Zeppa, P.; Marotta, V.; Faggiano, A.; Vitale, M. Benign thyroid nodules with RAS mutation grow faster. *Clin. Endocrinol.* **2016**, *84*, 736–740. [CrossRef]
8. The Cancer Genome Atlas Research Network: Integrated genomic characterization of papillary thyroid carcinoma. *Cell* **2014**, *159*, 676–690. [CrossRef]

9. Palos-Paz, F.; Perez-Guerra, O.; Cameselle-Teijeiro, J.; Rueda-Chimeno, C.; Barreiro-Morandeira, F.; Lado-Abeal, J.; Galician Group for the Study of Toxic Multinodular Goitre; Vilar, D.A.; Argueso, R.; Barca, O.; et al. Prevalence of mutations in TSHR, GNAS, PRKAR1A and RAS genes in a large series of toxic. *Eur. J. Endocrinol.* **2008**, *159*, 623–631. [CrossRef] [PubMed]
10. Ye, L.; Zhou, X.; Huan, F.; Wang, W.; Qi, Y.; Xu, H.; Yang, S.; Shen, L.; Fei, X.; Xie, J.; et al. The genetic landscape of benign thyroid nodules revealed by whole exome and transcriptome sequencing. *Nat. Commun.* **2017**, *8*, 15533. [CrossRef] [PubMed]
11. Kure, S.; Ohashi, R. Thyroid Hurthle Cell Carcinoma: Clinical, Pathological, and Molecular Features. *Cancers* **2020**, *13*, 26 [CrossRef]
12. Ganly, I.; Makarov, V.; Deraje, S.; Dong, Y.; Reznik, E.; Seshan, V.; Nanjangud, G.; Eng, S.; Bose, P.; Kuo, F.; et al. Integrated Genomic Analysis of Hürthle Cell Cancer Reveals Oncogenic Drivers, Recurrent Mitochondrial Mutations, and Unique Chromosomal Landscapes. *Cancer Cell* **2018**, *34*, 256–270. [CrossRef]
13. Nikiforov, Y.E.; Seethala, R.R.; Tallini, G.; Baloch, Z.W.; Basolo, F.; Thompson, L.D.R.; Barletta, J.A.; Wenig, B.M.; Ghuzlan, A.A.; Kakudo, K.; et al. Nomenclature Revision for Encapsulated Follicular Variant of Papillary Thyroid Carcinoma: A Paradigm Shift to Reduce Over- treatment of Indolent Tumors. *JAMA Oncol.* **2016**, *2*, 1023–1029. [CrossRef]
14. Carney, J.A.; Ryan, J.; Goellner, J.R. Hyalinizing trabecular adenoma of the thyroid gland. *Am. J. Surg. Pathol.* **1987**, *11*, 583–591 [CrossRef]
15. Carney, J.A.; Hirokawa, M.; Lloyd, R.V.; Papotti, M.; Sebo, T.J. Hyalinizing trabecular tumors of the thyroid gland are almost all benign. *Am. J. Surg. Pathol.* **2008**, *32*, 1877–1889. [CrossRef]
16. Nikiforova, M.N.; Nikitski, A.V.; Panebianco, F.; Kaya, C.; Yip, L.; Williams, M.; Chiosea, S.I.; Seethala, R.R.; Roy, S.; Condello, V.; et al. GLIS rearrangement is a genomic hallmark of hyalinizing trabecular tumors of the thyroid gland. *Thyroid.* **2019**, *29*, 161–173. [CrossRef]
17. Vuong, H.G.; Kondo, T.; Pham, T.Q.; Oishi, N.; Mochizuki, K.; Nakazawa, T.; Hassel, L.; Katoh, R. Prognostic significance of diffuse sclerosing variant papillary thyroid carcinoma: A systematic review and meta- analysis. *Eur. J. Endocrinol.* **2017**, *176*, 433–441. [CrossRef]
18. Volante, M.; Collini, P.; Nikiforov, Y.E.; Sakamoto, A.; Kakudo, K.; Katoh, R.; Lloyd, R.V.; LiVolsi, V.A.; Papotti, M.; Sobrinho-Simões, M.; et al. Poorly differentiated thyroid carcinoma: The Turin proposal for the use of uniform diagnostic criteria and an algorithmic diagnostic approach. *Am. J. Surg. Pathol.* **2007**, *31*, 1256–1264. [CrossRef]
19. Ito, Y.; Hirokawa, M.; Fukushima, M.; Inoue, H.; Yabuta, T.; Uruno, T.; Kihara, M.; Higashiyama, T.; Takamura, Y.; Miya, A.; et al. Prevalence and prognostic significance of poor differentiation and tall cell variant in papillary carcinoma. *World J. Surg.* **2008**, *32*, 1535–1543. [CrossRef]
20. Marotta, V.; Sciammarella, C.; Colao, A.; Faggiano, A. Application of molecular biology of differentiated thyroid cancer for clinical prognostication. *Endocr.-Relat. Cancer* **2016**, *23*, R499–R515. [CrossRef]
21. Liu, R.; Bishop, J.; Zhu, G.; Zhang, T.; Ladenson, P.W.; Xing, M. Mortality Risk Stratification by Combining BRAF V600E and TERT Promoter Mutations in Papillary Thyroid Cancer: Genetic Duet of BRAF and TERT Promoter Mutations in Thyroid Cancer Mortality. *JAMA Oncol.* **2017**, *3*, 202–208. [CrossRef] [PubMed]
22. Hirokawa, T.; Arimasu, Y.; Chiba, T.; Fujiwara, M.; Kamma, H. Clinicopathological significance of the single nucleotide polymorphism, rs2853669 within the TERT promoter in papillary thyroid carcinoma. *Pathol. Int.* **2020**, *70*, 217–223. [CrossRef] [PubMed]
23. Liu, R.; Zhu, G.; Tan, J.; Shen, X.; Xing, M. Genetic Trio of BRAF and TERT Mutations and rs2853669TT in Papillary Thyroid Cancer Aggressiveness. *J. Natl. Cancer Inst.* **2023**, *ahead of print*. [CrossRef] [PubMed]
24. Alzumaili, B.; Xu, B.; Spanheimer, P.M.; Tuttle, R.M.; Sherman, E.; Katabi, N.; Dogan, S.; Ganly, I.; Untch, B.R.; Ghossein, R.A. Grading of medullary thyroid carcinoma on the basis of tumor necrosis and high mitotic rate is an independent. *Mod. Pathol.* **2020**, *33*, 1690–1701. [CrossRef] [PubMed]
25. Fuchs, T.L.; Nassour, A.J.; Glover, A.; Sywak, M.S.M.F.; Sidhu, S.B.P.; Delbridge, L.W.M.; Clifton-Bligh, R.J.P.; Gild, M.L.P.; Tsang, V.P.; Robinson, B.G.M.; et al. A Proposed Grading Scheme for Medullary Thyroid Carcinoma Based on Proliferative Activity (Ki-67 and Mitotic Count) and Coagulative Necrosis. *Am. J. Surg. Pathol.* **2020**, *44*, 1419–1428. [CrossRef] [PubMed]

biomedicines

MDPI

Article

The Effect of Radioiodine Therapy on the Prognosis of Differentiated Thyroid Cancer with Lung Metastases

Shenghong Zhang [1,2,3,4], Mengqin Zhu [1,2,3,4,†], Han Zhang [3,4,†], Hanhui Liu [1,2,3,4], Xin Fan [3,4], Jiajia Zhang [3,4] and Fei Yu [1,2,3,4,*]

1 Shanghai Clinical College, Anhui Medical University, Shanghai 200040, China; hailee6677@163.com (S.Z.)
2 The Fifth Clinical Medical College, Anhui Medical University, Hefei 230032, China
3 Department of Nuclear Medicine, Shanghai Tenth People's Hospital, Tongji University School of Medicine, Shanghai 200040, China
4 Institute of Nuclear Medicine, Tongji University School of Medicine, Shanghai 200040, China
* Correspondence: yufei_021@163.com; Tel.: +86-021-66302721
† These authors contributed equally to this work.

Abstract: Lung metastasis substantially influences the survival of thyroid cancer (TC) patients. This study sought to investigate factors impacting the survival of differentiated thyroid cancer patients with lung metastases (DTC–LM) undergoing radioiodine therapy (RAI) after thyroid surgery. The retrospective study encompassed 609 TC patients with lung metastases. Survival outcomes—specifically, overall survival (OS) and thyroid cancer-specific survival (TCSS)—were examined through both univariate and multivariate Cox regression analyses. Radioiodine therapy (RAI)'s impact on DTC–LM patient survival was further assessed with the Kaplan–Meier survival curve. Of the 609 TC patients with lung metastases, 434 (71.3%) were found to have undergone thyroid surgery after a median follow-up of 59 months. Anaplastic thyroid cancer (ATC), stage IV, and lung metastases associated with other metastases were identified as risk factors for OS and TCSS in TCLM patients. RAI therapy significantly enhances survival in DTC–LM patients followed by primary site surgery under the age of 55, PTC patients, and those with single organ metastases at lung.

Keywords: lung metastasis; RAI; thyroid cancer; thyroid cancer-specific survival

1. Introduction

Thyroid cancer (TC) is the most prevalent malignant tumor in the head and neck region, originating from either the thyroid follicular epithelium or parafollicular epithelial cells [1,2]. According to the latest cancer report published in the Journal of the National Cancer Center (JNCC), the incidence of TC in China has increased 20-fold between 2000 and 2016 [3]. TC is histologically categorized into differentiated thyroid cancer (DTC), medullary thyroid cancer (MTC), and anaplastic thyroid cancer (ATC), based on differences in tumor origin and differentiation [4]. Papillary thyroid cancer (PTC) and follicular thyroid cancer (FTC) are two subtypes of DTC, with the former being the most common subtype, accounting for approximately 90% of all TC cases [5,6].

The overall prognosis for patients with DTC is favorable, while patients with distant metastases have a significantly poorer prognosis [7,8]. The lung is the most commonly affected site of distant metastases for DTC metastases, with an incidence rate of 2–20% [9,10]. Indeed, research indicated a higher incidence of lung metastasis compared to other organs in thyroid cancer patients with distant metastasis [11–13], likely due to the lungs' extensive vascularization and tumor-friendly microenvironment [14]. Of those with lung metastases, 50% of patients die within 10 years [9,15,16]. Several factors, including age, serum thyroglobulin levels, cumulative dose of radioiodine therapy (RAI), and tumor size, have been shown to influence the prognosis of patients with DTC correlated with pulmonary metastases [17,18]. Despite the considerable number of studies on patients with lung metastases from thyroid cancer, few studies have focused on the prognostic impact of all pathological types on thyroid cancer with lung metastasis (TCLM).

The therapeutic approaches for TC primarily comprise surgical intervention, RAI therapy, external radiotherapy, and chemotherapy, with targeted therapy and immunotherapy emerging as novel systemic treatment modalities in recent years [19,20]. The 2015 guidelines of the American Thyroid Association (ATA) highly endorse RAI therapy as the recommended treatment following thyroidectomy for stratified DTC patients at high risk of recurrence [21]. Additionally, patients with ^{131}Iodine-avid lung metastasis, smaller nodules, no other metastases, and younger age groups (<55 years) demonstrate favorable prognosis [22,23]. However, the factors influencing the survival of patients with TCLM who have undergone primary site surgery and RAI therapy necessitate further exploration.

In this study, our primary objective was to identify prognostic risk factors for TCLM patients who have undergone primary site surgery based on the Surveillance, Epidemiology, and End Results (SEER) database. The impact of RAI therapy on the survival of TCLM patients who have undergone primary site surgery was also evaluated through a stratified analysis based on age, histology, and other distant metastases. These findings could prove valuable in guiding clinical decision-making related to therapy.

2. Materials and Methods

2.1. Data Source

This retrospective study employed data from the SEER program, which covers around 30% of the entire U.S. population. We identified patients diagnosed with 87,737 cases of thyroid cancer between 2010 and 2017 using SEER*stat 8.3.5 software. The year 2010 was chosen as the starting point due to the availability of data on distant metastases beginning from that year. Furthermore, the American Joint Committee on Cancer (AJCC), 7th edition was utilized for the years 2010 to 2015. From 2016 to 2017, cancer registries in the United States transitioned from Collaborative Staging (CS) to SEER Combined Stage (2016–2017), which incorporates TNM categories, staging groups, and definitions based on the TNM Classification of Malignant Tumors, 7th edition. As such, all AJCCs from 2010 to 2017 are referred to as AJCC 7th. Given the variability of AJCC 8th and constraints on SEER data collection, there is currently no viable conversion method, and, hence, we opted for the unification of SEER data collection while utilizing AJCC 7th.

2.2. Patient Selection

The study retrieved data from the SEER database, which included variables such as race, sex, marital status, histological type ICD-O-3 [PTC (8050, 8260, 8340, 8341, 8342, 8343, 8344), MTC (8345, 8510), FTC (8330, 8331, 8332, 8335), ATC (8020, 8021)] [24], T stage, N stage, SEER-specific etiology of death classification, vital status, and survival time (months). Other races encompassed American Indian/Alaska Native, Asian or Pacific Islander, and unknown racial groups, due to their representation of only 1% of the SEER database. TNM staging and stage data were based on a combination of derived AJCC 7th (2010–2015) data and derived SEER combined TNM data due to constraints in the composition of the SEER database across years. Exclusions were made for TC patients with unknown demographic and clinicopathological information from 2010 to 2017. Despite marital status being a significant determinant in various cancers, its significance in thyroid cancer remains unknown. Therefore, patients with uncertain marital status were eliminated to investigate the impact of marital status on the prognosis of TC patients [25,26]. Thyroid cancer patients were classified into two groups: those with and without lung metastases. In TCLM patients, an additional distinction was made based on whether primary surgery was performed. The detailed screening process is illustrated in Figure 1.

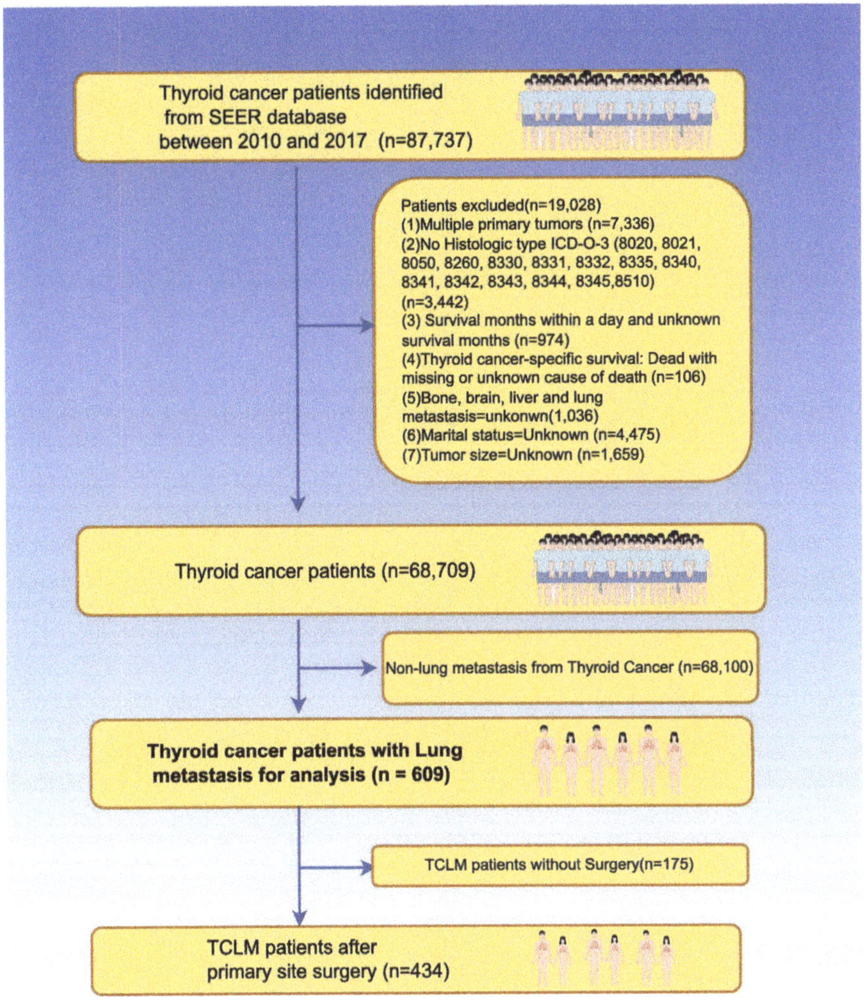

Figure 1. The schematic workflow of patient selection (By Figdraw). SEER: The Surveillance, Epidemiology, and End Results; TCLM: Thyroid cancer with lung metastasis.

As all data used in this study were obtained from the publicly available SEER database, no approval from a medical ethics committee was necessary since the database is accessible to the public free of charge. Therefore, the Ethics Committee of Shanghai Tenth People's Hospital deemed that no review of this study was required.

2.3. Statistical Analyses

First of all, the study employed the chi-square test to compare the demographic and clinical features of TCLM patients with and without radioiodine therapy. Secondly, univariate and multivariate Cox regression analyses were conducted to identify the factors that impact overall survival (OS) and thyroid cancer-specific survival (TCSS) in patients with TCLM, as well as the possible factors that affect prognosis in TCLM patients after primary site surgery. The results were presented as hazard ratio (HR), 95% confidence intervals (CI), and p-value. Finally, the stratified Kaplan–Meier survival curve was utilized to investigate the parameters that influence TCSS with RAI therapy in TCLM patients who underwent primary site surgery. A p-value of 0.05 was considered statistically significant. All data were analyzed using SPSS software (version 26; IBM Corp., Armonk, NY, USA).

3. Results

3.1. Demographic and Clinicopathologic Characteristics of Participants

This study involved 68,709 patients diagnosed with TC between 2010–2017. After a median follow-up of 59 months, the patients were categorized into two groups: those with pulmonary metastases and those without. The sex ratio was approximately 1:1, while the proportion of patients aged over 55 years was higher in the TC patients with lung metastasis compared to those without. More than half of the cases were classified as PTC and had a tumor size > 40 mm. Furthermore, the proportion of TC patients with lung metastasis who underwent primary site surgery was notably higher than those who did not receive surgery at the primary site, accounting for 71.3% and 28.7%, respectively. Additionally, among the TC patients with lung metastasis (LM), 36.6% underwent RAI treatment, while 63.4% did not (Supplementary Table S1). Among TCLM patients who underwent RAI treatment, 99.6% opted for surgical intervention at the primary site. Table 1 provides further details of the demographics and clinicopathologic characteristics of thyroid cancer patients with lung metastases.

Table 1. Demographic and clinicopathologic features of thyroid cancer patients with lung metastases.

	All		Radioiodine Therapy				p
			Absence		Presence		
	(n = 609)		(n = 386)		(n = 223)		
Sex							
Female (n,%)	317	52.1%	201	52.1%	116	52.0%	<0.001
Male (n,%)	292	47.9%	185	47.9%	107	48.0%	
Race							
White (n,%)	463	76.0%	288	774.6%	175	78.5%	0.443
Black (n,%)	42	6.90%	30	7.80%	12	5.40%	
Other (n,%)	104	17.1%	68	17.6%	36	16.1%	
Marital status							
Single (n,%)	133	21.8%	74	19.2%	59	26.5%	0.010
Married (n,%)	343	56.3%	214	55.4%	129	57.8%	
Divorced (n,%)	44	7.20%	29	7.50%	15	6.70%	
Widowed (n,%)	89	14.6%	69	17.9%	20	9.00%	
Age (years)							
<55 (n,%)	177	29.1%	87	22.5%	90	40.4%	<0.001
≥55 (n,%)	432	70.9%	299	77.5%	133	59.6%	
Histology							
PTC (n,%)	369	60.6%	176	45.6%	193	193%	
MTC (n,%)	25	4.10%	25	6.50%	0	0.00%	
FTC (n,%)	67	11.0%	38	9.80%	29	13.0%	<0.001
ATC (n,%)	148	24.3%	147	38.1%	1	0.40%	
Tumor size (mm)							
≤10 (n,%)	29	4.80%	15	3.90%	14	6.30%	
11–20 (n,%)	69	11.3%	27	7.00%	42	18.8%	
21–40 (n,%)	160	26.3%	82	21.2%	78	35.0%	<0.001
>40 (n,%)	351	57.6%	262	67.9%	89	39.9%	
Stage							<0.001
II (n,%)	79	13.0%	25	6.50%	54	24.4%	
IV (n,%)	529	86.9%	360	93.3%	169	75.8%	
Unknown (n,%)	1	0.20%	1	0.30%	0	0.00%	
T							
T1 (n,%)	41	6.70%	16	4.10%	25	11.2%	
T2 (n,%)	44	7.20%	24	6.20%	20	9.00%	
T3 (n,%)	160	26.3%	59	15.3%	101	45.3%	
T4 (n,%)	352	57.8%	279	72.3%	73	32.7%	<0.001
TX (n,%)	9	1.50%	6	1.60%	3	1.30%	
T0 (n,%)	3	0.50%	2	0.50%	1	0.40%	

Table 1. *Cont.*

	All (n = 609)		Radioiodine Therapy				p
			Absence (n = 386)		Presence (n = 223)		
N							
N0 (n,%)	163	26.8%	111	28.8%	52	23.3%	
N1 (n,%)	416	68.3%	253	65.5%	163	73.1%	<0.001
NX (n,%)	30	4.90%	22	5.70%	8	3.60%	
Surgery of primary site							
No (n,%)	175	28.7%	174	45.1%	1	0.40%	<0.001
Yes (n,%)	434	71.3%	212	54.9%	222	99.6%	
LM							
Only lung (n,%)	440	72.2%	250	64.8%	190	85.2%	<0.001
Lung + 1(n,%)	129	21.2%	99	25.6%	30	13.5%	
Lung + 2 (n,%)	40	6.60%	37	9.60%	3	1.30%	

TNM categories, stage groups, and definitions used by SEER are based on the AJCC 7th Edition; LM: lung metastasis; Only lung: TC patients with single organ metastases at lung; Lung + 1: TC patients combined with lung and other one distant metastasis; Lung + 2: TC patients combined with lung and other several distant metastases.

3.2. The Predictive Factors of Overall Survival and Thyroid Cancer-Specific Survival in Patients with TCLM

In the univariate Cox analysis, several factors emerged as significant risk factors for the OS of patients with TCLM. These factors included age ≥ 55 years (HR = 2.474, 95%CI: 1.885–3.246, $p < 0.001$), non-PTC (MTC vs. FTC vs. ATC, 2.233 (1.350–3.695) vs. 1.578 (1.118–2.229) vs. 10.827 (8.256–14.200), $p < 0.05$), tumor size > 40 mm (HR = 2.868, 95%CI: 1.566–5.252, $p < 0.05$), stage IV (HR = 7.143, 95%CI: 3.915–13.036, $p < 0.001$), T4 (HR = 4.238, 95%CI: 2.425–7.405, $p < 0.001$), and LM combined with other distant metastasis (Lung + 1 vs. Lung + 2, 1.635 (1.282–2.084) vs. 2.505 (1.741–3.604), $p < 0.001$). Moreover, surgical intervention at the primary site (HR = 0.223, 95%CI: 0.179–0.278, $p < 0.001$ for OS; HR = 0.224, 95%CI: 0.178–0.282, $p < 0.001$, for TCSS) was found to have a potentially positive effect on both OS and TCSS, while sex did not. RAI therapy (HR = 0.188, 95%CI: 0.142–0.248, $p < 0.001$, for OS; HR = 0.169, 95%CI: 0.124–0.229, $p < 0.001$, for TCSS) improved overall survival (OS) and thyroid cancer-specific survival (TCSS) of TCLM patient, which can effectively manage the progression of TCLM patients.

In the multivariate Cox analysis, three variables were identified as significant risk factors for the OS of TCLM patients. These variables included ATC (HR = 3.981, 95%CI: 2.876–5.512, $p < 0.001$, for OS; HR = 3.864, 95%CI: 2.763–5.403, $p < 0.001$, for TCSS), stage IV (HR = 2.794, 95%CI: 1.433–5.447, $p = 0.003$, for OS; HR = 2.768, 95%CI: 1.379–5.556, $p = 0.004$, for TCSS), and lung metastasis combined with other metastasis (Lung + 1, 1.299 (1.002–1.684), $p < 0.05$, for OS; Lung + 1,1.359 (1.039–1.779), $p < 0.05$, for TCSS). Conversely, both surgical intervention at the primary site (HR = 0.653, 95%CI: 0.506–0.842, $p = 0.001$, for OS; HR = 0.664, 95%CI: 0.510–0.864, $p = 0.002$, for TCSS) and RAI therapy (HR = 0.397, 95%CI: 0.283–0.558, $p < 0.001$, for OS; HR = 0.371, 95%CI: 0.257–0.535, $p < 0.001$, for TCSS) were considered protective factors for the OS and TCSS of TCLM patients. Table 2 presents the HR and 95%CI for each variable in both the univariate and multivariate Cox proportional hazard models.

Table 2. Univariate and multivariable Cox analysis of overall survival and thyroid cancer-specific survival in TCLM patients.

Variable	Univariate Analysis				Multivariate Analysis			
	Overall Survival		Specific Survival		Overall Survival		Specific Survival	
	HR (95%CI)	p	HR (95%CI)	p	HR (95%CI)	p	HR (95%CI)	p
Sex								
Female	Ref		Ref		/		/	
Male	1.027 (0.835–1.263)	0.802	0.980 (0.789–1.217)	0.855	/	/	/	/

Table 2. *Cont.*

Variable	Univariate Analysis				Multivariate Analysis			
	Overall Survival		Specific Survival		Overall Survival		Specific Survival	
	HR (95%CI)	*p*	HR (95%CI)	*p*	HR (95%CI)	*p*	HR (95%CI)	*p*
Race								
White	Ref		Ref		/		/	
Black	0.668 (0.419–1.063)	0.088	0.737 (0.463–1.175)	0.200	/	/	/	/
Other	0.908 (0.683–1.207)	0.506	0.908 (0.673–1.223)	0.524	/	/	/	/
Marital status								
Single	Ref		Ref		/		/	
Married	0.406 (0.287–0.576)	<0.001	1.593 (1.173–2.164)	0.003	/	/	/	/
Divorced	0.639 (0.485–0.843)	0.002	1.559 (0.969–2.509)	0.067	/	/	/	/
Widowed	0.633 (0.407–0.985)	0.043	2.660 (1.848–3.827)	<0.001	/	/	/	/
Age (years)								
<55	Ref		Ref		Ref		Ref	
≥55	2.474 (1.885–3.246)	<0.001	2.264 (1.715–2.988)	<0.001	1.343 (0.989–1.823)	0.059	1.225 (0.897–1.672)	0.201
Histology								
PTC	Ref		Ref		Ref		Ref	
MTC	2.233 (1.350–3.695)	0.002	2.333 (1.386–3.925)	0.001	0.892 (0.519–1.534)	0.680	0.917 (0.523–1.605)	0.761
FTC	1.578 (1.118–2.229)	0.010	1.425 (0.974–2.085)	0.068	1.231 (0.848–1.788)	0.275	1.124 (0.747–1.691)	0.575
ATC	10.827 (8.256–14.200)	<0.001	11.005 (8.316–14.564)	<0.001	3.981 (2.876–5.512)	<0.001	3.864 (2.763–5.403)	<0.001
Tumor size (mm)								
≤10	Ref		Ref		Ref		Ref	
11–20	1.265 (0.634–2.526)	0.505	1.044 (0.514–2.123)	0.905	1.462 (0.704–3.038)	0.308	1.222 (0.577–2.588)	0.601
21–40	1.381 (0.732–2.607)	0.319	1.193 (0.628–2.266)	0.590	1.117 (0.549–2.271)	0.761	1.023 (0.499–2.097)	0.952
>40	2.868 (1.566–5.252)	0.001	2.612 (1.425–4.786)	0.002	1.397 (0.708–2.756)	0.335	1.228 (0.618–2.437)	0.558
Stage								
II	Ref		Ref		Ref		Ref	
IV	7.143 (3.915–13.036)	<0.001	6.996 (3.724–13.144)	<0.001	2.794 (1.433–5.447)	0.003	2.768 (1.379–5.556)	0.004
Unknown	17.813 (2.210–133.618)	0.007	17.65 (2.251–138.415)	<0.001	1.698 (0.161–17.934)	0.660	2.087 (0.182–23.883)	0.554
T								
T1	Ref		Ref		Ref		Ref	
T2	1.212 (0.576–2.548)	0.612	0.947 (0.402–2.229)	0.900	1.068 (0.448–2.548)	0.881	0.791 (0.297–2.105)	0.639
T3	1.043 (0.569–1.914)	0.892	1.044 (0.540–2.018)	0.899	1.028 (0.517–2.043)	0.938	1.012 (0.482–2.127)	0.975
T4	4.238 (2.425–7.405)	<0.001	4.614 (2.519–8.451)	<0.001	1.798 (0.922–3.507)	0.085	1.868 (0.910–3.832)	0.088
TX	2.111 (0.752–5.926)	0.156	1.965 (0.625–6.177)	0.248	0.895 (0.272–2.947)	0.855	0.731 (0.190–2.817)	0.649
T0	0.874 (0.114–6.692)	0.897	1.076 (0.139–8.333)	0.944	0.663 (0.080–5.496)	0.703	0.734 (0.088–6.140)	0.775
N								
N0	Ref		Ref		Ref		Ref	
N1	1.061 (0.836–1.346)	0.627	1.083 (0.843–1.391)	0.533	1.260 (0.972–1.634)	0.081	1.225 (0.933–1.608)	0.144
NX	1.931 (1.224–3.048)	0.005	2.041 (1.276–3.264)	0.003	1.771 (1.084–2.895)	0.023	1.848 (1.114–3.066)	0.017
LM								
Only lung	Ref		Ref		Ref		Ref	
Lung + 1	1.635 (1.282–2.084)	<0.001	1.679 (1.304–2.162)	<0.001	1.299 (1.002–1.684)	0.048	1.359 (1.039–1.779)	0.025
Lung + 2	2.505 (1.741–3.604)	<0.001	2.622 (1.809–3.800)	<0.001	1.347 (0.917–1.978)	0.129	1.403 (0.948–2.076)	0.091

Table 2. *Cont.*

Variable	Univariate Analysis				Multivariate Analysis			
	Overall Survival		Specific Survival		Overall Survival		Specific Survival	
	HR (95%CI)	*p*	HR (95%CI)	*p*	HR (95%CI)	*p*	HR (95%CI)	*p*
Surgery of primary site								
No	Ref		Ref		Ref		Ref	
Yes	0.223 (0.179–0.278)	<0.001	0.224 (0.178–0.282)	<0.001	0.653 (0.506–0.842)	0.001	0.664 (0.510–0.864)	0.002
RAI								
No	Ref		Ref		Ref		Ref	
Yes	0.188 (0.142–0.248)	<0.001	0.169 (0.124–0.229)	<0.001	0.397 (0.283–0.558)	<0.001	0.371 (0.257–0.535)	<0.001

TNM categories, stage groups, and definitions used by SEER are based on the AJCC 7th Edition. LM: lung metastasis; Only lung: TC patients with single organ metastases at lung; Lung + 1: TC patients combined with lung and other one distant metastasis; Lung + 2: TC patients combined with lung and other several distant metastases; RAI: radioiodine therapy.

3.3. *The Predictive Factors of OS and TCSS in TCLM Patients following Primary Site Surgery*

To further investigate the prognostic factors of patients with TCLM who have undergone surgery at their primary site, a multivariate Cox analysis was conducted. The results of the analysis revealed that age (HR = 1.484, 95%CI: 1.018–2.165, $p < 0.05$, for OS), histology (ATC, 4.672 (2.964–7.366), $p < 0.001$, for OS; ATC, 4.626 (2.890–7.405), $p < 0.001$, for TCSS), stage (IV, 2.631 (1.238–5.592), $p < 0.05$, for OS; IV, 2.589 (1.170–5.728), $p < 0.05$, for TCSS), T stage (T4, 3.133 (1.366–7.187), $p < 0.01$, for OS; T4, 3.358 (1.386–8.133), $p < 0.01$, for TCSS), and other distant metastasis (Lung + 1 vs. Lung + 2, 1.551 (1.097–2.194) vs. 1.866 (1.064–3.274), $p < 0.05$, for OS; Lung + 1 vs. Lung + 2, 1.725 (1.207–2.464) vs. 1.837 (1.026–3.288), $p < 0.05$, for TCSS) were all significant predictors of OS in these patients. The risk of OS in TCLM patients who received RAI treatment after primary site surgery was 0.507 times that of no treatment (HR = 0.507, 95%CI: 0.350–0.733, $p < 0.001$). Total thyroidectomy, subtotal thyroidectomy or near-total thyroidectomy at the primary site accounted for 95.0% of TCLM patients treated with RAI therapy (Supplementary Table S2). Similarly, these same variables, with the exception of age ($p = 0.103$), were also found to be independent predictors of TCSS in TCLM patients following primary site surgery. As a result, TCLM patients who were older than 55 years, had an ATC subtype, were in stage IV, had T4 stage, had multiple distant metastases, and did not receive RAI treatment were shown to have a poorer prognosis (Table 3). TCLM patients who receive RAI therapy after primary site surgery are associated with a diminished risk of TCSS relative to their untreated counterparts (HR = 0.482, 95%CI: 0.323–0.718, $p < 0.001$).

Table 3. Multivariable Cox analysis of overall survival and thyroid cancer-specific survival in TCLM patients following surgery of primary site.

Variable	N (%)	Overall Survival		Specific Survival	
		HR (95%CI)	*p*	HR (95%CI)	*p*
Age (years)					
<55	156 (35.9%)	Ref		Ref	
≥55	278 (64.1%)	1.484 (1.018–2.165)	0.040	1.379 (0.937–2.028)	0.103
Histology					
PTC	316 (72.8%)	Ref		Ref	
MTC	13 (3.0%)	1.038 (0.485–2.220)	0.924	1.087 (0.505–2.342)	0.831
FTC	50 (11.5%)	1.396 (0.890–2.189)	0.146	1.284 (0.779–2.116)	0.328
ATC	55 (12.7%)	4.672 (2.964–7.366)	<0.001	4.626 (2.890–7.405)	<0.001
Tumor size (mm)					
≤10	25 (5.8%)	Ref		Ref	
11–20	61 (14.1%)	0.964 (0.421–2.211)	0.932	0.839 (0.358–1.962)	0.685
21–40	129 (29.7%)	0.781 (0.344–1.777)	0.556	0.673 (0.292–1.552)	0.354
>40	219 (50.5%)	0.952 (0.432–2.097)	0.903	0.808 (0.363–1.799)	0.602

Table 3. *Cont.*

Variable	N (%)	Overall Survival HR (95%CI)	Overall Survival p	Specific Survival HR (95%CI)	Specific Survival p
Stage					
II	77 (17.7%)	Ref		Ref	
IV	357 (82.3%)	2.631 (1.238–5.592)	0.012	2.589 (1.170–5.728)	0.019
T					
T1	36 (8.3%)	Ref		Ref	
T2	32 (7.4%)	1.213 (0.385–3.818)	0.742	0.836 (0.216–3.231)	0.795
T3	147 (33.9%)	1.516 (0.648–3.545)	0.337	1.501 (0.604–3.731)	0.382
T4	213 (49.1%)	3.133 (1.366–7.187)	0.007	3.358 (1.386–8.133)	0.007
TX	4 (0.9%)	2.892 (0.588–14.221)	0.191	1.757 (0.208–14.854)	0.605
T0	2 (0.5%)	0.000 (–)	0.951	0.000 (–)	0.955
LM					
Only lung	329 (75.8%)	Ref		Ref	
Lung + 1	85 (19.6%)	1.551 (1.097–2.194)	0.013	1.725 (1.207–2.464)	0.003
Lung + 2	20 (4.6%)	1.866 (1.064–3.274)	0.03	1.837 (1.026–3.288)	0.041
RAI					
No	212 (48.8%)	Ref		Ref	
Yes	222 (51.2%)	0.507 (0.350–0.733)	<0.001	0.482 (0.323–0.718)	<0.001

TNM categories, stage groups, and definitions used by SEER are based on the AJCC 7th Edition. LM: lung metastasis; Only lung: Thyroid cancer patients with single organ metastases at lung; Lung + 1: Thyroid cancer patients combined with lung and other one distant metastasis; Lung + 2: Thyroid cancer patients combined with lung and other several distant metastases; RAI: radioiodine therapy.

3.4. Effect of RAI on Survival in Subgroup

To analyze the difference in survival among TCLM patients who underwent surgery at the primary site, the Kaplan–Meier method and log-rank test were utilized. The Kaplan–Meier analysis was stratified based on RAI treatment, age, histology, and other distant metastases.

Firstly, improved TCSS was observed in patients with TCLM who underwent RAI treatment post-primary surgery compared to those who did not receive RAI, irrespective of age. In TCLM patients who underwent RAI treatment following primary surgery, younger patients (age < 55 years) exhibited considerably enhanced TCSS in contrast to their older counterparts (age ≥ 55 years) (Figures 2a and S1a,b).

Secondly, regardless of whether the histology is PTC or FTC (ATC and MTC were not considered because patients with them rarely received RAI treatment), TCLM patients who underwent surgery of the primary site followed by RAI treatment had significantly better prognosis compared to those without RAI. However, the histology did not affect the impact of RAI on the TCSS of TCLM patients following surgery at the primary site (Figures 2b and S1c,d).

Last but not least, the benefits of RAI therapy on the TCSS of TCLM patients following primary site surgery were observed in subgroups with only lung metastasis ($p < 0.001$) and those with a combination of lung and one other distant metastasis ($p < 0.001$). However, this effect was not observed in TCLM patients who had multiple distant metastases following primary site surgery. Notably, among TCLM patients who underwent primary site surgery and received RAI therapy, those with only lung metastasis exhibited superior TCSS compared to those with a combination of lung and one other distant metastasis (Figure 2c–e).

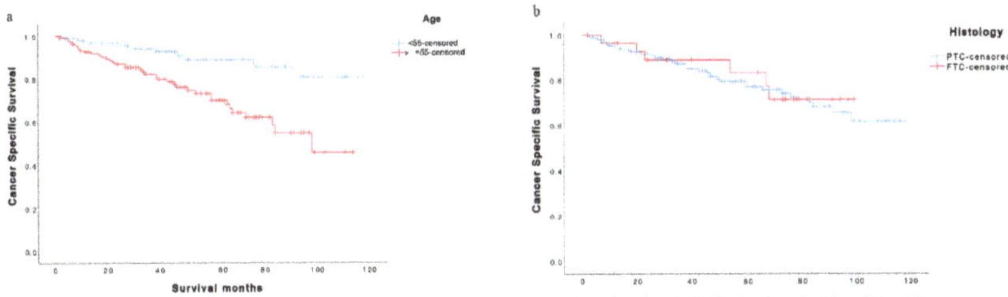

Age	Estimate	Mean 95% Confidence Interval Lower Bound	Upper Bound	p
<55	105.202	97.857	112.547	<0.001
>=55	81.520	73.354	89.687	

Histology	Estimate	Mean 95% Confidence Interval Lower Bound	Upper Bound	p
PTC	92.966	86.434	99.498	0.845
FTC	83.498	72.398	94.598	

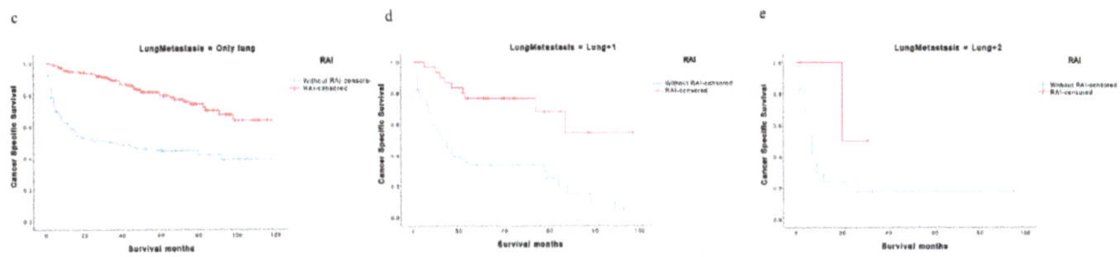

LungMetastasis	RAI	Estimate	Mean 95% Confidence Interval Lower Bound	Upper Bound	p
Only lung	Without RAI	56.895	47.546	66.244	<0.001
	RAI	94.955	88.669	101.241	
Lung+1	Without RAI	30.372	21.502	39.241	<0.001
	RAI	69.956	55.586	84.326	
Lung+2	Without RAI	22.000	5.775	38.225	0.216
	RAI	25.500	17.877	33.123	

Figure 2. Stratified Kaplan–Meier survival curves of TCSS based on subgroups of age, histology, and lung metastasis. (**a**) In TCLM patients who underwent RAI treatment following primary surgery, younger patients (age < 55 years) exhibited enhanced TCSS compared to older patients (age ≥ 55 years). (**b**) Among TCLM patients who underwent primary site surgery and received RAI therapy, no statistical difference in TCSS was observed between PTC patients and FTC patients. (**c**–**e**) Among TCLM patients who underwent primary site surgery and received RAI therapy, those with only lung metastasis exhibited superior TCSS compared to those with a combination of lung and one other distant metastasis. Only lung: Thyroid cancer patients with single organ metastases at lung; Lung + 1: Thyroid cancer patients combined with lung and one other distant metastasis; Lung + 2: Thyroid cancer patients combined with lung and other several distant metastases.

4. Discussion

The results of this study indicate that surgery at the primary site may serve as an independent prognostic factor to improve the OS and TCSS in patients with TCLM. A previous study reported that surgery at the primary site, whether for the primary or distant site, can prolong OS and TCSS in TCLM patients [27]. Additionally, our study suggests that combining surgery of the primary site with RAI therapy may further enhance the prognosis of patients with lung metastasis compared to surgery of the primary site alone. These findings underscore the importance for clinicians to carefully consider the appropriate surgical approach and adjuvant therapy for lung metastasis, factoring in the patient's overall condition.

RAI therapy has been identified as a highly efficacious intervention for the management of metastatic DTC, offering a substantial extension of life expectancy for patients [28]. Our results demonstrate that RAI therapy confers a significant improvement in both overall survival rate and thyroid cancer-specific survival rate for patients with TCLM compared to those who do not receive RAI therapy. Despite the considerable number of studies that examine the impact of RAI therapy on the prognosis of DTC patients with lung metastasis [11,29], few studies have reported the effect of RAI therapy on the prognosis of all histological types of thyroid cancer with lung metastasis. Therefore, this study provides a systematic analysis of the factors influencing the survival of patients with this condition.

Firstly, this study has revealed that nearly 50 percent of post-thyroidectomy patients with TCLM did not undergo RAI therapy, possibly due to the failure to meet therapeutic criteria, specifically, the lack of iodine uptake in metastatic lung lesions. In addition, the guidelines for RAI therapy of DTC [30] have indicated that ^{131}I treatment for pulmonary metastasis is largely dependent of iodine uptake, age, nodule size, and the presence of other distant metastatic lesions. Notably, Song et al. have suggested that DTC patients at <40 years old and with small and only lung metastases, without other organ metastases, had better outcomes with RAI therapy [23]. Similarly, our study has identified that age plays a significant role in the effectiveness of RAI therapy on the prognosis of patients with lung metastasis after thyroidectomy. Specifically, our results have demonstrated that patients under 55 years of age treated with RAI therapy have a more favorable prognosis compared to those aged 55 years and above. Moreover, the study has revealed that patients with lung metastasis alone had a better survival rate than those with lung and other distant metastases after RAI therapy. Conversely, there was no statistically significant difference in prognosis among patients with multiple distant metastases, which may be attributed to the small sample size of patients with lung and other metastases.

Additionally, it has been reported that some patients with thyroid carcinoma and lung metastases who either fail to uptake iodine or lose iodine uptake properties following RAI therapy eventually develop radioiodine-refractory thyroid cancer (RAIR-TC) over time [31]. The loss of iodine uptake may be consequent upon the dedifferentiation of malignant cells resulting in reduced expression of the sodium/iodide symporter (NIS) or clonal selection. One of the risk factors for the prognosis of these patients is the iodine uptake of distant metastases, Hong-Jun Song et al. found that, amongst TCLM patients, those unresponsive to RAI therapy bore a significantly lower 10-year survival rate [23]. However, only two-thirds of TCLM patients had ^{131}I uptake in their metastases [32]. Considering the adverse effects of other therapeutic modalities, it is necessary to strictly grasp the indications for application before deciding on further treatment options. Thus, this analysis of various risk factors may assist in identifying patients who are suitable candidates for RAI treatment.

Finally, our findings support the 2015 ATA recommendations for RAI therapy [21] as a post-thyroidectomy treatment. However, it is worth noting that, while the 2015 ATA guidelines [21] strongly recommend RAI treatment for TCLM patients with lung micrometastases, our study has provided further evidence in specific subgroups of TCLM patients and has expanded the clinical application of RAI therapy for TCLM patients following primary site surgery.

Li et al. have reported that RAI therapy should be precisely administered to young patients with well-differentiated tumors and may improve survival rates of lung metastases [11]. Consistent with these findings, our study has demonstrated that RAI therapy significantly enhances OS and TCSS in TCLM patients following primary site surgery under the age of 55, PTC patients, and those with single organ metastases at lung. Additionally, the results may assist clinicians in determining which patients will benefit from RAI therapy, thus providing new avenues for treatment.

However, this study is not without certain limitations. First of all, the number of patients with ATC and MTC in the histology sample is limited, leading to potential statistical bias. Secondly, this study relies on a public database, and further validation of clinical information for patients is required. Additionally, the dose and frequency of administration, as well as the route of administration, the time interval between primary surgery and RAI treatment, and other factors may also influence RAI treatment outcomes. Unfortunately, the SEER database does not contain sufficient data to thoroughly investigate these issues. Finally, it should be noted that the SEER database does not include information on iodine uptake rate, thyroid-stimulating hormone suppression therapy, or serological indicators of thyroid, including serum *BRAFV600E* mutation, progressive nodal burden, extrathyroidal extension, thoracic surgery for lung metastasis, and thyroxine kinase inhibitors

(TKI). Thoracic surgery for lung metastases can indeed potentially affect the efficacy of RAI treatment and may provide survival benefits for specific patients. Furthermore, postoperative survival rates depend highly on factors such as the primary tumor entity, histology and differentiation, absence of disease interval, and the number and size of metastatic lesions [33]. Research has demonstrated that targeted therapy with TKIs can improve clinical outcomes in TCLM patients [34,35]. These factors are essential for assessing the risk of thyroid cancer recurrence [36–38].

5. Conclusions

This study identified that, compared to primary site surgery alone, RAI in conjunction with surgery significantly improved TCSS for TCLM patients. Specifically, TCLM patients after thyroid surgery who are younger (<55 years), have PTC and metastases only in the lungs, and without involvement of other organs may benefit from RAI treatment. These results have important implications for identifying TCLM patients who have undergone primary site surgery that may be candidates for iodine therapy, as well as developing appropriate treatment regimens for them.

Supplementary Materials: The following supporting information can be downloaded at: https://www.mdpi.com/article/10.3390/biomedicines12030532/s1, Figure S1: Stratified Kaplan-Meier survival curves of TCSS based on subgroup of age and histology; Table S1: Demographic and clinicopathologic features of thyroid cancer patients with and without lung metastases; Table S2: Surgical types of primary site in TCLM patients.

Author Contributions: S.Z., M.Z. and H.Z. made substantial contributions to the acquisition, analysis, and interpretation of data. S.Z., M.Z. and X.F. all played a central role in the conception and design of the manuscript. The manuscript was written by S.Z. and M.Z. H.Z., X.F. and J.Z. were involved in critically revising it for important intellectual content. H.L. made significant contributions to supervision, review writing, and editing. F.Y. contributed massively to the conception, obtaining of funds, supervision, writing evaluations, and editing. All authors have read and agreed to the published version of the manuscript.

Funding: The study was supported by research grants from National Natural Science Foundation of China (82071956), Clinical Research Plan of SHDC (2020CR4065), National Key Research and Development Program of China (2020YFA0909000), National Natural Science Foundation of China (82127807), and Shanghai Key Laboratory of Molecular Imaging (18DZ2260400).

Institutional Review Board Statement: Not applicable.

Informed Consent Statement: Not applicable.

Data Availability Statement: These researchers analyzed publicly available datasets. This information can be found here: "https://seer.cancer.gov/".

Acknowledgments: The authors would like to thank all of the patients who participated in this study. The authors wish to thank everyone in Surveillance, Epidemiology, and End Results for their help in collecting medical records.

Conflicts of Interest: The authors have no relevant financial or non-financial interests to disclose.

Abbreviations

Thyroid cancer (TC); Differentiated thyroid cancer patients with lung metastasis (DTC–LM); Journal of the National Cancer Center (JNCC); differentiated thyroid cancer (DTC); medullary thyroid cancer (MTC); anaplastic thyroid cancer (ATC); Papillary thyroid cancer (PTC); follicular thyroid cancer (FTC); Radioiodine therapy (RAI); thyroid cancer with lung metastasis (TCLM); American Thyroid Association (ATA); The Surveillance, Epidemiology, and End Results (SEER); American Joint Committee on Cancer (AJCC); Collaborative Staging (CS); odds ratio (OR); overall survival (OS); thyroid cancer-specific survival (TCSS); hazard ratio (HR); lung metastasis (LM); confidence intervals (CI); radioiodine-refractory thyroid cancer (RAIR-TC); thyroxine kinase inhibitors (TKI).

References

1. Liu, S.; Zuo, R.; Yang, T.; Pang, H.; Wang, Z. A semiquantitative study of the optimal whole-body imaging time after 131I therap for differentiated thyroid cancer. *Front. Endocrinol.* **2022**, *13*, 955387. [CrossRef] [PubMed]
2. Bao, W.-Q.; Zi, H.; Yuan, Q.-Q.; Li, L.-Y.; Deng, T. Global burden of thyroid cancer and its attributable risk factors in 204 countrie and territories from 1990 to 2019. *Thorac. Cancer* **2021**, *12*, 2494–2503. [CrossRef] [PubMed]
3. Zheng, R.; Zhang, S.; Zeng, H.; Wang, S.; Sun, K.; Chen, R.; Li, L.; Wei, W.; He, J. Cancer incidence and mortality in China, 2016. *Natl. Cancer Cent.* **2022**, *2*, 1–9. [CrossRef]
4. Araque, K.A.; Gubbi, S.; Klubo-Gwiezdzinska, J. Updates on the Management of Thyroid Cancer. *Horm. Metab. Res.* **2020**, *5* 562–577. [CrossRef] [PubMed]
5. Fallahi, P.; Ferrari, S.M.; Galdiero, M.R.; Varricchi, G.; Elia, G.; Ragusa, F.; Paparo, S.R.; Benvenga, S.; Antonelli, A. Molecula targets of tyrosine kinase inhibitors in thyroid cancer. *Semin. Cancer Biol.* **2022**, *79*, 180–196. [CrossRef] [PubMed]
6. Raue, F.; Frank-Raue, K. Thyroid Cancer: Risk-Stratified Management and Individualized Therapy. *Clin. Cancer Res.* **2016**, *2* 5012–5021. [CrossRef] [PubMed]
7. Sheu, N.-W.; Jiang, H.-J.; Wu, C.-W.; Chiang, F.-Y.; Chiou, H.-Y.C.; Hsiao, P.-J. Lenvatinib complementary with radioiodine therap for patients with advanced differentiated thyroid carcinoma: Case reports and literature review. *World J. Surg. Oncol.* **2019**, *17*, 8 [CrossRef]
8. Cai, M.; Ni, W.-J.; Wang, Y.-H.; Wang, J.-J.; Zhou, H. Targeting TMEM88 as an Attractive Therapeutic Strategy in Malignan Tumors. *Front. Oncol.* **2022**, *12*, 906372. [CrossRef]
9. Maciel, J.; Cavaco, D.; Silvestre, C.; Pereira, J.S.; Vilar, H.; Leite, V. Clinical outcomes of a cohort of 271 patients with lun metastases from differentiated thyroid carcinoma. *Clin. Endocrinol.* **2022**, *97*, 814–821. [CrossRef]
10. Liu, W.; Wang, S.; Ye, Z.; Xu, P.; Xia, X.; Guo, M. Prediction of lung metastases in thyroid cancer using machine learning based o SEER database. *Cancer Med.* **2022**, *11*, 2503–2515. [CrossRef]
11. Li, C.; Wu, Q.; Sun, S. Radioactive Iodine Therapy in Patients With Thyroid Carcinoma With Distant Metastases: A SEER-Base Study. *Cancer Control* **2020**, *27*, 1–9. [CrossRef] [PubMed]
12. Nixon, I.J.; Whitcher, M.M.; Palmer, F.L.; Tuttle, R.M.; Shaha, A.R.; Shah, J.P.; Patel, S.G.; Ganly, I. The impact of distant metastase at presentation on prognosis in patients with differentiated carcinoma of the thyroid gland. *Thyroid* **2012**, *22*, 884–889. [CrossRef
13. Hirsch, D.; Levy, S.; Tsvetov, G.; Gorshtein, A.; Slutzky-Shraga, I.; Akirov, A.; Robenshtok, E.; Shimon, I.; Benbassat, C.A Long-term Outcomes and Prognostic Factors in Patients with Differentiated Thyroid Cancer and Distant Metastases. *Endoc Pract.* **2017**, *23*, 1193–1200. [CrossRef] [PubMed]
14. Altorki, N.K.; Markowitz, G.J.; Gao, D.; Port, J.L.; Saxena, A.; Stiles, B.; McGraw, T.; Mittal, V. The lung microenvironment: A important regulator of tumour growth and metastasis. *Nat. Rev. Cancer* **2019**, *19*, 9–31. [CrossRef] [PubMed]
15. Ferrari, S.M.; Fallahi, P.; Politti, U.; Materazzi, G.; Baldini, E.; Ulisse, S.; Miccoli, P.; Antonelli, A. Molecular Targeted Therapies o Aggressive Thyroid Cancer. *Front. Endocrinol.* **2015**, *6*, 176. [CrossRef] [PubMed]
16. Kondraciuk, J.D.; Rice, S.L.; Zhou, X.; Gharzeddine, K.; Knezevic, A.; Spratt, D.E.; Sabra, M.; Larson, S.M.; Grewal, R.K.; Osborne J.R. Thyroid Cancer Bone Metastasis: Survival and Genomic Characteristics of a Large Tertiary Care Cohort. *Clin. Nucl. Me* **2019**, *44*, e465–e471. [CrossRef] [PubMed]
17. Sohn, S.Y.; Kim, H.I.; Kim, Y.N.; Kim, T.H.; Kim, S.W.; Chung, J.H. Prognostic indicators of outcomes in patients with lung metastases from differentiated thyroid carcinoma during long-term follow-up. *Clin. Endocrinol.* **2018**, *88*, 318–326. [CrossRef]
18. Yang, J.; Zheng, R.; Liang, M.; Jia, Y.; Lin, L.; Geng, J.; Chen, S.; Li, Y.-X. Association of the Cumulative Dose of Radioactive Iodin Therapy With Overall Survival in Patients With Differentiated Thyroid Cancer and Pulmonary Metastases. *Front. Oncol.* **2019**, *9* 558. [CrossRef]
19. Lorusso, L.; Cappagli, V.; Valerio, L.; Giani, C.; Viola, D.; Puleo, L.; Gambale, C.; Minaldi, E.; Campopiano, M.C.; Matrone, A. et al. Thyroid Cancers: From Surgery to Current and Future Systemic Therapies through Their Molecular Identities. *Int. J. Mol Sci.* **2021**, *22*, 3117. [CrossRef]
20. NCCN Guidelines for Patients Thyroid Cancer. Thyroid Cancer. 2020. Available online: http://nccn.org/patients (accessed on 23 February 2024).
21. Haugen, B.R.; Alexander, E.K.; Bible, K.C.; Doherty, G.M.; Mandel, S.J.; Nikiforov, Y.E.; Pacini, F.; Randolph, G.W.; Sawka A.M.; Schlumberger, M.; et al. 2015 American Thyroid Association Management Guidelines for Adult Patients with Thyroid Nodules and Differentiated Thyroid Cancer: The American Thyroid Association Guidelines Task Force on Thyroid Nodules and Differentiated Thyroid Cancer. *Thyroid* **2016**, *26*, 1–133. [CrossRef]
22. Kim, M.; Kim, W.G.; Park, S.; Kwon, H.; Jeon, M.J.; Lee, J.J.; Ryu, J.-S.; Kim, T.Y.; Shong, Y.K.; Kim, W.B. Initial Size of Metastatic Lesions Is Best Prognostic Factor in Patients with Metastatic Differentiated Thyroid Carcinoma Confined to the Lung. *Thyroid* **2017**, *27*, 49–58. [CrossRef]
23. Song, H.-J.; Qiu, Z.-L.; Shen, C.-T.; Wei, W.-J.; Luo, Q.-Y. Pulmonary metastases in differentiated thyroid cancer: Efficacy of radioiodine therapy and prognostic factors. *Eur. J. Endocrinol.* **2015**, *173*, 399–408. [CrossRef]
24. National Cancer Institute. *International Classification of Diseases for Oncology*, 3rd ed.; Definitions; Qeios: London, UK, 2020.
25. Aizer, A.A.; Chen, M.-H.; McCarthy, E.P.; Mendu, M.L.; Koo, S.; Wilhite, T.J.; Graham, P.L.; Choueiri, T.K.; Hoffman, K.E.; Martin N.E.; et al. Marital status and survival in patients with cancer. *J. Clin. Oncol.* **2013**, *31*, 3869–3876. [CrossRef]

26. Ai, L.; Li, N.; Tan, H.-L.; Wei, B.; Zhao, Y.-X.; Chen, P.; Hu, H.-Y.; Liu, M.; Ou-Yang, D.-J.; Qin, Z.-E.; et al. Effects of marital status on survival of medullary thyroid cancer stratified by age. *Cancer Med.* **2021**, *10*, 8829–8837. [CrossRef] [PubMed]
27. Zhong, M.; Khan, F.Z.; He, X.; Cui, L.; Lei, K.; Ge, M. Impact of Lung Metastasis versus Metastasis of Bone, Brain, or Liver on Overall Survival and Thyroid Cancer-Specific Survival of Thyroid Cancer Patients: A Population-Based Study. *Cancers* **2022**, *14*, 3133. [CrossRef] [PubMed]
28. Colombo, C.; Minna, E.; Gargiuli, C.; Muzza, M.; Dugo, M.; De Cecco, L.; Pogliaghi, G.; Tosi, D.; Bulfamante, G.; Greco, A.; et al. The molecular and gene/miRNA expression profiles of radioiodine resistant papillary thyroid cancer. *J. Exp. Clin. Cancer Res.* **2020**, *39*, 245. [CrossRef] [PubMed]
29. Zhang, X.; Liu, D.-S.; Luan, Z.-S.; Zhang, F.; Liu, X.-H.; Zhou, W.; Zhong, S.-F.; Lai, H. Efficacy of radioiodine therapy for treating 20 patients with pulmonary metastases from differentiated thyroid cancer and a meta-analysis of the current literature. *Clin. Transl. Oncol.* **2018**, *20*, 928–935. [CrossRef] [PubMed]
30. Avram, A.M.; Zukotynski, K.; Nadel, H.R.; Giovanella, L. Management of Differentiated Thyroid Cancer: The Standard of Care. *J. Nucl. Med.* **2022**, *63*, 189–195. [CrossRef]
31. Moneke, I.; Kaifi, J.T.; Kloeser, R.; Samson, P.; Haager, B.; Wiesemann, S.; Diederichs, S.; Passlick, B. Pulmonary metastasectomy for thyroid cancer as salvage therapy for radioactive iodine-refractory metastases. *Eur. J. Surg.* **2018**, *53*, 625–630. [CrossRef]
32. Schlumberger, M.; Challeton, C.; De Vathaire, F.; Travagli, J.P.; Gardet, P.; Lumbroso, J.D.; Francese, C.; Fontaine, F.; Ricard, M.; Parmentier, C. Radioactive iodine treatment and external radiotherapy for lung and bone metastases from thyroid carcinoma. *J. Nucl. Med.* **1996**, *37*, 598–605.
33. Khan, J.H.; McElhinney, D.B.; Rahman, S.B.; George, T.I.; Clark, O.H.; Merrick, S.H. Pulmonary metastases of endocrine origin: The role of surgery. *Chest* **1998**, *114*, 526–534. [CrossRef] [PubMed]
34. Iwasaki, H.; Yamazaki, H.; Takasaki, H.; Suganuma, N.; Sakai, R.; Nakayama, H.; Hatori, S.; Toda, S.; Masudo, K. Treatment outcomes of differentiated thyroid cancer with distant metastasis improve by tyrosine kinase inhibitors. *Oncol. Lett.* **2019**, *17*, 5292–5300. [CrossRef] [PubMed]
35. Tahara, M.; Kiyota, N.; Hoff, A.O.; Badiu, C.; Owonikoko, T.K.; Dutcus, C.E.; Suzuki, T.; Ren, M.; Wirth, L.J. Impact of lung metastases on overall survival in the phase 3 SELECT study of lenvatinib in patients with radioiodine-refractory differentiated thyroid cancer. *Eur. J. Cancer* **2021**, *147*, 51–57. [CrossRef] [PubMed]
36. Leong, D.; Gill, A.J.; Turchini, J.; Waller, M.; Clifton-Bligh, R.; Glover, A.; Sywak, M.; Sidhu, S. The Prognostic Impact of Extent of Vascular Invasion in Follicular Thyroid Carcinoma. *World J. Surg.* **2022**, *47*, 412–420. [CrossRef]
37. Le, M.-K.; Kawai, M.; Odate, T.; Vuong, H.G.; Oishi, N.; Kondo, T. Metastatic Risk Stratification of 2526 Medullary Thyroid Carcinoma Patients: A Study Based on Surveillance, Epidemiology, and End Results Database. *Endocr. Pathol.* **2022**, *33*, 348–358. [CrossRef]
38. Ho, A.S.; Luu, M.; Shafqat, I.; Mallen-St Clair, J.; Chen, M.M.; Chen, Y.; Jain, M.; Ali, N.; Patio, C.; Filarski, C.F.; et al. Predictive Impact of Metastatic Lymph Node Burden on Distant Metastasis Across Papillary Thyroid Cancer Variants. *Thyroid* **2021**, *31*, 1549–1557. [CrossRef]

biomedicines

MDPI

Article

Association of *BRAF* V600E Mutant Allele Proportion with the Dissemination Stage of Papillary Thyroid Cancer

Ivan Blazekovic [1,2], Ivan Samija [1,3,*], Josipa Perisa [1], Koraljka Gall Troselj [4], Tihana Regovic Dzombeta [5,6], Petra Radulovic [5], Matija Romic [1], Roko Granic [1], Ines Sisko Markos [1,2], Ana Frobe [1,3], Zvonko Kusic [7] and Tomislav Jukic [1,6,8]

1 Department of Oncology and Nuclear Medicine, University Hospital Center Sestre Milosrdnice, 10 000 Zagreb, Croatia; blazekovic90@gmail.com (I.B.); jperisa92@gmail.com (J.P.); romicmatija1@gmail.com (M.R.); roko.granic@gmail.com (R.G.); inessisko@gmail.com (I.S.M.); ana.frobe@kbcsm.hr (A.F.); tomislav.jukic@kbcsm.hr (T.J.)
2 School of Medicine, Catholic University of Croatia, 10 000 Zagreb, Croatia
3 School of Dental Medicine, University of Zagreb, 10 000 Zagreb, Croatia
4 Laboratory for Epigenomics, Division of Molecular Medicine, Ruđer Bošković Institute, 10 000 Zagreb, Croatia; troselj@irb.hr
5 Department of Pathology Ljudevit Jurak, University Hospital Center Sestre Milosrdnice, 10 000 Zagreb, Croatia; tihana.dzombeta@mef.hr (T.R.D.); pradulovi@gmail.com (P.R.)
6 School of Medicine, University of Zagreb, 10000 Zagreb, Croatia
7 Croatian Academy of Science and Arts, 10000 Zagreb, Croatia; zaklada@hazu.hr
8 Faculty of Medicine Osijek, Josip Juraj Strossmayer University of Osijek, 31 000 Osijek, Croatia
* Correspondence: ivan.samija@kbcsm.hr

Abstract: The early identification of aggressive forms of cancer is of high importance in treating papillary thyroid cancer (PTC). Disease dissemination is a major factor influencing patient survival. Mutation status of *BRAF* oncogene, *BRAF* V600E, is proposed to be an indicator of disease recurrence; however, its influence on PTC dissemination has not been deciphered. This study aimed to explore the association of the frequency of *BRAF* V600E alleles in PTC with disease dissemination. In this study, 173 PTC samples were analyzed, measuring the proportion of *BRAF* V600E alleles by qPCR, which was then normalized against the proportion of tumor cells. Semiquantitative analysis of BRAF V600E mutant protein was performed by immunohistochemistry. The *BRAF* V600E mutation was present in 60% of samples, while the normalized frequency of mutated *BRAF* alleles ranged from 1.55% to 92.06%. There was no significant association between the presence and/or proportion of the *BRAF* V600E mutation with the degree of PTC dissemination. However, the presence of the *BRAF* mutation was significantly linked with angioinvasion. This study's results suggest that there is a heterogeneous distribution of the *BRAF* mutation and the presence of oligoclonal forms of PTC. It is likely that the *BRAF* mutation alone does not significantly contribute to PTC aggressiveness.

Keywords: papillary thyroid cancer; dissemination; *BRAF* V600E; tumor heterogeneity; qPCR

1. Introduction

Thyroid cancer is a common tumor with a significant increase in incidence. Croatia ranks 4th according to the age-standardized incidence rate in Europe [1,2]. In recent years, increased screening in the general population, primarily in developed countries, has led to an increase in the incidence of PTC [3,4]. According to the data from the Surveillance, Epidemiology, and End Results-9 (SEER-9) cancer registry program [5], the mortality rate for thyroid cancer is increasing as well. This suggests that the increase in incidence cannot solely be attributed to improvements in diagnostic methods, but also to changes in disease aggressiveness, likely caused by environmental factors [6,7].

Although considered to be an indolent tumor, that most often occurs as a localized disease or with lymphogenic metastases, PTC can still initially present with hematogenous metastases in approximately 4% of patients, leading to an increased risk of recurrence and an increased mortality rate [8–10]. It is crucial to differentiate the indolent type of PTC from the more aggressive forms as early as possible. The discovery of new subclinical cases and the treatment with long-term follow-up of patients with non-aggressive diseases represent a significant burden for the patient, as well as for the healthcare system. The discovery of molecular markers that would allow for early recognition of well-differentiated thyroid tumors with a higher potential of disease dissemination, would enable timely recognition of high-risk patients. Research on genetic changes, especially mutations that may affect the biological behavior of tumors, will allow for a better understanding of the fundamental molecular features that determine the aggressiveness of thyroid cancer [11,12].

Well-differentiated thyroid tumors, according to the standard accepted model of oncogenesis, arise from the gradual malignant transformation of thyroid cells [13]. The most common mutations in PTC affect *BRAF* (B-Raf proto-oncogene serine/threonine-protein kinase) and *RAS* genes. These mutations, as well as RET/PTC rearrangements, are considered to be driving mutations. There are also *TERT* (Telomerase Reverse Transcriptase) gene mutations that occur at a later stage of tumor development and additionally contribute to tumor aggressiveness [12,14,15]. Mutations in the aforementioned genes are present in approximately 70% of all thyroid cancers [16]. Recent data suggest that certain molecular profiles, such as the coexistence of *BRAF* with other oncogenic mutations, TERT promoter mutations, or TP53 mutations may be more specific markers of a less favorable outcome of PTC [17]. Diagnostic and predictive value of *RAS* mutation are limited in thyroid nodular disease [18]. However, the presence of *BRAF* or *RAS* mutations enhances the prognostic effects of *TERT* promoter mutations [19]. It has also been shown that *TERT* promoter mutations significantly increase the risk of both recurrence and mortality in high-risk (according to American Thyroid Association, ATA) and TNM stage III/IV groups [19]. Currently, ATA guidelines suggest high risk of recurrence in patients with both *BRAF* and *TERT* mutation. On the other hand, the presence of *BRAF* mutation is only associated with a low and intermediate risk of recurrence. Clinical significance of isolated *BRAF* mutation for risk stratification is not clear, and it is not routinely recommended in postoperative care of PTC [8].

Mutation *BRAF* V600E is the most common mutation in PTC, with an average incidence rate of approximately 45%, ranging from 27.3 to 87.1% [20,21]. This type of mutation has been discovered in more than 90% of PTCs with known *BRAF* mutations. If BRAF V600E is present, the activity of BRAF kinase is 480 times higher than in the BRAF wild-type cells [22]. The mutation is in the activating domain of the protein (CR3), which is composed of amino acids 457–717 [23]. The mutation itself results in constitutive activation of the MAP-kinase signaling pathway, which can result in aberrant gene expression, accelerated proliferation, and avoidance of apoptosis. Although extensively investigated, the clear association between the presence of the *BRAF* V600E mutation and clinicopathological prognostic factors of PTC has not yet been demonstrated [24]. Accordingly, mutation in the *BRAF* gene, as a prognostic factor in PTC, is still questionable [25,26]. Recent research has revealed the molecular mechanisms determining the progression and aggressiveness of PTC due to *BRAF* mutation [27,28]. These mechanisms include the down-regulation of major tumor suppressor genes and thyroid iodide-metabolizing genes, as well as the up-regulation of molecules that promote cancer, such as vascular endothelial growth factor (VEGF) A and its receptor VEGF receptor (VEGFR)-2, the main regulators of the angiogenic process [28].

The results of research based on the association of the mutation with the clinicopathological prognostic factors of PTC (bilaterality, multifocality, thyroid capsule infiltration, and lymph node metastases) remain controversial. While some studies show a connection between the presence of a mutation and the aforementioned factors [29,30], the results of other studies did not demonstrate such connection [26]. A study showed that presence of the *BRAF* mutation was significantly associated with increased cancer-related mortality in PTC patients [31]. The study found that the recurrence rates were higher in *BRAF* mutation-positive patients (47.71 per 1000 person-years) compared to those who were *BRAF* mutation-negative (26.03 per 1000 person-years). This difference was statistically significant ($p < 0.001$), with a hazard ratio (HR) of 1.82 (95% CI, 1.46 to 2.28). On the other hand, another study found that this difference remained significant even after adjusting for clinicopathogenic factors in a multivariable model [32]. In all studies cited, only the presence or absence of the *BRAF* V600E mutation was explored, without a further quantification of mutated alleles, in positive cases. However, *BRAF* mutation may only be present in a small proportion of cells. This is especially important when a large lymphocytic infiltrate is present, as in the case of Hashimoto's thyroiditis, where mutated, tumor-originating *BRAF* alleles become "diluted" by wild-type alleles originating from infiltrating lymphocytes [33]. Furthermore, the monoclonality of PTC has recently been questioned by multiple studies [34–37]. These studies claim that there is a heterogeneous distribution of cells containing mutation *BRAF* V600E, within the tumor [23–26]. The heterogenous distribution could be one of the proposed explanations for the unclear relationship between the presence of the *BRAF* V600E mutation and the prognostic factors that determine the aggressiveness of PTC [34–37]. It has been also suggested that *BRAF* V600E mutation is heterogeneously distributed and limited to part of the tumor cells in most PTC samples [35,38]. The aim of this research is to study the association of the proportion of tumor cells with *BRAF* V600E coding allele and the dissemination of the disease.

2. Materials and Methods

2.1. Participants

We retrospectively collected data from 173 adult patients diagnosed with PTC at the Department of Oncology and Nuclear Medicine of the University Hospital Center Sestre milosrdnice, Zagreb, Croatia. All procedures were in accordance with the 1964 Helsinki Declaration and its later amendments, or comparable ethical standards. The study was approved by the institutional Ethics Committee (University Hospital Center Sestre milosrdnice; approval No. EP-9941/19-7), and informed consent was obtained from all the patients. Paraffin blocks of the primary thyroid tumor after total thyroidectomy were collected. We also assessed data on the pathohistological (PH) characteristics of the tumor, clinical data, and data related to postoperative oncological treatment.

Based on the PH findings, the following data were collected: size of the primary tumor, area of thyroid involvement (left or right lobe, isthmus), dissemination within the thyroid gland, infiltration of the thyroid capsule, extrathyroidal expansion, and angioinvasion (i.e., tumor cells in vascular spaces determined by histopathologic examination).

Based on the findings of postoperative oncological treatment, as well as the findings of PH, it was established whether there were metastatic positive lymph nodes in the neck and distant metastases sites. With respect to positive lymph nodes, the largest metastatic lymph node was analyzed, and breakthrough of the lymph node capsule, if present, was noted.

2.2. Histological Analysis of the Primary Tumor

After fixation in 10% buffered formalin and dehydration in increasing concentrations of alcohol, the removed thyroid tissue was embedded in paraffin blocks. Paraffin sections were cut at 5 μm. Deparaffinization in xylene and hemalaun and eosin staining (H&E) was performed by the standard method. Sections were cut from each block in the following manner: the first section stained with H&E was used to assess the proportion of tumor cells expressed as a percentage in relation to all remaining cells in that section. The next few sections were then used for the extraction of genomic DNA for *BRAF* V600E mutation analysis. An additional section obtained from 45 selected paraffin blocks (positive and negative in relation to the presence of the mutation *BRAF* V600E) was used for analyzing BRAF on a protein level, by immunohistochemistry.

2.3. DNA Extraction and BRAF V600E Mutation Detection

DNA was extracted following the manufacturer's instructions using the QIAamp DNA FFPE Tissue kit (Qiagen, Hilden, Germany). The concentration and quality of the extracted DNA was determined using NanoDrop 2000 (Thermo Fisher Scientific, Waltham, MA, USA) spectrophotometer. Only DNA of OD (optical density coefficient, 260/280) 1.70 ± 20% was used for further experiments.

For mutation analysis, the target DNA was amplified and detected using TaqMan® Mutation Detection Assay (Applied Biosystems, Foster City, CA, USA) on 7500 Real-time PCR System (Applied Biosystems, Foster City, CA, USA) following the manufacturer's instructions. Each reaction was performed in triplicate, using 25 ng of DNA. In each reaction, a negative and a positive control were used.

Analysis of qPCR reaction data was performed with Mutation Detector software package (Applied Biosystems, Foster City, CA, USA). From the Ct values obtained with the TaqMan mutation detection probe and the TaqMan reference gene probe, the normalized ΔCt value was calculated. The percentage of mutated alleles was calculated from the normalized ΔCt according to the following Formula (1):

$$\%\text{mutation} = [1/2\Delta\text{Ct} \div (1/2\Delta\text{Ct} + 1)] \times 100\% \quad (1)$$

Since the assessment of genetic heterogeneity in tumor samples can be imprecise due to the presence of non-tumor cells, the data related to the percentage of mutation were normalized with respect to the previously determined percentage of tumor cells in the sample, according to the following Formula (2) as suggested by de Biase et al. [36]:

$$\text{Normalized \% mutation in tumor} = \text{\% mutation}/\text{\% tumor cells in the section of the preparation} \quad (2)$$

2.4. Immunohistochemical (IHC) Analysis

The presence of *BRAF* V600E mutation (Ventana anti-*BRAF* V600E/VE1, Roche, Mannheim, Germany) was determined in 45 tumor sections using the BenchMark GX automatic multifunctional IHC staining system (Roche, Basel, Switzerland) with the OptiView DAB Detection Kit (Ventana Medical Systems Inc., Oro Valley, AZ, USA), following the manufacturer's instructions. The antibody used was previously validated for detecting BRAF V600E protein in thyroid cancer [39]. Post-counterstaining was performed using Bluing Reagent, after Hematoxylin counterstaining. Metastatic melanoma tissue with a confirmed *BRAF* gene mutation was used as a positive control. In the case of a positive finding, the percentage of PTC cells with expressed altered protein in the analyzed sample was estimated.

2.5. Statistical Methods in Data Processing

The comparison of the clinicopathological features between the groups with and without *BRAF* V600E mutation was performed using the χ^2 test, Mann–Whitney, and *t*-test, while the association between the frequency of *BRAF* V600E mutated alleles and the extent of PTC was tested with a one-way ANOVA and Spearman test. A comparison of the concordance between the *BRAF* mutation results and the results obtained by immunohistochemistry was tested using Cohen's kappa method. Statistical analysis was performed using the Statistica program (StatSoft, Inc., Hamburg, Germany). A statistically significant result was considered to be $p < 0.05$.

3. Results

3.1. Association between BRAF Mutation with Disease Dissemination and Characteristics of the Disease

Patient and tumor characteristics are presented in Table 1. We analyzed the association between the existence of the *BRAF* V600E mutation as well as the normalized values of the proportion of the mutated allele *BRAF* V600E with disease dissemination, age, sex, tumor size, capsule breakthrough, angioinvasion, dissemination within the thyroid gland, extrathyroidal expansion and infiltration of the lymph node capsule, in case of local metastases.

Table 1. Sex and age of the patient, extent of the disease, and clinicopathological characteristics of the tumor.

Basic Characteristics of the Patient	All Patients		*BRAF* +	*BRAF* −	*p* Value
	Gender (n = 173); n (%)				
Women	109 (63.0)		62	47	$p = 0.257$ [a]
Men	64 (37.0)		42	22	
Age, mean ± SD, years	46.56 ± 16.62		49.58 ± 15.5	42.01 ± 17.3	$p = 0.003$ [*,b]
	Dissemination (n = 173); n (%)				
Confined to the thyroid	81 (46.8)		50 (61.7)	31 (38.3)	$p = 0.154$ [a]
Loco-regional involvement	61 (35.3)		40 (65.6)	21 (34.4)	
Distant metastases	31 (17.9)		14 (45.2)	17 (54.8)	
Tumor size, mean ± SD, mm	2.03 ± 1.33		1.84 ± 1.05	2.35 ± 1.60	$p = 0.09$ [b]
	Perforation of the thyroid capsule (n = 167); n (%)				
YES	37 (22.2)		21 (56.8)	16 (43.2)	$p = 0.541$ [a]
NO	130(77.8)		81 (62.3)	49 (37.7)	
	Dissemination within the thyroid gland (n = 169); n (%)				
YES	67(39.6)		38 (56.7)	29 (43.3)	$p = 0.433$ [a]
NO	102(60.4)		64 (62.7)	38 (37.3)	
	Extrathyroidal spreading (n = 164); n (%)				
YES	37	22.6	23(62.2)	14(37.8)	$p = 0.866$ [a]
NO	127	77.4	77 (60.6)	50 (39.4)	
	Angioinvasion (n = 132); n (%)				
YES	12 (9,1)		4(33.3)	8 (66.7)	$p = 0.043$ [*,a]
NO	120 (90.9)		76 (63.3)	44 (36.7)	
	Breakthrough of the lymph node capsule (n = 47); n (%)				
YES	6	12.8	3	3	$p = 0.309$ [a]
NO	41	87.2	29	12	

n = number of patients; [a]: Chi^2-test; [b]: Mann–Whitney test; * statistically significant *p* value.

There was no significant association between the existence of the *BRAF* V600E mutation and disease dissemination (χ^2 (1, N = 173) = 3.737; $p = 0.154$). The results of our study show a lack of association of the *BRAF* mutation status with gender ($\chi^2 = 1.2859$; $p = 0.257$), tumor size (Mann–Whitney U test; U = 2890.5, Z = −1.69, $p = 0.09$), extrathyroidal expansion (χ^2 (1, N = 164) = 0.028; $p = 0.866$), capsule infiltration (χ^2 (1, N = 167) = 0.373; $p = 0.541$), or dissemination within the thyroid gland (χ^2 (1, N = 169) = 0.614; p = 0.433). There was a statistically significant association between the presence of *BRAF* V600E and angioinvasion (χ^2 (1, N = 132) = 4.112; $p = 0.043$). Also, age at diagnosis was significantly higher in the group with *BRAF* V600E mutation (Mann–Whitney U test; U = 2613.5, Z = 3.02, $p = 0.03$). If lymphatic metastases were present, the relationship between the lymph node capsule infiltration and the existence of the *BRAF* V600E mutation was analyzed, but no statistically significant association was found (χ^2 (1, N = 47) = 1.035; p = 0.309).

Further analysis of the association of the normalized frequency of mutated allele *BRAF* with disease dissemination, presented in Table 2, did not show a statistically significant association (ANOVA test, F(2, 97)=0.28287, p = 0.754). No statistically significant association of heterogeneity with dissemination was shown, even when patients were divided into those with a frequency of tumor cells below 40%, 40 to 60%, and those above 60% (Table 3; χ^2 (4, N = 100) = 3.257; p = 0.515). There was also no statistically significant association with thyroid capsule infiltration (Mann–Whitney U test; U = 808, Z = 0, p = 1.000), tumor angioinvasion (Mann–Whitney U test; U = 72, Z = −1.663, p = 0.096), dissemination in the thyroid gland (Mann–Whitney U test; U = 1052, Z = 0.557, p = 0.576), and extrathyroidal expansion (Mann–Whitney U test, U = 776, Z = 0.54, p = 0.589). Although the age at the time of diagnosis was significantly higher in the group with *BRAF* mutation, further analysis of the group with *BRAF* mutation showed no statistically significant correlation between the percentage of mutated allele and age at diagnosis (Spearman's test, N = 100; t = 0.311; p = 0.756). There was also no statistically significant correlation between the percentage of mutated allele and tumor size (Spearman's test, N = 98, R = 0.0196; t = 0.192; p = 0.847).

Table 2. Association of the frequency of the *BRAF* V600E mutated allele and dissemination status.

Normalized Percentage of *BRAF V600E* Allele				
Disease dissemination	Arithmetic mean (%)	CI− 95.00%	CI+ 95.00%	N
Confined to the thyroid	29.63	22.99	36.27	47
Loco-regional involvement	28.23	20.94	35.52	39
Distant metastases	33.61	21.44	45.78	14
ANOVA test, F(2, 97) = 0.28287, p = 0.754				

N = number of patients; χ^2 = Chi^2-test.

Table 3. Distribution of patients according to the frequency of the mutation allele *BRAF* V600E.

Number of Patients					
		Groups according to the normalized percentage of *BRAF V600E* allele			Total number
		Up to 40%	40% to 60%	More than 60%	
Disease dissemination	Confined to the thyroid	36 (74.5%)	7 (14.9%)	5 (10.6%)	47
	Loco-regional involvement	30 (76.9%)	5 (12.8%)	4 (10.3%)	39
	Distant metastases	11 (78.6%)	0 (0%)	3 (21.4%)	14
Total		76	12	12	100
(χ^2 (4, N = 100) = 3.257; p = 0.515)					

N = number of patients; χ^2 = Chi^2-test; N = 100 including only *BRAF* V600E positive patients with data on normalized percentage of *BRAF* V600E allele.

3.2. *Heterogeneity of Mutated BRAF V600E Allele (qPCR)*

The mutation *BRAF* V600E in primary tumors was detected in 104 (60.1%) of a total of 173 tumors. The percentage of *BRAF* V600E alleles assessed with qPCR ranged from 0.5% to 41.6%, with a median of 5.91%. The estimated proportion of tumor cells in the sample ranged from 5% to 90% with a median of 30%. The normalized proportion of mutated *BRAF* V600E allele ranged from 1.55% to 92.06%, with a median of 23.33% (Figure 1). We observed a wide range of values of the normalized proportion but noticed that the majority of tumors (76%) had less than 40% mutated *BRAF* alleles (Table 3).

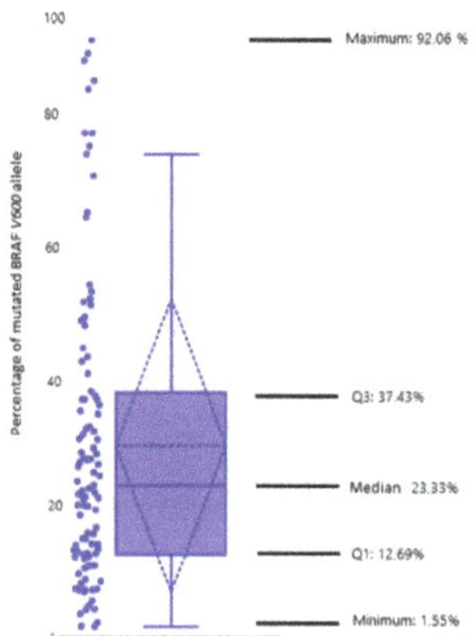

Figure 1. Box-plot showing the proportion of mutated allele in the primary tumor of all *BRAF* V600E positive patients. A single dot indicates the percentage of mutated allele for each individual *BRAF* positive patient. Marked on the picture: median, maximum, and minimum value, first and third quartile.

3.3. Comparison of qPCR and Immunohistochemistry Method

Staining of BRAF V600E mutated protein by IHC (Figure 2) was performed on 45 samples, 43 of which were included in further analysis. The two remaining samples were not further analyzed due to unspecific cytoplasmic staining of tumor cells and staining of stromal cells. Of 43 samples, 13 were negative for the presence of BRAF-mutated protein. The same samples were also negative when analyzed by qPCR. Of a total of 30 IHC-positive samples, 29 were positive by qPCR analysis. The only sample that was negative for the presence of the *BRAF* V600E by qPCR and positive by immunohistochemical staining had a percentage of BRAF mutated protein-containing cells of only 5%. Cohen's kappa test showed a very good agreement between the results of BRAF mutation analysis obtained by two methods (Cohen's Kappa = 0.9460; % of agreement: 97.67).

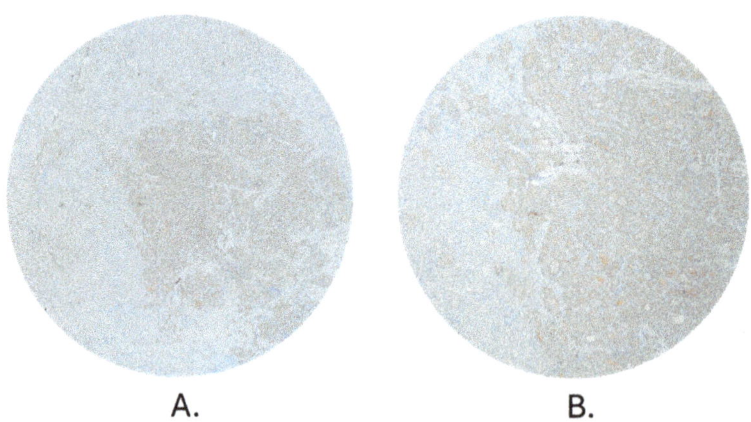

Figure 2. *Cont.*

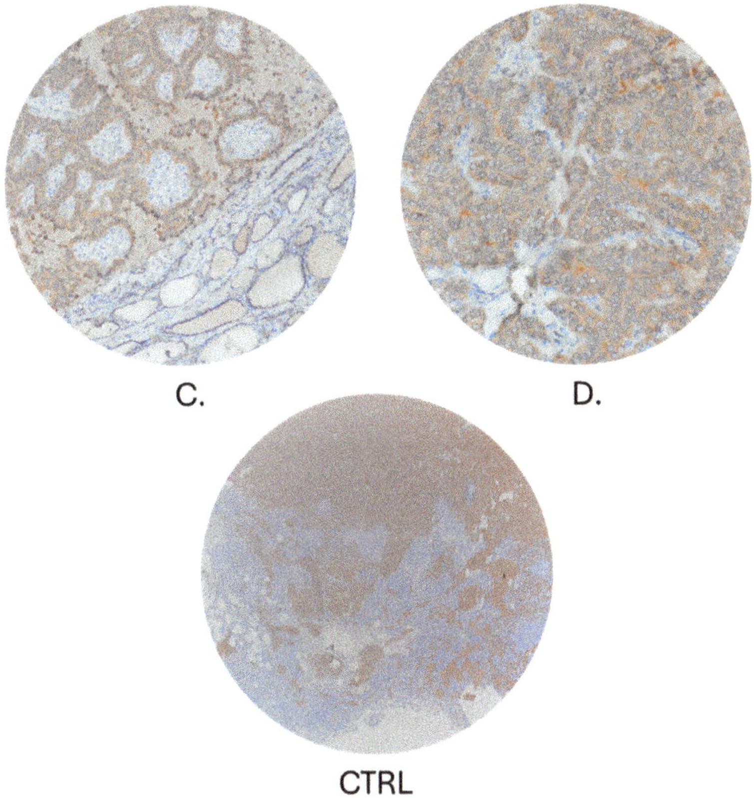

Figure 2. Staining of *BRAF* V600E mutated protein by IHC in tumors of different heterogeneity. Magnifications: (**A**) 40×; (**B**) 100×; (**C**) 200×; (**D**) 400×. CTRL Lymph node with metastatic melanoma showing positive immunohistochemical reaction to BRAF, positive control (100×).

4. Discussion

Due to the fact that the mutation *BRAF* V600E presents the most common mutation in PTC, it is not surprising that numerous studies are exploring the association between *BRAF* mutation and prognostic factors of the disease. So far, published studies have shown inconsistent results, and further analyses, based on the association of allele mutation frequency and tumor characteristics, are needed. In our PTC study, the proportion of *BRAF* V600E positive samples was 60%, which is within the expected, previously described range of approximately 45% [21,27]. We analyzed the association between the existence of mutation *BRAF* V600E and the normalized values of mutated alleles with all available PTC features. Our results show no statistically significant association between the existence of mutation *BRAF* V600E and metastatic spreading of PTCs ($p = 0.154$) nor pathohistological features of the primary tumor, except for tumor angioinvasion ($p = 0.043$). There was no significant difference in gender distribution between the groups. Still, the *BRAF* V600E-positive patients were significantly older at the time of diagnosis ($p = 0.003$), although there was no statistically significant correlation between the percentage of mutated allele and the age at diagnosis ($p = 0.756$). In several previous studies, a statistically significant association between the presence of the *BRAF* V600E mutation and distant PTC metastases was described [40,41]. On the other hand, the impact of *BRAF* V600E mutation on lymphogenic local metastases has been investigated in several studies with contradictory results. Some of them describe a statistically significant association between the presence of *BRAF* V600E mutation and the existence of local metastases [40,42–44]. However, a study performed by

Sapio et al. reports a statistically significant association of mutation *BRAF* V600E with the absence of local metastases (χ^2, N = 43; p = 0.011) [45]. Further on, a study conducted by Gandolfi and colleagues did not find an association of *BRAF* mutation with either local or distant metastases [37]. In their study, the mutation *BRAF* V600E was found in 18 of 37 PTCs without metastasis (48.6%) and in 40 of 95 PTCs with local metastases (42.1%). The mutation was also detected in 33.3% of PTCs with distant metastases [37]. The results reported by Kim et al. and Finkel et al. present a higher percentage of mutated alleles in patients with local metastases [46,47]. Kim found that lymph node metastases were more common in PTCs with a high abundance ($\geq$20%) of mutant alleles than in those with a low abundance of mutant alleles (p = 0.010) [47]. Although we noticed a trend of higher frequency of *BRAF* V600E alleles in patients with distant metastases, compared to patients without metastases as well as to patients with local metastases, there was no statistical significance (p = 0.515). To further examine the clinical importance of the *BRAF* gene mutation, Cheng et al. investigated the association between the frequency of mutated alleles and clinicopathological features and showed a significantly higher frequency of mutated alleles in larger tumors (p = 0.0001) and tumors with infiltration of the thyroid capsule (p = 0.034) [38]. Our results show no such association between the frequency of mutated alleles and tumor size (p = 0.847), thyroid capsule infiltration (p = 1.000), tumor angioinvasion (p = 0.096), dissemination in the thyroid gland (p = 0.576), or extrathyroidal expansion (p = 0.589).

According to our results, there is a heterogeneous distribution of *BRAF*-mutated alleles in the PTC tissue. Normalized frequency values of the *BRAF* gene allele ranged from 1.55% to 92.06%, with a median of 23.33%, indicating oligoclonal development. The oligoclonal pattern of BRAF mutation presence strongly indicates a heterogenous cellular composition of the PTC, at the time of surgical extirpation. This, of course, does not exclude monoclonal origin of the tumor. These results are in accordance with the results of Guerra and colleagues who described the oligoclonal existence of the mutation in most of the analyzed PTC samples [35]. They demonstrated that only in 4/41 PTC samples did mutation *BRAF* V600E range from 44.7 to 43.7%, and in 27/41 samples ranged from 25 to 5.1%. This means that 66% of PTCs with *BRAF* mutation had the frequency of the mutation alleles less than 25%, suggesting that *BRAF* mutation is often an oligoclonal event [35]. Similar results were reported by Kim et al., who found that the median frequency of the *BRAF* V600E mutated allele was 20%. Similarly so, Finkel et al. described the range of *BRAF* mutated allele frequency from 12% to 39% [46,47]. Research by Gandolfi et al. and De Biase et al. also showed the presence of heterogeneity of *BRAF* mutation and confirmed the results obtained by pyrosequencing, allele-specific locked nucleic acid PCR, and next-generation sequencing by immunohistochemical analysis of the mutated BRAF protein [36,37]. Gandolfi et al. demonstrated that BRAF mutation is frequently an oligoclonal event, present in 58.6% (34 out of 58) of PTCs, with a mutation percentage ranging between 20% and 35% [37]. On the other hand, not all studies are showing results in line with PTC heterogeneity.

Colombo et al. showed the existence of *BRAF* mutation heterogeneity only in a small number of cases (10/87) presenting a mean normalized allelic frequencies of 49.91 $\pm$ 11.22 (mode: 51, range 22–100) for mutation *BRAF* V600E [25]. In our study, the heterogeneity was clearly presented by the results of qPCR, but the number of positive *BRAF* V600E cells determined by IHC seemed higher than one would expect based on qPCR analysis. In other words, the results obtained on the protein level did not support the concept of heterogeneity and further suggested a homogeneous distribution of the mutation, which is in accordance with the results of Ghosein and colleagues [48].

Limitations

The research was performed on consecutive slides of the paraffin block, obtained from the area with the largest diameter of the tumor. Although the slides were only 5 μm-thick, there is still a possibility that the section(s) used for DNA isolation differed with respect to the proportion of tumor cells which were estimated in the first slide cut off.

However, the average diameter range of the nucleus of PTC is up to 5.92 μm [49] or in the range of 4.7–9.6 μm [50]. The next possible drawbacks are the decision on the optimal section of the tumor for the H&E staining, and presence of DNA degradation. The assumption is that the site of the largest diameter of the primary tumor is the best for analysis. This is where we expect the most tumor cells and a representative sample for detecting mutations of interest. However, if there is a heterogenous distribution of *BRAF* mutated allele in PTC tissue, a late mutation can occur in any part of the tumor, including its periphery.

5. Conclusions

This study demonstrates that neither the presence of the *BRAF* V600E mutation nor the proportion of cells with a mutated allele is significantly linked to the aggressiveness of PTC. These findings suggest that the role of the *BRAF* V600E mutation as a negative prognostic marker in PTCs needs to be reevaluated. According to the data available, heterogeneity of mutations in PTC are not as common as in other types of cancer such as melanoma, but it still exists. Thus, the potential multifocal growth of tumors with mutation *BRAF* V600E should be considered. However, even the demonstrated heterogeneity is not sufficient for explaining the ambiguous role of *BRAF* V600E mutation as a prognostic marker which may have a potential to affect important clinical decision. It seems that it still represents a hardly understandable influence on the clinical and pathological presentation of PTC. Furthermore, as expected, the proportion of patients with a mutation increases with age, and this factor should also be considered when evaluating clinical significance of the *BRAF* V600E mutation.

Author Contributions: Conceptualization, I.B., K.G.T., I.S. and T.J.; methodology I.B., J.P., T.R.D. and P.R.; data collection I.B., M.R., I.S., I.S.M. and R.G.; resources A.F. and Z.K.; writing—original draft preparation, I.B.; writing—review and editing, K.G.T., I.S. and T.J.; visualization I.B., M.R. and I.S. All authors have read and agreed to the published version of the manuscript.

Funding: This work was supported by the Croatian Science Foundation project: Genetic and epigenetic markers as indicators of aggressiveness of differentiated thyroid cancer (IP-2019-04-1130).

Institutional Review Board Statement: The study was conducted in accordance with the Declaration of Helsinki, and approved by the institutional Ethics Committee (University Hospital Center Sestre milosrdnice; approval No. EP-9941/19-7).

Informed Consent Statement: Informed consent was obtained from all subjects involved in this study.

Data Availability Statement: The data presented in this study are available on request from the corresponding author.

Conflicts of Interest: The authors declare no conflicts of interest.

References

1. GLOBOCAN. n.d. Available online: https://gco.iarc.fr/today/ (accessed on 15 May 2022).
2. HZJZ. Hrvatsku Zavod za Javno Zdravstvo. Available online: http://www.hzjz.hr/wp-content/uploads/2021/12/Bilten44_2019.pdf (accessed on 16 May 2022).
3. Dal Maso, L.; Tavilla, A.; Pacini, F.; Serraino, D.; Dijk, B.A.C.; Chirlaque, M.D.; Capocaccia, R.; Larrañaga, N.; Colonna, M.; Agius, D.; et al. Survival of 86,690 patients with thyroid cancer: A population-based study in 29 European countries from EUROCARE-5. *Eur. J. Cancer* **2017**, *77*, 140–152. [CrossRef]
4. Li, M.; Brito, J.P.; Vaccarella, S. Long-Term Declines of Thyroid Cancer Mortality: An International Age–Period–Cohort Analysis. *Thyroid* **2020**, *30*, 838–846. [CrossRef] [PubMed]
5. Lim, H.; Devesa, S.S.; Sosa, J.A.; Check, D.; Kitahara, C.M. Trends in Thyroid Cancer Incidence and Mortality in the United States, 1974–2013. *JAMA* **2017**, *317*, 1338. [CrossRef]
6. Pellegriti, G.; Frasca, F.; Regalbuto, C.; Squatrito, S.; Vigneri, R. Worldwide Increasing Incidence of Thyroid Cancer: Update on Epidemiology and Risk Factors. *J. Cancer Epidemiol.* **2013**, *2013*, 965212. [CrossRef]
7. Liu, Y.; Su, L.; Xiao, H. Review of Factors Related to the Thyroid Cancer Epidemic. *Int. J. Endocrinol.* **2017**, *2017*, 5308635. [CrossRef]

8. Haugen, B.R.; Alexander, E.K.; Bible, K.C.; Doherty, G.M.; Mandel, S.J.; Nikiforov, Y.E.; Pacini, F.; Randolph, G.W.; Sawka, A.M.; Schlumberger, M.; et al. 2015 American Thyroid Association Management Guidelines for Adult Patients with Thyroid Nodules and Differentiated Thyroid Cancer: The American Thyroid Association Guidelines Task Force on Thyroid Nodules and Differentiated Thyroid Cancer. *Thyroid* **2016**, *26*, 1–133. [CrossRef] [PubMed]
9. Tuttle, R.M.; Haugen, B.; Perrier, N.D. Updated American Joint Committee on Cancer/Tumor-Node-Metastasis Staging System for Differentiated and Anaplastic Thyroid Cancer (Eighth Edition): What Changed and Why? *Thyroid* **2017**, *27*, 751–756. [CrossRef]
10. Shaha, A.R.; Ferlito, A.; Rinaldo, A. Distant Metastases from Thyroid and Parathyroid Cancer. *ORL* **2001**, *63*, 243–249. [CrossRef] [PubMed]
11. Masoodi, T.; Siraj, A.K.; Siraj, S.; Azam, S.; Qadri, Z.; Albalawy, W.N.; Parvathareddy, S.K.; Al-Sobhi, S.S.; Al-Dayel, F.; Alkuraya, F.S.; et al. Whole-Exome Sequencing of Matched Primary and Metastatic Papillary Thyroid Cancer. *Thyroid* **2020**, *30*, 42–56 [CrossRef]
12. Agrawal, N.; Akbani, R.; Aksoy, B.A.; Ally, A.; Arachchi, H.; Asa, S.L.; Auman, J.T.; Balasundaram, M.; Balu, S.; Baylin, S.B.; et al Integrated Genomic Characterization of Papillary Thyroid Carcinoma. *Cell* **2014**, *159*, 676–690. [CrossRef]
13. Nowell, P.C. The Clonal Evolution of Tumor Cell Populations: Acquired genetic lability permits stepwise selection of variant sublines and underlies tumor progression. *Science* **1976**, *194*, 23–28. [CrossRef]
14. Abuali, I.; Lee, C.-S.; Seetharamu, N. A narrative review of the management of BRAF non-V600E mutated metastatic non-small cell lung cancer. *Precis. Cancer Med.* **2022**, *5*, 13. [CrossRef]
15. McKelvey, B.A.; Umbricht, C.B.; Zeiger, M.A. Telomerase Reverse Transcriptase (TERT) Regulation in Thyroid Cancer: A Review *Front. Endocrinol.* **2020**, *11*, 485. [CrossRef]
16. Nikiforov, Y.E. Thyroid carcinoma: Molecular pathways and therapeutic targets. *Mod. Pathol.* **2008**, *21*, S37–S43. [CrossRef]
17. Xing, M.; Liu, R.; Liu, X.; Murugan, A.K.; Zhu, G.; Zeiger, M.A.; Pai, S.; Bishop, J. *BRAF* V600E and *TERT* Promoter Mutations Cooperatively Identify the Most Aggressive Papillary Thyroid Cancer With Highest Recurrence. *JCO* **2014**, *32*, 2718–2726 [CrossRef] [PubMed]
18. Marotta, V.; Bifulco, M.; Vitale, M. Significance of RAS Mutations in Thyroid Benign Nodules and Non-Medullary Thyroid Cancer *Cancers* **2021**, *13*, 3785. [CrossRef] [PubMed]
19. Song, Y.S.; Lim, J.A.; Choi, H.; Won, J.; Moon, J.H.; Cho, S.W.; Lee, K.E.; Park, Y.J.; Yi, K.H.; Park, D.J.; et al. Prognostic effects of *TERT* promoter mutations are enhanced by coexistence with *BRAF* or *RAS* mutations and strengthen the risk prediction by the ATA or TNM staging system in differentiated thyroid cancer patients. *Cancer* **2016**, *122*, 1370–1379. [CrossRef] [PubMed]
20. Argyropoulou, M.; Veskoukis, A.S.; Karanatsiou, P.-M.; Manolakelli, A.; Kostoglou-Athanassiou, I.; Vilaras, G.; Karameris, A., Liadaki, K. Low Prevalence of TERT Promoter, BRAF and RAS Mutations in Papillary Thyroid Cancer in the Greek Population *Pathol. Oncol. Res.* **2020**, *26*, 347–354. [CrossRef]
21. Nikiforov, Y.E.; Nikiforova, M.N. Molecular genetics and diagnosis of thyroid cancer. *Nat. Rev. Endocrinol.* **2011**, *7*, 569–580 [CrossRef]
22. Wan, P.T.C.; Garnett, M.J.; Roe, S.M.; Lee, S.; Niculescu-Duvaz, D.; Good, V.M.; Project, C.G.; Jones, C.M.; Marshall, C.J.; Springer C.J.; et al. Mechanism of Activation of the RAF-ERK Signaling Pathway by Oncogenic Mutations of B-RAF. *Cell* **2004**, *116*, 855–867 [CrossRef]
23. Mayank, M.; Kaur, N.; Singh, N. Structural insights and influence of V599 mutations on the overall dynamics of *BRAF* protein against its kinase domains. *Integr. Biol.* **2018**, *10*, 646–657. [CrossRef]
24. Gouveia, C.; Can, N.T.; Bostrom, A.; Grenert, J.P.; Zante, A.; Orloff, L.A. Lack of Association of *BRAF* Mutation With Negative Prognostic Indicators in Papillary Thyroid Carcinoma: The University of California, San Francisco, Experience. *JAMA Otolaryngol. Head Neck Surg.* **2013**, *139*, 1164. [CrossRef] [PubMed]
25. Colombo, C.; Muzza, M.; Proverbio, M.C.; Tosi, D.; Soranna, D.; Pesenti, C.; Rossi, S.; Cirello, V.; De Leo, S.; Fusco, N.; et al Impact of Mutation Density and Heterogeneity on Papillary Thyroid Cancer Clinical Features and Remission Probability. *Thyroid* **2019**, *29*, 237–251. [CrossRef] [PubMed]
26. Walczyk, A.; Kowalska, A.; Kowalik, A.; Sygut, J.; Wypiórkiewicz, E.; Chodurska, R.; Pięciak, L.; Góźdź, S. The *BRAF*^{V600E} mutation in papillary thyroid microcarcinoma: Does the mutation have an impact on clinical outcome? *Clin. Endocrinol.* **2014**, *80*, 899–904. [CrossRef] [PubMed]
27. Xing, M. BRAF Mutation in Papillary Thyroid Cancer: Pathogenic Role, Molecular Bases, and Clinical Implications. *Endocr. Rev* **2007**, *28*, 742–762. [CrossRef] [PubMed]
28. Marotta, V.; Sciammarella, C.; Capasso, M.; Testori, A.; Pivonello, C.; Chiofalo, M.G.; Gambardella, C.; Grasso, M.; Antonino A.; Annunziata, A.; et al. Germline Polymorphisms of the VEGF Pathway Predict Recurrence in Nonadvanced Differentiated Thyroid Cancer. *J. Clin. Endocrinol. Metab.* **2017**, *102*, 661–671. [CrossRef] [PubMed]
29. Zheng, X.; Wei, S.; Han, Y.; Li, Y.; Yu, Y.; Yun, X.; Ren, X.; Gao, M. Papillary Microcarcinoma of the Thyroid: Clinical Characteristics and BRAFV600E Mutational Status of 977 Cases. *Ann. Surg. Oncol.* **2013**, *20*, 2266–2273. [CrossRef] [PubMed]
30. Rossi, E.D.; Martini, M.; Capodimonti, S.; Lombardi, C.P.; Pontecorvi, A.; Vellone, V.G.; Zannoni, G.F.; Larocca, L.M.; Fadda, G *BRAF* (V600E) mutation analysis on liquid-based cytology-processed aspiration biopsies predicts bilaterality and lymph node involvement in papillary thyroid microcarcinoma: *BRAF* Mutation in Micro-PTC on LBC. *Cancer Cytopathol.* **2013**, *121*, 291–297 [CrossRef]

31. Xing, M.; Alzahrani, A.S.; Carson, K.A.; Viola, D.; Elisei, R.; Bendlova, B.; Yip, L.; Mian, C.; Vianello, F.; Tuttle, R.M.; et al. Association Between BRAF V600E Mutation and Mortality in Patients With Papillary Thyroid Cancer. *JAMA* **2013**, *309*, 1493. [CrossRef]
32. Xing, M.; Alzahrani, A.S.; Carson, K.A.; Shong, Y.K.; Kim, T.Y.; Viola, D.; Elisei, R.; Bendlová, B.; Yip, L.; Mian, C.; et al. Association Between *BRAF* V600E Mutation and Recurrence of Papillary Thyroid Cancer. *JCO* **2015**, *33*, 42–50. [CrossRef]
33. Guerra, A.; Di Stasi, V.; Zeppa, P.; Faggiano, A.; Marotta, V.; Vitale, M. BRAF V600E assessment by pyrosequencing in fine needle aspirates of thyroid nodules with concurrent Hashimoto's thyroiditis is a reliable assay. *Endocrine* **2014**, *45*, 249–255. [CrossRef] [PubMed]
34. Guerra, A.; Fugazzola, L.; Marotta, V.; Cirillo, M.; Rossi, S.; Cirello, V.; Forno, I.; Moccia, T.; Budillon, A.; Vitale, M. A High Percentage of BRAFV600E Alleles in Papillary Thyroid Carcinoma Predicts a Poorer Outcome. *J. Clin. Endocrinol. Metab.* **2012**, *97*, 2333–2340. [CrossRef]
35. Guerra, A.; Sapio, M.R.; Marotta, V.; Campanile, E.; Rossi, S.; Forno, I.; Fugazzola, L.; Budillon, A.; Moccia, T.; Fenzi, G.; et al. The Primary Occurrence of *BRAF* ^{V600E} Is a Rare Clonal Event in Papillary Thyroid Carcinoma. *J. Clin. Endocrinol. Metab.* **2012**, *97*, 517–524. [CrossRef] [PubMed]
36. Biase, D.; Cesari, V.; Visani, M.; Casadei, G.P.; Cremonini, N.; Gandolfi, G.; Sancisi, V.; Ragazzi, M.; Pession, A.; Ciarrocchi, A.; et al. High-Sensitivity *BRAF* Mutation Analysis: *BRAF* V600E Is Acquired Early During Tumor Development but Is Heterogeneously Distributed in a Subset of Papillary Thyroid Carcinomas. *J. Clin. Endocrinol. Metab.* **2014**, *99*, E1530–E1538. [CrossRef] [PubMed]
37. Gandolfi, G.; Sancisi, V.; Torricelli, F.; Ragazzi, M.; Frasoldati, A.; Piana, S.; Ciarrocchi, A. Allele Percentage of the *BRAF* V600E Mutation in Papillary Thyroid Carcinomas and Corresponding Lymph Node Metastases: No Evidence for a Role in Tumor Progression. *J. Clin. Endocrinol. Metab.* **2013**, *98*, E934–E942. [CrossRef] [PubMed]
38. Cheng, S.-P.; Hsu, Y.-C.; Liu, C.-L.; Liu, T.-P.; Chien, M.-N.; Wang, T.-Y.; Lee, J.-J. Significance of Allelic Percentage of BRAF c.1799T > A (V600E) Mutation in Papillary Thyroid Carcinoma. *Ann. Surg. Oncol.* **2014**, *21*, 619–626. [CrossRef] [PubMed]
39. Bullock, M.; O'Neill, C.; Chou, A.; Clarkson, A.; Dodds, T.; Toon, C.; Sywak, M.; Sidhu, S.B.; Delbridge, L.W.; Robinson, B.G.; et al. Utilization of a MAB for BRAFV600E detection in papillary thyroid carcinoma. *Endocr.-Relat. Cancer* **2012**, *19*, 779–784. [CrossRef] [PubMed]
40. Namba, H.; Nakashima, M.; Hayashi, T.; Hayashida, N.; Maeda, S.; Rogounovitch, T.I.; Ohtsuru, A.; Saenko, V.A.; Kanematsu, T.; Yamashita, S. Clinical Implication of Hot Spot *BRAF* Mutation, V599E, in Papillary Thyroid Cancers. *J. Clin. Endocrinol. Metab.* **2003**, *88*, 4393–4397. [CrossRef]
41. Kebebew, E.; Weng, J.; Bauer, J.; Ranvier, G.; Clark, O.H.; Duh, Q.-Y.; Shibru, D.; Bastian, B.; Griffin, A. The Prevalence and Prognostic Value of BRAF Mutation in Thyroid Cancer. *Ann. Surg.* **2007**, *246*, 466–471. [CrossRef]
42. Lee, X.; Gao, M.; Ji, Y.; Yu, Y.; Feng, Y.; Li, Y.; Zhang, Y.; Cheng, W.; Zhao, W. Analysis of Differential BRAFV600E Mutational Status in High Aggressive Papillary Thyroid Microcarcinoma. *Ann. Surg. Oncol.* **2009**, *16*, 240–245. [CrossRef]
43. Kim, J.; Giuliano, A.E.; Turner, R.R.; Gaffney, R.E.; Umetani, N.; Kitago, M.; Elashoff, D.; Hoon, D.S.B. Lymphatic Mapping Establishes the Role of BRAF Gene Mutation in Papillary Thyroid Carcinoma: *Ann. Surg.* **2006**, *244*, 799–804. [CrossRef]
44. Frasca, F.; Nucera, C.; Pellegriti, G.; Gangemi, P.; Attard, M.; Stella, M.; Loda, M.; Vella, V.; Giordano, C.; Trimarchi, F.; et al. BRAF(V600E) mutation and the biology of papillary thyroid cancer. *Endocr. Relat. Cancer* **2008**, *15*, 191–205. [CrossRef] [PubMed]
45. Sapio, M.R.; Posca, D.; Troncone, G.; Pettinato, G.; Palombini, L.; Rossi, G.; Fenzi, G.; Vitale, M. Detection of BRAF mutation in thyroid papillary carcinomas by mutant allele-specific PCR amplification (MASA). *Eur. J. Endocrinol.* **2006**, *154*, 341–348. [CrossRef] [PubMed]
46. Finkel, A.; Liba, L.; Simon, E.; Bick, T.; Prinz, E.; Sabo, E.; Ben-Izhak, O.; Hershkovitz, D. Subclonality for *BRAF* Mutation in Papillary Thyroid Carcinoma Is Associated With Earlier Disease Stage. *J. Clin. Endocrinol. Metab.* **2016**, *101*, 1407–1413. [CrossRef] [PubMed]
47. Kim, M.-H.; Bae, J.S.; Lim, D.-J.; Lee, H.; Jeon, S.R.; Park, G.S.; Jung, C.K. Quantification of BRAF V600E alleles predicts papillary thyroid cancer progression. *Endocr.-Relat. Cancer* **2014**, *21*, 891–902. [CrossRef] [PubMed]
48. Ghossein, R.A.; Katabi, N.; Fagin, J.A. Immunohistochemical Detection of Mutated BRAF V600E Supports the Clonal Origin of BRAF-Induced Thyroid Cancers Along the Spectrum of Disease Progression. *J. Clin. Endocrinol. Metab.* **2013**, *98*, E1414–E1421. [CrossRef] [PubMed]
49. Seok, J.Y.; An, J.; Cho, H.Y.; Kim, Y.; Ha, S.Y. Nuclear features of papillary thyroid carcinoma: Comparison of Core needle biopsy and thyroidectomy specimens. *Ann. Diagn. Pathol.* **2018**, *32*, 35–40. [CrossRef]
50. Lee, T.-K.; Myers, R.T.; Bond, M.G.; Marshall, R.B.; Kardon, B. The significance of nuclear diameter in the biologic behavior of thyroid carcinomas: A retrospective study of 127 cases. *Hum. Pathol.* **1987**, *18*, 1252–1256. [CrossRef]

biomedicines

MDPI

Article

Minimal Extrathyroid Extension (mETE) as the Only Risk Factor in Patients with Papillary Thyroid Carcinoma (PC): Its Clinical Impact on Recurrence and Outcome during Long-Term Follow-Up

Andrea Marongiu [1], Susanna Nuvoli [1], Andrea De Vito [2], Sonia Vargiu [1], Angela Spanu [1,*] and Giuseppe Madeddu [1]

1 Unit of Nuclear Medicine, Department of Medicine, Surgery and Pharmacy, University of Sassari, 07100 Sassari, Italy; amarongiu2@uniss.it (A.M.); smfnuvoli@uniss.it (S.N.); sovargiu@tiscali.it (S.V.); giuseppe.madeddu@email.it (G.M.)

2 Unit of Infectious Diseases, Department of Medicine, Surgery and Pharmacy, University of Sassari, 07100 Sassari, Italy; andreadevitoaho@gmail.com

* Correspondence: aspanu@uniss.it

Abstract: Minimal extrathyroid extension (mETE) effect on papillary thyroid carcinoma (PC) prognosis is still debated even more so now that this factor has been removed in the 8th AJCC Edition, supporting the hypothesis that mETE is not associated with aggressive tumors. We retrospectively enrolled 91 PC patients (Group 1) submitted to total thyroidectomy and radioiodine ablation. At the time of the primary tumor surgery, mETE was ascertained in all patients with no other risk factors, such as multifocality, vascular invasion, neck and distant metastases, and aggressive histological variants. As controls, 205 consecutive matched PC patients (Group 2) without mETE and the aforementioned risk factors were enrolled. During the follow-up (average 8 years), 16/91 (17.58%) Group 1 patients and 15/205 (7.32%) Group 2 patients developed metastases ($p = 0.0078$). Cox regression analysis showed an increased risk of metastases in patients with mETE (HR: 2.58 (95% CI 1.28–5.22) $p = 0.008$). Disease-free survival (DFS) was significantly lower in patients with mETE than in controls ($p = 0.0059$). The present study seems to demonstrate that mETE can be associated with an aggressive PC and can be considered, even alone without other risk factors, an independent factor of unfavorable DFS. Thus, by excluding mETE in the 8th AJCC Edition, patient care and management could be compromised.

Keywords: papillary thyroid carcinoma; risk factors; minimal extrathyroid extension; follow-up; neck lymph node metastasis; distant metastasis; ^{131}I SPECT/CT

1. Introduction

The extrathyroid extension (ETE) in patients with differentiated thyroid carcinoma (DTC) has been defined as when tumor cells invade tissues and structures near the gland. In particular, extended ETE (eETE) represents the macroscopic tumor extension to subcutaneous soft tissue, trachea, larynx, esophagus, or recurrent laryngeal nerve, while in the minimal ETE (mETE) condition, extension to thyroid capsule, perithyroid soft tissue, and/or sternothyroid muscle invasion are microscopically detected at histology.

While the eETE is recognized as a predicted factor for tumor recurrence and mortality, the role of mETE as a risk factor for developing metastases and its impact on clinical outcomes during follow-up after thyroidectomy and radioiodine ablation is still a matter of debate [1–12]. Some authors retain that mETE has no impact on the disease behavior and prognosis, not representing a risk factor for developing metastases during the follow-up [11,13–24]. However, others do not agree with this interpretation and reported that mETE could play an important role in PTC patients, suggesting that this factor is associated with an increased risk for a poor outcome [10,25–30]. Moreover, mETE, in particular in patients with primary tumor $\geq$ 1 cm, can be considered a significant factor in the management of cervical lymph node (LN) metastasis in patients with PTC [31].

The risk stratification according to the ATA guidelines [32] considers the patients with mETE as patients with intermediate risk for developing metastases during the follow-up. In the face of this risk, the major guidelines for thyroid cancer suggest in these patients a more aggressive treatment such as total thyroidectomy, prophylactic dissection of LN of the central compartment, and subsequent radioiodine therapy.

However, recently, the 8th Edition of the American Joint Committee on Cancer (AJCC) [33] removed mETE from the definition of T3 disease when it is only detected on histological examination. This is in contrast to what has been reported in both the seventh and sixth editions, where mETE was categorized as T3, as well as in the fifth edition, where ETE, including both eETE and mETE, had been categorized as T4. Thus, the conflict remains whether the presence of mETE may still have significant importance in specifying TNM stage in patients operated for DTC and its impact on the management and outcome of the patients as a predictor of prognosis.

In light of controversial data reported in the literature, the present study aimed to further investigate the impact of mETE, ascertained microscopically at histology, on metastasis development and outcome during long-term follow-up. The study was carried out in a group of patients with papillary carcinoma (PC) with mETE, but without risk factors at the surgery of the primary tumor, such as eETE, vascular invasion, multifocality/multicentricity, neck and distant metastases, and aggressive histological PC variants. The data obtained in the patients with mETE have been compared with those observed in a control group of thyroidectomized PC patients without mETE and the same risk factors as above.

2. Materials and Methods

2.1. Patients

Among a large PC patient group submitted to total thyroidectomy and radioiodine ablation therapy, 91 consecutive patients (Group 1) were retrospectively enrolled. In all of them, mETE had been ascertained at histological microscopic exam after surgery. The inclusion criteria were that the patients had no risk factors, such as eETE, vascular invasion, multifocality/multicentricity, neck LN metastases both in the central compartment and in the lateral cervical regions, distant metastases, and aggressive histological PC variants.

Table 1 illustrates the characteristics of 91 patients at the time of the primary tumor surgery: 69/91 patients were females, 22/91 were males, 48 were aged <55 years, and 43 were aged $\geq$55 years. The size of carcinomas was $\leq$10 mm (microcarcinomas-PTMC) in 20 patients (5 $\leq$ 5 mm and 15 > 5 mm) and >10 mm in 71 patients. According to the risk stratification system, based on the most recent American Thyroid Association (ATA) guidelines [32], these 91 patients with mETE were classified as intermediate risk. Based on the TNM system, considering the AJCC 8th [33], 20 patients were T1aN0M0, 33 T1bN0M0, 29 T2N0M0, and 9 T3aN0M0.

Two hundred and five PC consecutive patients (Group 2) shown in the same Table 1, were also retrospectively enrolled as controls, and these were matched for sex, age, and tumor size with Group 1 patients. All patients had undergone total thyroidectomy and radioiodine ablation in the same period as PC patients with mETE. In all cases, neither mETE nor the risk factors previously mentioned were ascertained in histology. Based on the TNM system, considering the AJCC 8th, 60 patients were T1aN0M0, 78 T1bN0M0, 51 T2N0M0, and 16 T3aN0M0.

Table 1. Demographic and histological characteristics of 91 patients with papillary carcinoma (PC) with minimal extrathyroid extension (mETE) and 205 patients with PC without mETE who served as controls, at the time of the primary tumor surgery.

	PC Patients with mETE (91 Patients)	PC Patients without mETE as Controls (205 Patients)	p-Value
Age (years)	48 (52.75%) < 55 43 (47.25%) ≥ 55	124 (60.49%) < 55 81 (39.51%) ≥ 55	0.213
Age (years), mean ± SD	52.79 ± 14.09	49.90 ± 14.64	0.110
Sex (F/M)	69 (75.82%)/22 (24.18%)	159 (77.56%)/46 (22.44%)	0.743
Histology	Classic variant 82 (90.1%) Follicular variant 9 (9.9%)	Classic variant 175 (85.37%) Follicular variant 30 (14.63%)	0.265
Tumor size (mm)	20 (21.98%) ≤ 10 71 (78.02%) > 10	60 (29.27%) ≤ 10 145 (70.73%) > 10	0.193
Tumor size (mm), mean ± SD	20.08 ± 11.87	17.49 ± 12.42	0.090
Thyroid nodule (*n.*) **Multinodular goiter (*n.*)**	64 (70.33%) 27 (29.67%)	124 (60.49%) 81 (39.51%)	0.105
TNM (AJCC 8th)			0.431
T1a N0 M0 T1b N0 M0 T2 N0 M0 T3a N0 M0	20 (22.0%) 33 (36.2%) 29 (31.9%) 9 (9.9%)	60 (29.3%) 78 (38.0%) 51 (24.9%) 16 (7.8%)	

In 64/91 patients of Group 1, surgery was performed because the presence of thyroid nodules was highly suspect for DTC at fine needle aspiration biopsy (FNAB) and was confirmed at histology (10 PTMC), while the remaining 27/91 patients were operated on for multinodular goiter and carcinomas identified only at the time of histology (10 PTMC).

In Group 2 patients, the cause of the surgery in 124/205 patients was the presence of predominant thyroid nodules suspect for cancer at FNAB, 19 of these PTMC. The reason for the surgery in the other 81/205 patients was the abnormal growth of multinodular goiter, and the carcinoma foci were identified only microscopically at histology and 41 of these were PTMC.

Thyroid antibodies (AbTg, AbTPO, and TRABs) were absent or under cut-off in the serum of the two patient groups, and histological abnormalities from thyroid autoimmune diseases in association with PC were not ascertained. Moreover, all patients were on euthyroid clinical status, thus excluding hyper or hypothyroidism current conditions, no patients being on specific pharmacological therapy before surgery.

The total thyroidectomies were performed according to the therapeutic strategy of choice in the University Surgery Department, and no patient had postoperative complications, such as recurrent laryngeal nerve invasion, hypocalcemia, etc. After surgery, the patients underwent radioiodine ablation.

Globally, removal of central neck LN was performed in 41 patients (19 in Group 1 and 22 in Group 2) and lateral LN in 9 patients (5 in Group 1 and 4 in Group 2) when these were suspected of cancer during imaging procedures before surgery or during operation, but metastases had not been revealed.

As shown in Table 1, the patients of the two PC groups with and without mETE are comparable and no statistical difference was ascertained.

Histology confirmed the diagnosis of suspected metastases during follow-up. In some instances, the absence of histopathological findings for suspected lesions was observed due to the difficulty in reaching the potential site of the lesions. When histology was unavailable, the diagnosis has been validated through close follow-up for about 120 months and an average of 96 months with clinical and imaging procedures as well as traditional periodic assessment of thyroglobulin serum levels. The lesions thus ascertained were considered recurrent metastases and not as persistent disease when they appeared at least 18 months after radioiodine ablation.

2.2. Methods

All patients were monitored in a long-term follow-up after thyroidectomy and subsequent radioiodine ablation. In particular, PC patients with mETE were followed-up for 96.42 ± 31.03 months and control patients without mETE for a mean period of 95.10 ± 33.39 months; the difference is not statistically significant (p = 0.749).

During follow-up, to evaluate metastasis status, the patients were monitored with common diagnostic procedures, such as clinical exams, neck ultrasound, ^{131}I-Whole Body Scan (WBS), and single photon emission computerized tomography/computerized tomography (SPECT/CT). The latter two procedures were performed 24–48 h, and 72 h if necessary, after 185 MBq radioiodine diagnostic dose using a hybrid dual-head gamma camera in patients with hypothyroidism after L-thyroxine withdrawal or after recombinant thyroid stimulating hormone (rhTSH). Serum TSH levels were always over 50 μU/mL. Some patients, as complementary examinations, underwent CT or MRI and ^{18}F-FDG PET/CT, and, when the lesions were accessible, FNABs by ultrasound were practiced. Sequential serum thyroglobulin and AbTg levels were assayed, at intervals of 6–9 months, by chemiluminescent immunoassay method; the detection limit of thyroglobulin assay is 0.1 ng/mL. The cut-off was considered <0.2 ng/mL during suppressive therapy and <1 ng/mL after TSH stimulation. The AbTg cut-off was 100 IU/mL.

By chemiluminescent immunoassay method, AbTPO (cut-off: 16 IU/mL) and TRABs (cut-off: 1.75 IU/L) were also assayed. The values of cut-off of all the antibodies do represent the upper limit of the normal levels, and the values are considered positive if above that limit.

All radioisotopic instrumental examinations were performed in the Nuclear Medicine Center of the University Hospital, the site of the present study. Four nuclear medicine physicians (A.M., S.N., A.S., and G.M.), were aware of the reason for the exams but unaware of the results of the other previous investigations. Interobserver variability was very low, and disagreements were resolved by consensus. The other imaging exams were performed in the Radiologic Center and the "in vitro" tests in the Central Endocrinological Laboratory of the same University Hospital.

2.3. Statistics

The normality of quantitative data was evaluated by the Shapiro–Wilk test. Quantitative variables were summarized with mean ± standard deviation (SD) or medians and 25–75° percentiles (IQR), whereas qualitative ones were by absolute and relative (percentages) frequencies. The Mann–Whitney test or Student t-test evaluated the quantitative variable subgroup differences. The differences for qualitative variables were evaluated by Pearson chi-square or Fisher exact tests. Categorical variables were assessed by the Fisher chi-squared test.

A Cox regression analysis was performed to test the association between the collected variables and the risk of metastasis. Metastases were considered a dependent variable. The significance was fixed as $p < 0.05$.

Kaplan–Meier curves were plotted to visually assess 10-year disease-free survival, using the log-rank test to assess the statistical difference between mETE and non-mETE patients. A two-tailed $p < 0.05$ was considered statistically significant. All statistical analyses were performed with STATA version 16.1 (StataCorp. LLC, College Station, TX, USA).

3. Results

The results of the long-term follow-up after surgery and radioiodine ablation therapy in both Group 1 and Group 2 PC patients who developed metastases are illustrated in Table 2.

Table 2. Demographic and histological characteristics of 16/91 patients with mETE of Group 1 and 15/205 patients without mETE of Group 2 who developed metastases during long-term follow-up after surgery and radioiodine ablation therapy. All patients with mETE were classified as intermediate risk according to ATA classification and TNM according to AJCC 8th at the surgery of the primary tumor.

	16 PC Patients with mETE (Group 1)	15 PC Patients without mETE (Group 2)	*p*-Value
Age (years)	$(9 < 55/7 \geq 55)$	$(8 < 55/7 \geq 55)$	0.870
Age (years) mean± SD	54.50 ± 13.35	50.67 ± 15.68	0.469
Sex (M/F)	6/10	5/10	0.809
Tumor size (mm)	$(4 \leq 10/12 > 10)$	$(5 \leq 10/10 > 10)$	0.704
Tumor size (mm) mean± SD	20.56 ± 13.00	14.73 ± 8.98	0.159
Histology	16 classic variant	15 classic variant	
TNM (AJCC 8th)			
T1a N0M0 T1b N0M0 T2 N0M0 T3a N0M0	4 (25.0%) 6 (37.5%) 4 (25.0%) 2 (12.5%)	5 (33.3%) 7 (46.7%) 3 (20.0%) 0	0.747
Metastatic lesions (*n*.)	33	23	
Neck LN metastases (*n*.) LTC PT SM SC Mediastinal LN metastases	 9 12 3 0 2	 6 6 4 3 1	
Distant metastases			
Lung Bone	3 4 (1 spine, 1 skull, 1 homerus, 1 femur)	1 2 (1 spine, 1 sternum)	

LN: lymph node; LTC: laterocervical LN metastasis; PT: paratracheal LN metastasis; SM: submandibular LN metastasis; SC: supraclavicular LN metastasis.

In total, 16/91 (17.58%) patients of Group 1 developed metastases; 10/16 patients were females and 6/16 males, 9/16 were aged <55 years, and 7/16 $\geq$ 55 years; 4/16 patients had a tumor size $\leq$ 10 mm (PTMC), all of these with a size > 5 mm, and 12/16 with a size > 10 mm.

As illustrated in Table 2, as regards TNM, the comparison of the percentages of patients with metastases compared exclusively to the total number of patients (Group 1 and Group 2) who developed metastases with the same TNM category did not show statistical significance ($p = 0.747$). Even when the percentages of patients with metastases mentioned above were correlated to the total number of patients with the same TNM (not reported in the table), the comparison excluded a statistically significant difference ($p = 0.829$).

Thirty-three metastases were ascertained in the 16 patients of Group 1 during the follow-up. In 15/16 cases, 24 LN metastases were in the neck, 9 of which were laterocervical (LTC), 12 paratracheal (PT), and three submandibular (SM), including the four patients with PTMC, while in the remaining 1/16 patients, only one bone metastasis (cervical spine) was found. Two of the 15/16 patients, besides neck LN metastases, also had distant metastases. In particular, in one of these with LTC metastasis, one LN metastatic lesion in the superior mediastinum was ascertained; in the other patient, besides seven neck LN metastases, three lung and three bone metastatic lesions (one skull, one homerus and one femur) were found. This patient was the only one of 16 patients who had thyroid cancer-specific death, despite a second surgery on the neck and two further radioiodine ablations for both local and distant metastases during follow-up.

In 205 Group 2 patients, metastases occurred in 15/201 (7.32%) cases, ten females and eight males, eight aged <55 years and seven $\geq$ 55 years. Ten patients had tumor size >10 mm, while 5 $\leq$ 10 mm, two of the latter $\leq$ 5 mm.

Globally, 23 metastases were identified in 15 patients: two for each patient were found in the neck in four cases, one for each patient in the neck in nine cases, and one lesion in the neck together with one in the lung and one in the bone (sternum) in another case. In the remaining patient, one lesion in the neck, one in the superior mediastinum and one in the bone (spine) were ascertained.

The patients of Group 1 with mETE had a higher age and tumor size with respect to the patients of Group 2 without mETE, but the difference was not statistically significant.

The difference in the percentage of patients who developed metastases between Group 1 and Group 2 was statistically significant (p = 0.0078).

Except for the aforementioned patient who died of thyroid cancer, all the other patients of both groups are still alive and remain under observation.

As shown in Table 3, comparing the different variables of these patients, only mETE, at Cox regression analysis showed an increased risk of metastasis appearance during follow-up: HR: 2.58 (95% CI 1.28–5.22), p = 0.008.

Table 3. Cox regression analysis to assess the relationship between demographic and histological characteristics and 120 months of metastasis development.

	HR (95% CI)	p-Value
Age (years)	1.01 (0.98–1.03)	0.473
Age < 55	0.87 (0.43–1.77)	0.711
Female gender	0.52 (0.25–1.09)	0.086
Tumor size	1.00 (0.97–1.03)	0.821
Carcinoma $\leq$ 10 mm	1.06 (0.49–2.30)	0.882
mETE	2.58 (1.28–5.22)	0.008

Furthermore, in the mETE patients, metastasis appearance occurred in a shorter time in comparison with the control patients without mETE; however, the difference between median values of the two groups was not statistically significant (24 (IQR 22.5–35) months vs. 28 (IQR 24–34) months, p = 0.378).

Evaluating the disease-free survival (DFS) after ten years, this was significantly lower in the patients with mETE with respect to the patients without mETE (82% vs. 92%, p = 0.0059), as reported in Figure 1.

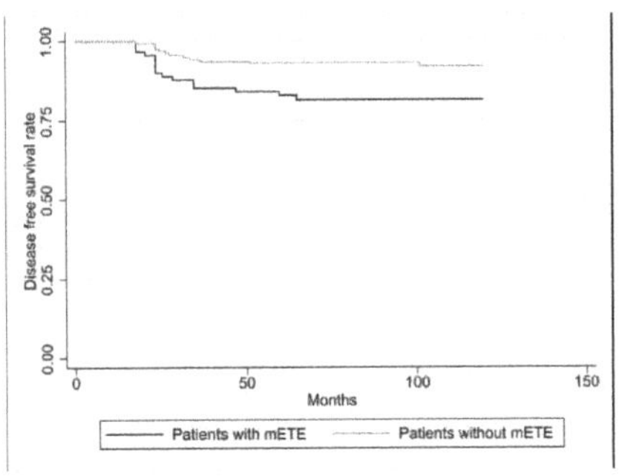

Figure 1. Disease-free survival (DFS) in PC patients with mETE (n. 91) and in PC patients without mETE (n. 205). According to the log-rank test, the difference was statistically significant (p = 0.0059).

As illustrated in Figure 2, evaluating DFS of both Group 1 and Group 2 patients with tumor size > 10 mm, this parameter was significantly reduced ($p = 0.0181$) according to the log-rank test, while in the patients with PTMC, this parameter showed no statistically significant difference ($p = 0.1526$).

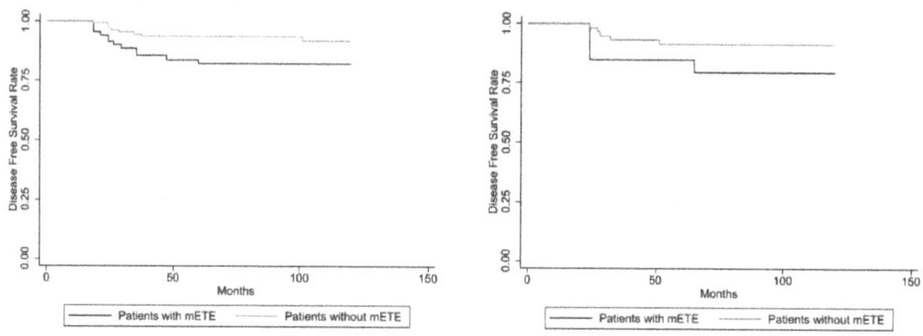

Figure 2. At (**left**): disease-free survival (DFS) in the 71 PC patients with mETE and in the 145 PC control patients with carcinoma >10 mm showed a statistical difference ($p = 0.0181$, calculated with log-rank test). At (**right**): disease-free survival (DFS) in the 20 PC patients with mETE and in the 60 PC control patients with PTMC ($\leq$10 mm) did not show statistical difference ($p = 0.1526$, calculated with log-rank test).

Subdividing the patients with PTMC according to the different sizes $\leq$ 5 and >5 mm, DFS was significantly ($p = 0.034$) reduced in the patients with size > 5 mm, but it was not significantly ($p = 0.370$) reduced in those with size $\leq$ 5 mm.

4. Discussion

The studies reported in the literature on the role of mETE during the follow-up of patients thyroidectomized for papillary thyroid carcinoma underline that this aspect is still strongly debated. In particular, microscopic extrathyroid extension in peri-thyroidal soft tissue is not explicitly mentioned in the AJCC 8th Edition [33] notwithstanding this infiltration is relatively frequent, since some authors retain that it does not represent a relevant prognostic factor [34], thus not justifying its inclusion in a separate category. This viewpoint had been confirmed by other authors before the 8th Edition of the TNM classification was published [7,11,18,34] but not accepted by others [31,35].

After the publication of the AJCC 8th Edition, many authors reported the results of their studies that still underlined the controversies on this problem.

According to a study conducted to comment on the stringent criteria proposed by the 8th Edition of the AJCC Staging System Manual, these were considered appropriate, supporting what was reported in the AJCC. These stringent criteria could decrease variability between observers and increase consistency in the diagnosis and staging of thyroid carcinoma [36].

In further support of what is reported in AJCC 8th Edition on the absence of mETE in the manual, some authors reported that the tumor size might be considered a more important factor than the presence of mETE in disease recurrence. Additionally, mETE was not a significant predictor of DFS, locoregional recurrences, and distant metastasis detection on multivariate analysis [22]. Another study showed that patients with mETE and those without mETE had the same recurrence rate or metastasis development, suggesting that intensive treatment may not be necessary for patients with mETE [23]. In particular, the study showed that age > 55 years did not have a significant impact on the risk of disease. In other studies, it has been observed that radioiodine therapy had a similar response rate in PTC patients regardless of the presence of mETE, although there was a high frequency of LN metastases [37]. According to the results obtained by other authors who reported that mETE increases the risk of recurrence in DTC patients, it has been observed that the absolute increase is small and, in addition, mETE has no impact on disease-related mortality [38]. Although in some studies mETE with an invasion of strap muscles did not seem to be a marker for poor prognosis, in other series of patients with age $\geq$ 55 years and large tumor size (>2 cm), the overall survival was impaired [39]. It has also been reported that mETE is a poor prognostic factor in tumors larger than 15 mm, but not in those smaller, which, without other unfavorable characteristics, should be classified as low risk [40].

However, based on the results obtained in other studies, mETE seems to represent an independent intermediate risk factor for recurrence except when it is identified in PTMC without LN metastases [12]. Other authors have reported that mETE may be associated with an increased risk of poor cancer-specific survival and overall survival, suggesting that it should be further investigated whether removing mETE from the last AJCC Staging System Manual is correct [25]. Furthermore, in other research, mETE was significantly linked to poor outcomes and the authors concluded that the TNM Staging System may need to be modified in the future due to this result [41]. It has been reported that even a small increase in thyroidal extension can lead to a significant increase in the risk of compromised survival. Therefore, mETE seems to be a reliable indicator of relapse-free survival and should be incorporated into the therapeutic thyroid cancer protocol [28] and thus included in a new AJCC Staging System Manual.

Considering the currently hot topic of debate, in the present retrospective study, the relationship between mETE and the prognosis of PC has been further evaluated during long-term follow-up of the affected patients after thyroidectomy and radioiodine ablation. A group of PC patients with no mETE was also included as controls, all of whom had been submitted to total thyroidectomy during the same period as patients with mETE.

Both groups of patients were exempted from the risk factors previously mentioned at the time of the primary tumor surgery, and age, gender, tumor size, histology, anatomic structure, and TNM did not differ significantly between patients with or without mETE.

During follow-up, it has been found that PC patients with mETE had a significantly higher rate of disease progression than PC matched control patients without mETE, even though their tumor characteristics were similar.

Compared to control patients, those with mETE had a significantly higher percentage of LN metastases. In addition, three patients with mETE and two belonging to the control group had distant metastases.

Moreover, patients with mETE had a significantly shorter DFS after ten years than those who did not have mETE. Additionally, patients with mETE experienced a faster occurrence of metastases than those without mETE. However, the difference in median values between both groups was not statistically significant.

The identification of metastases during follow-up is typically achieved through the use of traditional and highly sophisticated diagnostic imaging procedures, and in all patients, ^{131}I SPECT/CT has been included with high performance, confirming the reliable results of this procedure reported in the literature [42–45] also in patients with PC associated to thyroid autoimmune diseases [46,47].

Furthermore, in PC patients with mETE who had metastases, it may not be excluded that mETE alone could be a predictive risk factor for the development of metastases, potentially leading to worse disease prognosis and undesirable outcomes. Confirmation of these data was achieved through a Cox regression analysis that compared patients with and without mETE.

PC with mETE was found to be more aggressive than PC without mETE in the series of patients in the present study. Despite this, during the study period, only one patient of mETE died from a thyroid tumor, but otherwise, there was no relationship between cancer mortality and mETE.

Other authors also observed the same results obtained in this study regarding the aggressiveness of PC in patients with mETE [25,28,41]. However, the information obtained was in opposition to what was observed by others in several studies, which indicated an excellent prognosis and favorable disease-free survival for the patients [22,23,37–40] regardless of the presence of mETE. The exact reason for these contradicting results remains unclear.

The majority of PC patients with mETE who developed metastases were women, aged <55 years, and had a carcinoma size that was above 10 mm. The patients were also represented by PTMC in 25% of patients, and all of these were larger than 5 mm.

Regarding PTMC, it is widely known that this type of tumor is a disease with minimal invasiveness and a favorable long-term prognosis; however, PTMC has the potential to be more aggressive in certain patients, particularly when it involves multifocal and bilateral involvement, metastases in the neck LN, and distant metastases [48]. Thus, PTMC identification is necessary for the earliest treatment, and long follow-up surveillance is appropriate given that the recurrence rate lasts for many years, as validated in previous studies on this type of tumor [48].

Like classic PC with size > 10 mm, the role of mETE in PTMC as a risk factor is unclear and it is still debated with controversial results. Some authors [49] have reported that mETE did not show any impact on recurrences in patients with PTMC and there was no difference in DFS between patients with or without mETE ($p = 0.671$). No significant effect on recurrence rate in patients with PTMC has been also confirmed in a meta-analysis [38]. Moreover, patients with less than 5 mm have been reported to be associated with a low recurrence risk, leading to a better prognosis, which may allow clinicians to select less aggressive management strategies [50].

However, other authors [51] consider mETE as a factor in worsening prognosis with the presence of metastatic LN and a lower rate of DFS ($p = 0.034$). Moreover, mETE was reported as an independent risk factor for cancer recurrence for both neck LN and distant metastases in PTMC [52]. Still, other authors observed that mETE was independently related to LN metastases compared to patients without mETE, thus suggesting that this factor should be considered in the management of patients with single PTMC [53]. In the present study, mETE in patients with carcinomas smaller than 10 mm appeared not to influence DFS, unlike carcinomas over 10 mm. However, when the sizes were considered in the patients with PTMC, it was observed that those larger than 5 mm seemed to significantly affect the patient outcomes when compared to the carcinomas smaller than 5 mm. However, these data must be considered with caution due to the small number of patients.

Despite the absence of several risk factors at the time of the primary tumor surgery, as mentioned earlier, there were 17.58% of patients with mETE who underwent metastases; this percentage was significantly ($p = 0.0078$) higher than that of patients without mETE (7.32%).

Understanding tumor aggressiveness in certain instances, like those observed in this study, may require more research into a large number of PC patients with mETE. This latter factor alone appears to be the responsible one in these patients where other risk factors are absent, but the mechanism remains unclear.

Some limitations must be evidenced in the study:

The study is retrospective and only involves one center, which is the first thing to note. In addition, some information can be lost, and the study involves a modest number of patients because the exclusion criteria were very narrow, with only patients with mETE excluding the other aggressive risk factors.

Second, even though the average follow-up period is long, it may not be sufficient to detect occult metastasis if these only emerge during clinical and imaging examinations because metastases may occur later.

Third, the absence of histological findings in certain metastases is a limitation due to either the challenge of finding their sites or the unavailability of invasive intervention because of ethical reasons. The nature of the metastases can only be validated through long-term follow-up that includes clinical and imaging procedures performed sequentially, along with thyroglobulin changes, in these patients.

5. Conclusions

The results of the present study suggest that mETE may have an unfavorable effect on the outcome of the patients during the follow-up after thyroidectomy and radioiodine ablation, with a significantly different disease progression in patients with mETE than PC cases without mETE, and with a significantly lower DFS. These data, which have been confirmed by some authors, but not by others, suggest that even mETE alone may be a significant predictor factor for an increase in the risk of developing metastases in the future and hold greater significance since other risk factors were not found during the surgery of the primary tumor.

However, given the multiple contradictory findings on these issues, it is necessary to conduct more research on a larger number of patients, perhaps in prospective studies, to elucidate the various pathological mechanisms involved in the relationship between mETE and the prognosis of PC.

In closing, the present investigation demonstrates that mETE by itself is linked to an aggressive PC and is an independent factor of unfavorable DFS. Thus, excluding mETE in the 8th AJCC Edition could compromise patient care and management. Therefore, our data support the inclusion of mETE in the risk stratification model, such as in the previous 7th AJCC Edition, and, in addition, suggest carefully observing and following up in PC patients with mETE. In particular, a close observation of the patients with PTMC would also be necessary, especially those with a size over 5 mm, which was identified in a significant number of patients who developed metastases in the present casuistry.

Author Contributions: Conceptualization, A.S., A.M., S.N. and G.M.; methodology, A.S., A.M., S.N., A.D.V., S.V. and G.M.; statistical analysis, A.M. and A.D.V.; validation, A.S., A.M., S.N. and G.M.; formal analysis, A.S., A.M., S.N. and G.M.; investigation, A.M., S.N., A.D.V., S.V., A.S. and G.M.; data curation, A.M., S.N., A.D.V., S.V., A.S. and G.M.; writing—original draft preparation, A.M., S.N., A.S. and G.M.; writing—review and editing, A.M., S.N., A.S. and G.M.; visualization, A.M., S.N., A.S. and G.M.; supervision, A.S. and G.M.; project administration, A.S. and G.M. All authors have read and agreed to the published version of the manuscript.

Funding: No funding was received for the research.

Institutional Review Board Statement: The study was conducted for clinical purposes in accordance with the Helsinki Doctrine (as amended in 2013) and its amendments or ethical standards. Ethical approval was waived because the retrospective study involved data analysis in an anonymous form. All patient data were treated carefully following the Local Privacy Rules and Regulations.

Informed Consent Statement: Before scintigraphy, all subjects involved in the study routinely gave informed written consent. The patients have given their written informed consent for the paper publication for research purposes.

Data Availability Statement: The data that have been presented in this study are available on reasonable request from the corresponding author.

Conflicts of Interest: The authors declare no conflict of interest. The authors declare that they have not received any administrative or technical contributions or donations in kind.

References

1. Cady, B.; Rossi, R. An Expanded View of Risk-Group Definition in Differentiated Thyroid Carcinoma. *Surgery* **1988**, *104*, 947–953.
2. Andersen, P.E.; Kinsella, J.; Loree, T.R.; Shaha, A.R.; Shah, J.P. Differentiated Carcinoma of the Thyroid with Extrathyroidal Extension. *Am. J. Surg.* **1995**, *170*, 467–470. [CrossRef]
3. Ortiz, S.; Rodríguez, J.M.; Soria, T.; Pérez-Flores, D.; Piñero, A.; Moreno, J.; Parrilla, P. Extrathyroid Spread in Papillary Carcinoma of the Thyroid: Clinicopathological and Prognostic Study. *Otolaryngol.-Head Neck Surg.* **2001**, *124*, 261–265. [CrossRef]
4. Hay, I.D.; McConahey, W.M.; Goellner, J.R. Managing Patients with Papillary Thyroid Carcinoma: Insights Gained from the Mayo Clinic's Experience of Treating 2512 Consecutive Patients during 1940 through 2000. *Trans. Am. Clin. Climatol. Assoc.* **2002**, *113*, 241–260.
5. Hay, I.D. Papillary Thyroid Carcinoma. *Am. J. Surg. Pathol.* **2003**, *27*, 65–123.

6. Sugitani, I.; Kasai, N.; Fujimoto, Y.; Yanagisawa, A. A Novel Classification System for Patients with PTC: Addition of the New Variables of Large (3 Cm or Greater) Nodal Metastases and Reclassification during the Follow-up Period. *Surgery* **2004**, *135* 139–148. [CrossRef] [PubMed]
7. Ito, Y.; Tomoda, C.; Uruno, T.; Takamura, Y.; Miya, A.; Kobayashi, K.; Matsuzuka, F.; Kuma, K.; Miyauchi, A. Prognostic Significance of Extrathyroid Extension of Papillary Thyroid Carcinoma: Massive but Not Minimal Extension Affects the Relapse Free Survival. *World J. Surg.* **2006**, *30*, 780–786. [CrossRef]
8. Ito, Y.; Fukushima, M.; Kihara, M.; Takamura, Y.; Kobayashi, K.; Miya, A.; Miyauchi, A. Investigation of the Prognosis of Patients with Papillary Thyroid Carcinoma by Tumor Size. *Endocr. J.* **2012**, *59*, 457–464. [CrossRef]
9. Verburg, F.A.; Mäder, U.; Tanase, K.; Thies, E.-D.; Diessl, S.; Buck, A.K.; Luster, M.; Reiners, C. Life Expectancy Is Reduced in Differentiated Thyroid Cancer Patients $\geq$ 45 Years Old with Extensive Local Tumor Invasion, Lateral Lymph Node, or Distant Metastases at Diagnosis and Normal in All Other DTC Patients. *J. Clin. Endocrinol. Metab.* **2013**, *98*, 172–180. [CrossRef] [PubMed]
10. Yin, D.-T.; Yu, K.; Lu, R.-Q.; Li, X.; Xu, J.; Lei, M. Prognostic Impact of Minimal Extrathyroidal Extension in Papillary Thyroid Carcinoma. *Medicine* **2016**, *95*, e5794. [CrossRef] [PubMed]
11. Al-Qurayshi, Z.; Shama, M.A.; Randolph, G.W.; Kandil, E. Minimal Extrathyroidal Extension Does Not Affect Survival of Well-Differentiated Thyroid Cancer. *Endocr.-Relat. Cancer* **2017**, *24*, 221–226. [CrossRef]
12. Danilovic, D.L.S.; Castroneves, L.A.; Suemoto, C.K.; Elias, L.O.; Soares, I.C.; Camargo, R.Y.; Correa, F.A.; Hoff, A.O.; Marui, S. Is There a Difference Between Minimal and Gross Extension into the Strap Muscles for the Risk of Recurrence in Papillary Thyroid Carcinomas? *Thyroid* **2020**, *30*, 1008–1016. [CrossRef]
13. Nixon, I.J.; Ganly, I.; Patel, S.; Palmer, F.L.; Whitcher, M.M.; Tuttle, R.M.; Shaha, A.R.; Shah, J.P. The Impact of Microscopic Extrathyroid Extension on Outcome in Patients with Clinical T1 and T2 Well-Differentiated Thyroid Cancer. *Surgery* **2011**, *150* 1242–1249. [CrossRef]
14. Hotomi, M.; Sugitani, I.; Toda, K.; Kawabata, K.; Fujimoto, Y. A Novel Definition of Extrathyroidal Invasion for Patients with Papillary Thyroid Carcinoma for Predicting Prognosis. *World J. Surg.* **2012**, *36*, 1231–1240. [CrossRef]
15. Shin, J.H.; Ha, T.K.; Park, H.K.; Ahn, M.S.; Kim, K.H.; Bae, K.B.; Kim, T.H.; Choi, C.S.; Kim, T.K.; Bae, S.K.; et al. Implication of Minimal Extrathyroidal Extension as a Prognostic Factor in Papillary Thyroid Carcinoma. *Int. J. Surg.* **2013**, *11*, 944–947 [CrossRef]
16. Ito, Y.; Miyauchi, A.; Kihara, M.; Kobayashi, K.; Miya, A. Prognostic Values of Clinical Lymph Node Metastasis and Macroscopic Extrathyroid Extension in Papillary Thyroid Carcinoma. *Endocr. J.* **2014**, *61*, 745–750. [CrossRef]
17. Chéreau, N.; Buffet, C.; Trésallet, C.; Tissier, F.; Golmard, J.-L.; Leenhardt, L.; Menegaux, F. Does Extracapsular Extension Impact the Prognosis of Papillary Thyroid Microcarcinoma? *Ann. Surg. Oncol.* **2014**, *21*, 1659–1664. [CrossRef] [PubMed]
18. Jin, B.J.; Kim, M.K.; Ji, Y.B.; Song, C.M.; Park, J.H.; Tae, K. Characteristics and Significance of Minimal and Maximal Extrathyroidal Extension in Papillary Thyroid Carcinoma. *Oral. Oncol.* **2015**, *51*, 759–763. [CrossRef] [PubMed]
19. Woo, C.G.; Sung, C.O.; Choi, Y.M.; Kim, W.G.; Kim, T.Y.; Shong, Y.K.; Kim, W.B.; Hong, S.J.; Song, D.E. Clinicopathological Significance of Minimal Extrathyroid Extension in Solitary Papillary Thyroid Carcinomas. *Ann. Surg. Oncol.* **2015**, *22* (Suppl. S3) S728–S733. [CrossRef]
20. Hay, I.D.; Johnson, T.R.; Thompson, G.B.; Sebo, T.J.; Reinalda, M.S. Minimal Extrathyroid Extension in Papillary Thyroid Carcinoma Does Not Result in Increased Rates of Either Cause-Specific Mortality or Postoperative Tumor Recurrence. *Surgery* **2016**, *159*, 11–19. [CrossRef] [PubMed]
21. Kim, J.W.; Roh, J.-L.; Gong, G.; Cho, K.-J.; Choi, S.-H.; Nam, S.Y.; Kim, S.Y. Extent of Extrathyroidal Extension as a Significant Predictor of Nodal Metastasis and Extranodal Extension in Patients with Papillary Thyroid Carcinoma. *Ann. Surg. Oncol.* **2017** *24*, 460–468. [CrossRef]
22. Tam, S.; Amit, M.; Boonsripitayanon, M.; Busaidy, N.L.; Cabanillas, M.E.; Waguespack, S.G.; Gross, N.D.; Grubbs, E.G.; Williams M.D.; Lai, S.Y.; et al. Effect of Tumor Size and Minimal Extrathyroidal Extension in Patients with Differentiated Thyroid Cancer *Thyroid* **2018**, *28*, 982–990. [CrossRef]
23. Weber, M.; Binse, I.; Oebbecke, K.; Brandenburg, T.; Herrmann, K.; Theurer, S.; Weber, F.; Ehrlich, A.-K.; Schmid, K.W.; Führer-Sakel, D.; et al. Analysis of Risk Factors and Prognosis in Differentiated Thyroid Cancer with Focus on Minimal Extrathyroidal Extension. *BMC Endocr. Disord.* **2021**, *21*, 161. [CrossRef]
24. He, Q.; Ji, F.; Fu, X.; Li, Z.; Qiu, X. "Micro" Extrathyroidal Extension in Risk Stratification for Papillary Thyroid Carcinoma Should It Be in the Intermediate-Risk or High-Risk Group? A Single-Center Retrospective Study. *Cancer Manag. Res.* **2022**, *14* 3181–3190. [CrossRef] [PubMed]
25. Liu, Z.; Huang, Y.; Chen, S.; Hu, D.; Wang, M.; Zhou, L.; Zhou, W.; Chen, D.; Feng, H.; Wei, W.; et al. Minimal Extrathyroidal Extension Affects the Prognosis of Differentiated Thyroid Cancer: Is There a Need for Change in the AJCC Classification System? *PLoS ONE* **2019**, *14*, e0218171. [CrossRef] [PubMed]
26. Ozorio de Almeida, M.F.; Couto, J.S.; Ticly, A.L.T.; Guardia, V.C.; Marone, M.M.S.; Scalissi, N.M.; Cury, A.N.; Ferraz, C.; Padovani R.d.P. The Impact of Minimal Extrathyroidal Extension in the Recurrence of Papillary Thyroid Cancer Patients. *Arch. Endocrinol Metab.* **2020**, *64*, 251–256. [CrossRef] [PubMed]
27. Bortz, M.D.; Kuchta, K.; Winchester, D.J.; Prinz, R.A.; Moo-Young, T.A. Extrathyroidal Extension Predicts Negative Clinical Outcomes in Papillary Thyroid Cancer. *Surgery* **2021**, *169*, 2–6. [CrossRef] [PubMed]

28. Parvathareddy, S.K.; Siraj, A.K.; Qadri, Z.; DeVera, F.; Siddiqui, K.; Al-Sobhi, S.S.; Al-Dayel, F.; Al-Kuraya, K.S. Microscopic Extrathyroidal Extension Results in Increased Rate of Tumor Recurrence and Is an Independent Predictor of Patient's Outcome in Middle Eastern Papillary Thyroid Carcinoma. *Front. Oncol.* **2021**, *11*, 724432. [CrossRef] [PubMed]
29. Youngwirth, L.M.; Adam, M.A.; Scheri, R.P.; Roman, S.A.; Sosa, J.A. Extrathyroidal Extension Is Associated with Compromised Survival in Patients with Thyroid Cancer. *Thyroid* **2017**, *27*, 626–631. [CrossRef] [PubMed]
30. Al-Qurayshi, Z.; Sullivan, C.B.; Pagedar, N.; Lee, G.S.; Tufano, R.; Kandil, E. Prevalence and Risk of Metastatic Thyroid Cancers and Management Outcomes: A National Perspective. *Laryngoscope* **2021**, *131*, 237–244. [CrossRef] [PubMed]
31. Lee, H.S.; Park, C.; Kim, S.W.; Park, T.; Chun, B.K.; Hong, J.C.; Lee, K.D. Correlation of Minimal Extrathyroidal Extension with Pathologic Features of Lymph Node Metastasis in Patients with Papillary Thyroid Carcinoma: Minimal Exathyroidal Extension of PTC. *J. Surg. Oncol.* **2015**, *112*, 592–596. [CrossRef]
32. Haugen, B.R.; Alexander, E.K.; Bible, K.C.; Doherty, G.M.; Mandel, S.J.; Nikiforov, Y.E.; Pacini, F.; Randolph, G.W.; Sawka, A.M.; Schlumberger, M.; et al. 2015 American Thyroid Association Management Guidelines for Adult Patients with Thyroid Nodules and Differentiated Thyroid Cancer: The American Thyroid Association Guidelines Task Force on Thyroid Nodules and Differentiated Thyroid Cancer. *Thyroid* **2016**, *26*, 1–133. [CrossRef]
33. Amin, M.B.; Edge, S.; Greene, F.; Byrd, D.R.; Brookland, R.K.; Washington, M.K. *AJCC Cancer Staging Manual*, 8th ed.; American Joint Commission on Cancer; Springer: New York, NY, USA, 2017.
34. Mete, O.; Rotstein, L.; Asa, S.L. Controversies in Thyroid Pathology: Thyroid Capsule Invasion and Extrathyroidal Extension. *Ann. Surg. Oncol.* **2010**, *17*, 386–391. [CrossRef]
35. Radowsky, J.S.; Howard, R.S.; Burch, H.B.; Stojadinovic, A. Impact of Degree of Extrathyroidal Extension of Disease on Papillary Thyroid Cancer Outcome. *Thyroid* **2014**, *24*, 241–244. [CrossRef]
36. Turk, A.T.; Asa, S.L.; Baloch, Z.W.; Faquin, W.C.; Fellegara, G.; Ghossein, R.A.; Giordano, T.J.; LiVolsi, V.A.; Lloyd, R.; Mete, O.; et al. Interobserver Variability in the Histopathologic Assessment of Extrathyroidal Extension of Well Differentiated Thyroid Carcinoma Supports the New American Joint Committee on Cancer Eighth Edition Criteria for Tumor Staging. *Thyroid* **2019**, *29*, 619–624. [CrossRef] [PubMed]
37. Ahmaddy, F.; Wenter, V.; Ilhan, H.; Wacker, D.; Unterrainer, M.; Knösel, T.; Bartenstein, P.; Spitzweg, C.; Lehner, S.; Todica, A. Effects of the Minimal Extrathyroidal Extension on Early Response Rates after (Adjuvant) Initial Radioactive Iodine Therapy in PTC Patients. *Cancers* **2020**, *12*, 3357. [CrossRef] [PubMed]
38. Diker-Cohen, T.; Hirsch, D.; Shimon, I.; Bachar, G.; Akirov, A.; Duskin-Bitan, H.; Robenshtok, E. Impact of Minimal Extrathyroid Extension in Differentiated Thyroid Cancer: Systematic Review and Meta-Analysis. *J. Clin. Endocrinol. Metab.* **2018**, *103*, 2100–2106. [CrossRef]
39. Xu, M.; Xi, Z.; Zhao, Q.; Yang, W.; Tan, J.; Yi, P.; Zhou, J.; Huang, T. Causal Inference between Aggressive Extrathyroidal Extension and Survival in Papillary Thyroid Cancer: A Propensity Score Matching and Weighting Analysis. *Front. Endocrinol.* **2023**, *14*, 1149826. [CrossRef]
40. Castagna, M.G.; Forleo, R.; Maino, F.; Fralassi, N.; Barbato, F.; Palmitesta, P.; Pilli, T.; Capezzone, M.; Brilli, L.; Ciuoli, C.; et al. Small Papillary Thyroid Carcinoma with Minimal Extrathyroidal Extension Should Be Managed as ATA Low-Risk Tumor. *J. Endocrinol. Investig.* **2018**, *41*, 1029–1035. [CrossRef] [PubMed]
41. Xiang, J.; Wang, Z.; Sun, W.; Zhang, H. The New T3b Category Has Clinical Significance? SEER-Based Study. *Clin. Endocrinol.* **2021**, *94*, 449–459. [CrossRef]
42. Spanu, A.; Solinas, M.E.; Chessa, F.; Sanna, D.; Nuvoli, S.; Madeddu, G. 131I SPECT/CT in the Follow-up of Differentiated Thyroid Carcinoma: Incremental Value versus Planar Imaging. *J. Nucl. Med.* **2009**, *50*, 184–190. [CrossRef]
43. Xue, Y.-L.; Qiu, Z.-L.; Song, H.-J.; Luo, Q.-Y. Value of ^{131}I SPECT/CT for the Evaluation of Differentiated Thyroid Cancer: A Systematic Review of the Literature. *Eur. J. Nucl. Med. Mol. Imaging* **2013**, *40*, 768–778. [CrossRef] [PubMed]
44. Spanu, A.; Nuvoli, S.; Marongiu, A.; Gelo, I.; Mele, L.; Piras, B.; Madeddu, G. Neck Lymph Node Metastasis Detection in Patients with Differentiated Thyroid Carcinoma (DTC) in Long-Term Follow-up: A 131I-SPECT/CT Study. *BMC Cancer* **2020**, *20*, 239. [CrossRef]
45. Spanu, A.; Nuvoli, S.; Marongiu, A.; Gelo, I.; Mele, L.; De Vito, A.; Rondini, M.; Madeddu, G. The Diagnostic Usefulness of 131I-SPECT/CT at Both Radioiodine Ablation and during Long-Term Follow-up in Patients Thyroidectomized for Differentiated Thyroid Carcinoma: Analysis of Tissue Risk Factors Ascertained at Surgery and Correlated with Metastasis Appearance. *Diagnostics* **2021**, *11*, 1504. [CrossRef]
46. Marongiu, A.; Nuvoli, S.; De Vito, A.; Rondini, M.; Spanu, A.; Madeddu, G. A Comparative Follow-Up Study of Patients with Papillary Thyroid Carcinoma Associated or Not with Graves' Disease. *Diagnostics* **2022**, *12*, 2801. [CrossRef] [PubMed]
47. Marongiu, A.; Nuvoli, S.; De Vito, A.; Vargiu, S.; Spanu, A.; Madeddu, G. Hashimoto's Thyroiditis and Papillary Thyroid Carcinoma: A Follow-Up Study in Patients with Absence of Aggressive Risk Factors at the Surgery of the Primary Tumor. *Diagnostics* **2023**, *13*, 3068. [CrossRef] [PubMed]
48. Spanu, A.; Nuvoli, S.; Gelo, I.; Mele, L.; Piras, B.; Madeddu, G. Role of Diagnostic 131I SPECT/CT in Long-Term Follow-up of Patients with Papillary Thyroid Microcarcinoma. *J. Nucl. Med.* **2018**, *59*, 1510–1515. [CrossRef] [PubMed]
49. Moon, H.J.; Kim, E.-K.; Chung, W.Y.; Yoon, J.H.; Kwak, J.Y. Minimal Extrathyroidal Extension in Patients with Papillary Thyroid Microcarcinoma: Is It a Real Prognostic Factor? *Ann. Surg. Oncol.* **2011**, *18*, 1916–1923. [CrossRef]

50. Kaliszewski, K.; Diakowska, D.; Wojtczak, B.; Rudnicki, J. Cancer Screening Activity Results in Overdiagnosis and Overtreatment of Papillary Thyroid Cancer: A 10-Year Experience at a Single Institution. *PLoS ONE* **2020**, *15*, e0236257. [CrossRef]
51. Ruiz Pardo, J.; Ríos Zambudio, A.; Rodríguez González, J.M.; Paredes Quiles, M.; Soriano Giménez, V.; Oviedo Ramírez, M.I.; Hernández Martínez, A.M.; Parrilla Paricio, P. Papillary Thyroid Microcarcinoma with Minimal Extrathyroidal Extension. Is Its Course so Indolent That It Requires a Less Aggressive Treatment? *Rev. Clin. Esp.* **2021**, *221*, 131–138. [CrossRef]
52. Seifert, R.; Schäfers, M.; Heitplatz, B.; Kerschke, L.; Riemann, B.; Noto, B. Minimal Extrathyroidal Extension in Papillary Thyroid Microcarcinoma Is an Independent Risk Factor for Relapse Through Lymph Node and Distant Metastases. *J. Nucl. Med.* **2021**, *62*, 1702–1709. [CrossRef] [PubMed]
53. Song, R.-Y.; Kim, H.S.; Kang, K.H. Minimal Extrathyroidal Extension Is Associated with Lymph Node Metastasis in Single Papillary Thyroid Microcarcinoma: A Retrospective Analysis of 814 Patients. *World J. Surg. Oncol.* **2022**, *20*, 170. [CrossRef] [PubMed]

MDPI AG
Grosspeteranlage 5
4052 Basel
Switzerland
Tel.: +41 61 683 77 34

Biomedicines Editorial Office
E-mail: biomedicines@mdpi.com
www.mdpi.com/journal/biomedicines

www.ingramcontent.com/pod-product-compliance
Lightning Source LLC
Chambersburg PA
CBHW062057220926
51850CB00010B/2804
* 9 7 8 3 7 2 5 8 4 7 1 5 0 *